ANTIAGING 101:
COURSE MANUAL

ANTIAGING 101:
COURSE MANUAL
A Proactive Preventive Health Care Program

FRANK COMSTOCK, MD

authorHOUSE®

AuthorHouse™
1663 Liberty Drive
Bloomington, IN 47403
www.authorhouse.com
Phone: 1-800-839-8640

First published by AuthorHouse 8/27/2010

ISBN: 978-1-4389-8850-4 (sc)
ISBN: 978-1-4389-8851-1 (hc)
ISBN: 978-1-4389-8852-8 (e)

Library of Congress Control Number: 2010912307

Printed in the United States of America

This book is printed on acid-free paper.

To the memory of:

Howard C. Comstock, MD
My father, my role model, and the world's best pediatrician
Howard loved the Michigan Wolverines, family, and life, in that order.

William Zarifi
Our dear friend and valedictorian at University of Southern California
William fought cancer with an insurmountable spirit and willpower.

CONTENTS

INTRODUCTION

What is antiaging medicine?

Antiaging medicine is a program of optimal diet, nutraceuticals (nutritional supplementation), exercise, bioidentical hormone therapy, and stress management directed at optimizing health and slowing, even reversing, the aging process.

Each element of the antiaging program contributes to improved health and well-being. All components of the program work synergistically to optimize health, slow aging, and dramatically improve quality of life.

This is a medical program with an implicit goal of improving your quality of life! What a contrast from traditional medical care, which excels at acute medical and acute trauma care but focuses on disease care instead of health care. Indeed, we usually don't enter the current health-care arena unless we are ill or injured.

We definitely want access to state-of-the-art medical care to put out our acute medical "fires" and tame our chronic medical conditions, but we need to take advantage of lifestyle interventions that can significantly decrease our risk of disease and improve the quality of our health. This strategy becomes the ultimate preventive care.

Antiaging programs differ from traditional "preventive medicine." Most traditional preventive medicine programs are simply screening tools to find disease soon after it develops to allow the initiation of treatment at the earliest possible time. For example, colonoscopies, mammograms, and Pap smears are used to screen for cancer so treatment can be rendered before cancer progresses. While this is certainly a reasonable approach, it is not part of an antiaging program.

With antiaging, we look at how lifestyle interventions can impact our health to potentially decrease the chances that we do get ill. We focus on true prevention of disease.

When we combine age management medicine with traditional medicine, we are able to improve our health and vitality while simultaneously taking advantage of world-class medical and trauma care when necessary. If we are successful with our age management program, we may not need traditional medical therapy very often, but if we do, we have access to outstanding care.

This approach offers us the best of both worlds. It also allows each of us to take more personal responsibility for our own health and life. When we become empowered to take personal responsibility for our health and wellness, we can attain true health reform.

Can we slow aging?

I will answer the question with another question: *Can we accelerate aging?* The answer, of course, is a resounding yes!

In medical practice, every day we see patients with accelerated aging: young men and women with hypertension, elevated cholesterol, and cardiovascular disease; children with type 2 diabetes previously seen only in adults; and young adults with altered metabolism leading to obesity, depression, fatigue, arthritis, and many other conditions typically associated with the aging process, yet seen way too early in their lives. We see smokers with accelerated wrinkling of the skin; sugar addicts with advanced dental decay and dental loss; teenagers with gallbladder disease and gastric esophageal reflux disease; young adults with colitis, diverticulitis, and irritable bowel syndrome. The list of examples is endless.

Despite impressive advances in medicine, we see more and more patients on prescription medications at younger and younger ages. We see the majority of our population on multiple prescription medications. This isn't "health care"; this becomes "disease care."

With antiaging medicine, we strive to restore your health so you do not require multiple prescriptions. We improve your metabolism so you have energy and healthy body composition. We slow and even reverse the changes seen with the aging process. You will become chronologically older at the same time you become biologically younger.

Why is our health deteriorating if we live in a country with the best medical care in the world? Is it from some type of genetic mutation? Can we blame our genes? Our parents?

As it turns out, the more we learn about the genome and our "biological blueprint," the better we understand two important factors:

1) Our genes have changed less than 0.1 percent since our ancestors began walking upright millions of year's before.[1-4]

2) Most diseases, including many cancers, are the result of lifestyle, not genetics. Our genes represent potential, both good and bad. By improving our lifestyles with diet, nutrient supplementation, exercise, and stress reduction, and by maintaining hormone balance, we initiate positive genetic outcomes and limit the negative genetic possibilities. In scientific terms, this means we alter our "genetic expression."

Each cell in a person's body contains all his genes; however, not all the genes are "turned on" at all times. Via influence from our lifestyle choices and things we can control—our diets, exercise, supplements, stress reduction, and hormone levels—we can influence which genes are activated and which genes are turned off. In other words, which genes are "expressed."

Even our thoughts influence gene expression.[5-13] This is often referred to as "mind-body medicine." Our thoughts impact cell function via modification of gene activity. Our thoughts set the stage for positive or negative cell functions. We are all familiar with how effective a placebo, or sugar pill, can be in medical studies and in clinical practice. We know that when a patient has confidence in his surgeon, or in his specific medical therapy, this positively influences his outcome. So don't blame Mom and Dad! Instead, adopt a healthy lifestyle. Eat well, exercise efficiently, supplement with necessary and powerful nutraceuticals, and utilize stress reduction and bioidentical hormone therapy as needed to optimize health.

Live young and become younger!

Read this course manual, learn the material in *Antiaging 101*, and start slowing the aging process for the rest of your life. Let the class begin!

- Accelerated aging is avoidable
- Healthy aging is attainable
- Read on

Warning!

Remember the expression "Old age ain't for sissies"? Well, the opposite is also true; getting younger is not for sissies!

In this course, you will learn what steps to take to dramatically improve your health and flatten the slope of your aging curve. Be forewarned that it takes effort and commitment. This is not a quick fix or simple solution.

By learning this material, you will empower yourself and your family to make intelligent choices that will affect your health immediately. After this course, you will know what foods to eat, what supplements to take, what exercise to do, how to lower stress, and what hormones to utilize.

Yes, the program takes sacrifice and commitment, but in return you will have more energy, strength, and stamina. You will look better, and you will be healthier.

You will realize that each day, instead of being another step toward getting older, is actually an opportunity to get younger! Best of all, once you live this program, you will never want to stop. It is not a temporary program—it is a lifestyle.

Remember, it took a lot of time to gain that extra weight or to develop diabetes or high blood pressure. It takes time to lose the extra weight, to reverse your diabetes, and to reverse your high blood pressure.

Stay positive and focused, and your health will improve.

CHAPTER 1

GOALS OF ANTIAGING 101

As we begin our journey to optimal health, let's examine our goals. In the business world, this would be labeled a "business plan." A business plan outlines how to make a business successful. It is a set of blueprints to guide the vision of the business. It keeps the business running efficiently, economically, and profitably. The business plan ensures longevity of the business.

Our "health plan" is the same. It identifies specific goals and a framework to follow to ensure success and longevity.

It is interesting to note that many people spend more time planning a weekend getaway than planning a healthy lifestyle. People often joke that antiaging programs don't extend your life; they just make you feel as if you are living longer! This implies such sacrifice that the agony of it all just drags on.

Sure, our program takes effort, but you will find that you feel better and that your energy is enhanced—and the entire program actually becomes easier the longer you are on it. As unbelievable as it sounds, in time you won't even consider stopping the program. It really does become a way of life.

So let's develop our health plan by asking this question: *What are our goals for health?* As we discuss this, you should be forewarned that learning our goals leads to some scientific discussion. However, understanding the science behind the specific goals is pivotal because it allows you to appreciate why each of our goals is important, and how to reach each goal efficiently and effectively. You will become empowered to make healthy decisions for the rest of your long life. So let's start.

> Aging well improves your health. By improving your health, you enhance your vitality. When you enhance your vitality, you improve your life. Age well to live well.

Goal #1 CONTROL INSULIN LEVELS

Insulin control ... not just for diabetics.

The pancreas secretes the hormone insulin, primarily after we eat in response to elevation of our blood glucose (sugar) level. Insulin is essential for life. Insulin has multiple functions, primarily dealing with "storage" in the body. Insulin allows us to transport glucose from the bloodstream into cells for energy production. Insulin stores excess glucose in the body as fat.[1-2]

Patients who don't produce insulin require frequent daily injections of insulin to live. Most of us, however, produce way too much insulin, largely because of high-carbohydrate diets. When we lose control of our insulin levels, we set ourselves up for many adverse health consequences and accelerated aging.

When insulin levels are consistently elevated, the cells become resistant to the insulin "message." Because the insulin level is too high for too long, the cells become tired of hearing from insulin. The cells become resistant to insulin. To overcome this insulin resistance, the pancreas has to secrete even more insulin. This, of course, leads to even higher insulin levels.[3-5]

This insulin resistance problem is analogous to parents communicating with their teenagers. The more they hear parental advice, the more they become resistant to their parents' voices, and the louder their parents have to speak to get the message across!

With insulin resistance, the pancreas speaks louder by releasing higher levels of insulin in an attempt to get the insulin message across to the cells. When this happens, the elevated insulin levels lead us down a path of accelerated aging.[6-10]

Elevated insulin levels lead to obesity, hypertension, elevated cholesterol levels, and type 2 diabetes.[11-12]

Prolonged elevated insulin levels set the stage for the development of metabolic syndrome. Metabolic syndrome is a cluster of disorders including obesity, elevated cholesterol, hypertension, and insulin resistance. Gerald Reaven, a Stanford University diabetologist, initially identified metabolic syndrome in 1987. Metabolic syndrome greatly increases the risk for diabetes and cardiovascular disease.[13-15]

In addition, high insulin levels disrupt hormone balance throughout the body. Elevated insulin levels increase the risk for cardiovascular disease such as heart attacks and have been shown to increase the risk of cancer. High insulin levels increase inflammation throughout the body, which also adversely affects our health.[16-23] Insulin increases inflammation primarily by promoting fat storage and escalating the production of inflammatory cell hormones. (More on inflammation coming up.)

Let me recap the main points for you:

- High glucose (sugar) levels result in high insulin levels.
- High insulin levels produce insulin resistance.
- Insulin resistance leads to metabolic syndrome.
- Metabolic syndrome leads to poor health and accelerated aging.

In the current health-care model, the multiple conditions precipitated by elevated insulin are labeled metabolic syndrome. As we have discussed, patients with this syndrome are usually obese, hypertensive, have high cholesterol readings, and are at a dramatically increased risk of having a heart attack. They also have dramatically shortened lifespan (accelerated aging.)[24-32]

If you don't make the necessary lifestyle changes, your metabolic syndrome will likely be treated with prescriptions for blood pressure, high cholesterol, and high blood sugar; even diet pills may be necessary.

A much healthier approach is to deal with the underlying problem of metabolic syndrome: insulin control. *How?* By following the programs outlined in *Antiaging 101*.

We monitor goal #1 with a blood test called "fasting insulin level." Healthy-aging goal: fasting insulin level less than 5.

A thought provoker: cancer cells have twenty times more insulin receptors than normal cells because cancer cells live and thrive on sugar.[33-37]

HEALTH PROBLEMS ASSOCIATED WITH HIGH INSULIN LEVELS

- Obesity
- Diabetes
- Heart disease
- Cancer
- Dementia
- Elevated cholesterol
- Hypertension

- Increased inflammation
- Hormone imbalances
- Accelerated aging
- Osteoarthritis
- Polycystic ovarian syndrome
- Fatty liver
- Metabolic syndrome

You must maintain stable and low insulin levels to slow the aging process.

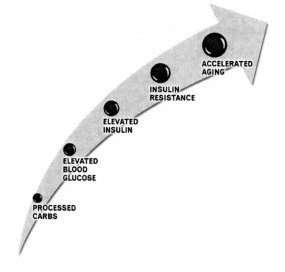

Goal #2 CONTROL BLOOD GLUCOSE LEVELS

Sugar is not so sweet.

Our cells utilize glucose for energy production. Our brains depend on a constant supply of glucose to function. We think and feel better when blood glucose levels are controlled.[38-40]

In contrast, elevated glucose levels damage the body. High glucose levels damage cells via a process called glycation. Glycation occurs when glucose combines with proteins in cells and disrupts cell function. This combination of glucose with proteins produces advanced glycation end products, which are extremely destructive to the body. The advanced glycation end products have been given the acronym AGEs because of their role in the aging process. AGEs accelerate your rate of aging.

The glaze on a honey-baked ham is an example of the glycation process. Physical examples of glycation include wrinkling and cataracts (the cloudy haze of the lens). AGEs accumulate everywhere in the body and injure all cells and organs.

Excessive glucose literally "gums up the works," and by doing so, increases the risk of many disease processes and greatly accelerates the aging process.[41-43] The glycation process results in injury to blood vessels throughout the body. The organs supplied by these injured blood vessels will suffer damage in the form of heart attacks, strokes, kidney failure, and blindness.

In addition to direct injury to cells and blood vessels, high glucose levels leads to high insulin levels and all the aforementioned health problems.

The main culprits in elevated glucose levels are diets high in processed carbohydrates.[44]

Virtually any carbohydrate that is not a whole fruit or vegetable is processed. Processed carbohydrates cause the blood glucose to soar to excessive levels in the blood. The body has difficulty processing these elevated glucose levels and is forced to store excess glucose as fat.

It is important to realize that excess sugar becomes excess body fat. Before you reach for the processed carbohydrates and candy, remember that it will damage your cells, increase your body fat, and accelerate the aging process. They aren't so sweet after all!

For healthy aging, it is imperative that we control our blood glucose levels. All the information you need to maintain stable and controlled glucose levels will be covered in the upcoming lectures on diet, exercise, supplements, and hormone therapy.

- High glucose levels lead to glycation.
- Glycation injures cells throughout the body.
- Glycation produces Advanced Glycation End Products "AGEs"
- "AGEs" result in accelerated aging.

We monitor goal #2 with blood tests called "fasting glucose level" and "hemoglobin A1C." Healthy-aging goal: fasting glucose level between 70–90 mg/dl; hemoglobin A1C less than 5mU/L.

A thought provoker: cancer cells require high glucose levels to survive.[45-47]

HEALTH PROBLEMS ASSOCIATED WITH HIGH GLUCOSE LEVELS:

- Obesity
- Heart disease
- Cancer
- Dementia
- Elevated cholesterol

- Cataracts
- Kidney disease
- Stroke
- Peripheral vascular disease
- Inability to pass this course

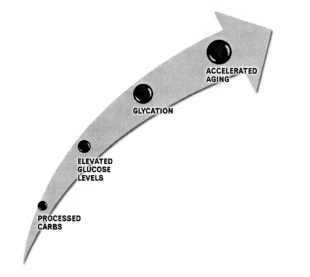

ACCELERATED AGING

GLYCATION

ELEVATED GLUCOSE LEVELS

PROCESSED CARBS

Goal #3 CONTROL CORTISOL LEVELS

Stress ages ... and kills.

Cortisol is known as the stress hormone since it is released during times of continued stress.[48] It functions to assist us in dealing with stressful situations. The adrenal glands, small organs on top of our kidneys, release the cortisol. The inner core of the adrenal gland, the medulla, releases the hormones epinephrine and norepinephrine to assist the body's fight-or-flight stress response. The initial, acute response to the stressor is dependent on epinephrine and norepinephrine. In essence, epinephrine and norepinephrine heighten our senses to meet whatever challenges we face. If the stress continues, the outer surface of the adrenal glands, the cortex, releases cortisol.

Cortisol helps us mobilize energy and slow down or even shut off non-vital systems in the body so we can deal with the stressful situation at hand. Cortisol breaks down protein to supply glucose to the brain and to the muscles. The production of glucose from protein is called gluconeogenesis. The cortisol-induced gluconeogenesis allows a continual energy supply to our cells for as long as the stressful conditions persist. Unfortunately, continued release of cortisol comes at a price to our health.

Without cortisol, we would die. If we have insufficient cortisol production, a condition called Addison's disease, we succumb to stress because we are unable to mobilize the necessary physiologic response that is required to survive. However (here we go again!), persistently elevated cortisol levels are damaging to our cells and to our metabolism.

Elevated cortisol levels develop when our bodies are under constant stress, whether that stress is psychological from worry over work, finances, or family issues, or whether it's physical, from unhealthy diet, nutritional deficiencies, excessive exercise or sleep deprivation.

High cortisol levels alter our metabolism and body composition.[49] Elevated cortisol levels lead to muscle loss, bone loss, and increased body fat.[50-52] Elevated cortisol levels disrupt our immune systems, putting us at increased risk of disease.[53] Excessive cortisol is also damaging to brain cells and leads to memory loss and increased risk of dementia.[54-57]

High cortisol is another frequently seen cause of accelerated aging. So we need to control our cortisol levels by following healthy lifestyles and by learning some easy-to-follow stress-reduction techniques. (Or you can stay away from your mother-in-law, get a new job, win the lottery …)

- Stress raises cortisol levels.
- High cortisol levels accelerates aging.

We monitor goal #3 with a blood test called "AM cortisol level." Healthy-aging goal: AM cortisol level 9–14 mcg/dl.

> A thought provoker: high cortisol levels make you gain fat, impair your memory and intellect, and make you weak and sick.

HEALTH PROBLEMS ASSOCIATED WITH HIGH CORTISOL LEVELS

- Obesity/weight gain
- Cancer
- Immune system dysfunction

- Muscle loss (sarcopenia)
- Bone loss (osteoporosis)
- Dementia/memory loss

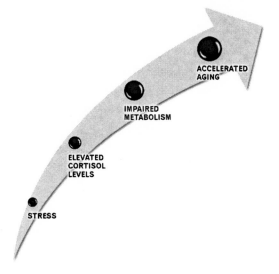

Goal #4 OPTIMIZE CELL FUNCTION

Healthy aging ... one cell at a time.

We have trillions of cells in the human body.[58] Each cell contributes to the health of a specific organ, and each organ contributes to the health of the body. So what's good for the cells is good for the organs is good for the body.

By taking care of our cells, we take care of our overall health. Cells spend considerable time taking in nutrients to produce energy in the form of ATP, adenosine triphosphate. ATP is known as the energy currency of the cell.[59] Cell energy production is what allows organs to function. For example, cell energy production keeps our hearts beating, lungs breathing, kidneys filtering, brains thinking, and the uvula (that thing hanging down in the back of our throats) doing whatever it does.

Needless to say, cell energy production is crucial to our health. Suboptimal cell production leads to fatigue and organ dysfunction.

Every cell in your body is surrounded by a cell membrane. The cell membrane envelopes the cell and allows the cell to interact with hormones, to communicate with other cells, and to assist the cell in bringing nutrients in and getting toxins out.[60-61] The quality of the cell membrane is critical to the quality of cell function. Having a healthy **brain** requires healthy "mem**branes**."

You will learn how the quality of the cell membrane is determined primarily by the quality and type of fats in your diet. By eating well and taking appropriate supplements, we can maintain healthy cell membranes while simultaneously supplying the cells with nutrients needed for healthy cell function and optimal cell energy production.

- There are trillions of cells in the body, all surrounded by cell membranes.
- Healthy cells require healthy cell membranes.
- Healthy cell membranes require healthy diet (and healthy fats).

> A thought provoker: cancer begins when one cell malfuntions.[62]

We monitor goal #4 with a blood test called a "fatty acid profile." Healthy-aging goal: omega 6 to omega 3 ratio of two to one (more on this later).

Goal #5 CONTROL FREE RADICALS

And radically improve your health.

Free radicals! *What is this, some sort of political statement?* Rest assured that this book is completely nonpartisan.

Free radicals are unstable molecules. They are by-products of our oxygen-based metabolism.[63] If you live and breathe, you are producing free radicals, so whatever you do, don't stop producing your free radicals!

However, excessive free radicals are damaging to our cells and even our DNA (yes, our genes). Since free radicals are unstable, they steal electrons from other molecules to stabilize themselves. They act like little Robin Hoods and steal from rich molecules, like cell membranes, and DNA. This process of stealing electrons damages cells and contributes to disease and accelerated aging.

Free radicals damage cells by a process called oxidation. Examples of oxidation include rust on metals or the brown discoloration of sliced apples. In essence, our cells are rusting because of oxidative damage.

We control free radicals with antioxidants. Our bodies have intrinsic antioxidants, but their effect can decrease with age.[64-65] It is important that we supply the body with additional antioxidants via supplementation, combined with a healthy diet. Well-known examples of antioxidants are vitamin C and vitamin E. Vitamin C is a water-soluble vitamin that provides antioxidant protection to the "water" portions of our cells. Vitamin E is a fat-soluble vitamin that offers protection to the "fat" portions of our cells. In class, we will expand on the role of antioxidants in healthy aging.

In addition, we learn to decrease exposure to additional oxidative stress by minimizing or avoiding suppliers of excessive free radicals, e.g., sugar, smoking, trans fats, toxins, pollution, lawyers …

- Free radicals lead to excessive oxidation.
- Oxidation leads to disease and accelerated aging.

We monitor goal #5 by measuring levels of antioxidants in the body.

A thought provoker: sugar intake produces high levels of free radicals. People with high blood sugar levels have excessive oxidation and significantly increased risk of cancer.[66-69]

HEALTH PROBLEMS ASSOCIATED WITH EXCESSIVE FREE RADICALS "OXIDATION"

- Cancer
- Dementia
- Accelerated aging
- Degenerative diseases

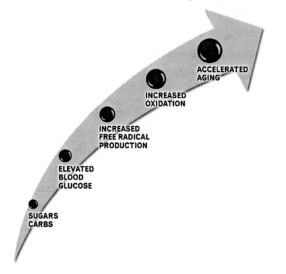

Goal #6 CONTROL HORMONE LEVELS

And I don't mean your teenagers.

We have addressed insulin hormone and cortisol hormone in previous goals, so you are probably wondering why more discussion about hormones. Controlling hormone levels refers to what are called sex steroid hormones (oh, now you are listening!) Sex steroid hormones such as testosterone, estrogen, and progesterone decline with age.

Hormones are chemical messengers that control all the body's functions. Many scientists feel that our hormone levels don't decline with age, but rather we age *because* our hormone levels decline.[70]

These hormones have diverse functions throughout the body. They support brain function, cardiac function, skin health, and influence cell function and cell communication.

They support healthy body composition by their effect on bone density, muscle mass, and fat distribution. Oh, I almost forgot: they also influence libido and sexual function. Hormone balance supports a healthy libido in numerous ways, primarily by supporting brain function, improving psychological status, and by optimizing circulation and blood flow.

In reality, hormones control our metabolism and run our bodies. We cannot optimize our health without optimal levels of these hormones because we will not have optimal cell function, and organ function will suffer.

Although there is debate about hormone replacement therapy options in medicine, there is no debate regarding the adverse effects throughout the body when hormone deficiencies exist.

Given the myriad of actions that these hormones exhibit in our bodies, it becomes evident that quality of health and quality of life suffer when hormones are deficient.

Fortunately, by enrolling in this class, you won't have to worry about how your health could suffer with hormone deficiencies. In *Antiaging 101*, you will learn how to improve your hormone profile with diet, exercise, and supplements. You will also learn about the extraordinary benefits of bioidentical hormone therapy.

We monitor goal #6 with blood levels of each hormone. Our healthy-aging goals include optimal ranges for each of the major hormones.

For estradiol levels in women, we maintain estradiol levels of greater than 90 pg/ml (pg/ml means picograms per milliliter; a picogram is one-trillionth of a gram). FSH (follicle stimulating hormone) less than 20 mIU/ml is optimal (mIU/ml means milli-international units per milliliter). In women, we maintain testosterone levels over 50 ng/dl (ng/dl means nanogram per deciliter; a nanogram is one-billionth of a gram). For men, we aim for testosterone levels of 700–900 ng/dl.

> A thought provoker: nursing home patients are models of hormone deficiencies.

HEALTH PROBLEMS ASSOCIATED WITH HORMONE DEFICIENCIES

- Weight gain/obesity
- Dementia
- Accelerated skin aging
- Sexual dysfunction
- Muscle loss (sarcopenia)
- Bone loss (osteoporosis)
- Cardiovascular disease
- Depression
- Fatigue
- Low libido

Goal #7 OPTIMIZE METABOLISM

Your body ... the best chemistry set you'll ever own.

Metabolism is the net result of all the chemical reactions taking place in the human body. Chemical reactions occur in our cells to produce energy as well as to break down and repair tissues.

Your body is extremely dynamic (contrary to what your spouse may say.) Our bodies are constantly breaking down and constantly rebuilding. Millions of cells are replaced every day.

Much like a house being remodeled, sections are being gradually destroyed while other sections are gradually being built up. In the body, we refer to these opposing forces as anabolic forces and catabolic forces.

Our metabolism is composed of both anabolic (buildup and repair) and catabolic (breakdown) forces at all times. When we are young (lets say less than forty years old, for illustration) anabolic forces exceed catabolic forces so the net result is growth and repair.

With aging, catabolic forces exceed anabolic forces, so we start to break down. So if you feel as if you are "breaking down," it may be because you are! To avoid this rapid deterioration, we must support metabolism as well as anabolic forces with all of our antiaging programs.

As we age, our body compositions change; we tend to gain fat and lose muscle and bone. With healthy diet, supplements, exercise, stress reduction, and hormone therapy, we reverse these age-associated changes in body composition.

All components of our antiaging program support and enhance our metabolism to slow the rate of breakdown and aging.

Anabolic metabolism repairs and regenerates the body

We monitor goal #7 with a DEXA scan that measures body composition, including body fat, bone density, and muscle mass.

DEXA stands for dual energy X-ray absorptiometry. It is quick, painless, and extremely safe. DEXA scans use a low dose of radiation to obtain accurate body composition measurements. You simply lie still while the scanner passes over you from head to toe. Within approximately ten minutes, we will know your bone density, body fat percentage, and your muscle mass. The scans usually cost between $150 and $250.

Healthy-aging goal for women is 20 to 25 percent body fat. For men, it is 15 to 20 percent body fat. Bone density T-score should be higher than -0.1 (The T-score is a universal scoring system that compares your bone density to a thirty-year-old healthy adult.)

A thought provoker: many people report success with deprivation diets that promote "weight loss." The weight loss with many deprivation or unbalanced diets is primarily muscle loss. This leads to accelerated aging and is detrimental to your metabolism.[71-75]

Goal #8 CONTROL INFLAMMATION

Burn, baby, burn

Inflammation is part of your immune system and is required for healing and tissue repair. For example, with an injury, inflammation results in increased blood supply to the area, increased white blood cell production and release, and chemicals released to improve the healing response.

The inflammatory response is represented in the swelling, redness, heat, and pain at the injured region of the body. Without a healthy inflammatory response, we would quickly succumb to viruses, bacteria, injury, and other threats.

Problems develop when we have excessive levels of inflammation in the body. This leads to a silent deterioration of organ function. Virtually every disease process has excessive inflammation at its core.

For example, plaque buildup in our arteries that leads to heart attacks and strokes is the result of excessive inflammation.[76] In addition, any disease process that ends with "itis" is disease fueled by inflammation: colitis, dermatitis, and arthritis are common examples.

Research has revealed that this silent inflammation not only increases our risk for disease but also accelerates the aging process.

As it turns out, many of us have excessive inflammation because of unbalanced diets and a deficiency of healthy fats. Quit adding gasoline to the fire! Learn how to eat and supplement well to control inflammation.

- Unhealthy diets lead to excessive inflammation
- Excessive inflammation leads to accelerated aging
- Inflammation ages the nation

We monitor goal #8 with a blood test called CRP (C-reactive protein). Healthy-aging goal: CRP less than 1.0.

A thought provoker: elevated inflammation is a much more dangerous cardiac risk factor than high cholesterol.[77-85]

HEALTH PROBLEMS ASSOCIATED WITH CHRONIC INFLAMMATION

- Obesity
- Heart disease
- Cancer
- Dementia
- Arthritis

- Chronic dermatitis
- Colitis
- All degenerative diseases
- Asthma
- Affinity toward rap music

So there you have it—eight goals for healthy aging. You will learn more about each of these goals, why they are crucial to strive for, and how to reach them as you continue with *Antiaging 101*.

By the end of the course, you will understand how all of them are interrelated. Reaching any one of the goals will help you on the road to reaching the other seven. The more you reach, the easier the remaining goals will become.

All of them are interrelated so your results are amplified when you accomplish subsequent goals. Once you reach all eight, you will be well on your way to optimal health and slower aging.

Enjoy the journey. I promise you will feel better, look better, and significantly decrease your risk of multiple diseases associated with the aging process.

EXAMPLE OF RELATIONSHIP BETWEEN OUR ANTIAGING GOALS:

Glucose control leads to insulin control. Insulin control leads to lowered inflammation.

Lowered inflammation leads to optimal cell function. Optimal cell function leads to improved metabolism.

Improved metabolism leads to lower free radicals. All the preceding goals lead to better hormonal control.

Hormone control leads to improved metabolism. Optimal metabolism leads to better body composition and cell energy production.

Indeed, our goals represent a web of interrelation leading to health and slowed aging.

Not reaching our goals accelerates aging

- Poor glucose control accelerates glycation, which occurs when glucose combines with proteins in cells and disrupts cell function.
- Glycation accelerates oxidation, essentially the rusting of our cells from unstable molecules called free radicals.
- Oxidation accelerates inflammation, which is the equivalent of our immune system attacking cells throughout our bodies, leading to silent deterioration of organ function.
- Inflammation accelerates aging.

Follow our antiaging program and get your foot off that aging accelerator!

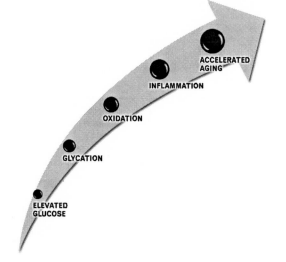

EIGHT GOALS FOR HEALTHY AGING:

1) Control glucose levels.

2) Control insulin levels.

3) Control cortisol levels.

4) Optimize cell function.

5) Control free radicals.

6) Control hormone levels.

7) Optimize metabolism.

8) Control inflammation.

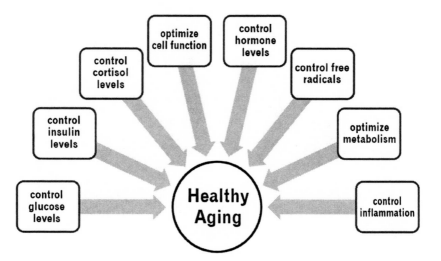

DON'T JOIN THE "AA CLUB"

The "AA Club" is the Accelerated Aging Club. The clubhouse entrance is enticing. The clubhouse is full of sugary treats, tobacco, and alcohol. The pantry is stocked with an endless supply of processed foods that never spoil. There are big-screen TVs, computers, video games. There is so much to do that you'll never want to sleep. You will never have to exercise. And there is no cover charge.

So what's the problem?

Once you step into the clubhouse, you'll start on a slippery slope toward a life of disability, pain, obesity, fatigue, and early death. You will never reach any of our healthy-aging goals.

So forget about it—stay away from the AA Club. Stay on the road to health and vitality.

CHAPTER 1
QUESTIONS

Student:

We always read and hear about the importance of low cholesterol for decreasing risk of heart disease, yet low cholesterol is not one of your healthy-aging goals. Why?

Professor:

Great question. It is important to realize that cholesterol is crucial for life. Cholesterol is needed by every cell in the human body. Cholesterol is not a villain. Without cholesterol, you would die.

Sure, very high levels of cholesterol can cause health problems; however, low cholesterol is associated with Parkinson's disease, cancer, depression, and many other conditions.

Like everything in the body, balance is best—not too high and not too low. The best way to achieve cholesterol balance is by following the *Antiaging 101* program.

Student:

When I go to the doctor, he always checks my blood pressure. Shouldn't good blood pressure be one of the healthy aging goals?

Professor:

In most people following the *Antiaging 101* program, blood pressure improves or normalizes. If you follow the program, you will most likely experience stable blood pressure, healthy body weight, and balanced cholesterol without medications.

However, don't stop current medications without physician supervision.

Student:

Aren't longevity and health determined by are genes?

Professor:

Your genes represent a potential, not an absolute. You must realize that we communicate with our genes via diet, hormones, exercise, stress management, and supplements. By improving our lifestyles, we can improve our genetic expression and improve our health.

This concept is pivotal in understanding the impact of lifestyle modifications on our health and longevity.

Student:

Which antiaging goals are most important?

Professor:

They are all important. If I had to choose only one, I would recommend controlling your glucose level.

Stable glucose levels results in stable insulin levels. Stable insulin levels improve cell function, decrease inflammation, help balance hormones, and improve metabolism. Stable glucose levels also lower free radical burden and improve cortisol levels.

The opposite is also true. High glucose results in high insulin, high inflammation, excessive free radical production, high cortisol, disrupted cell function, altered metabolism, and finally, poor hormone balance.

All eight goals are interconnected. Poor health choices have a negative cascade effect throughout the body. Healthy choices have a positive cascade effect throughout the body.

Student:

How often do you recommend the blood tests to monitor the eight antiaging goals?

Professor:

Usually at the start of the program, every six months until stable, then annually.

Student:

Six of the eight healthy aging goals are about control. Are you some sort of control freak?

Professor:

Control is part of our healthy aging goals because problems develop when there are excesses or deficiencies in our body. The body seeks balance at all levels. It maintains balance through a process called homeostasis.

The body is able to maintain remarkably consistent levels of chemicals, fluids, hormones, and temperature—in fact, everything in the body. This consistency and balance is constant unless we disrupt the balance of the body.

We are most guilty of disrupting balance because of lifestyle decisions regarding diets, supplements, exercise, stress, and changes that occur with the aging process.

Ironically, many of the disruptive lifestyle decisions are well intentioned and meant to improve our health. For example, a low-fat diet is a well-intentioned diet with a goal of decreasing body fat. Seems logical enough. However, a low-fat diet typically results in fat, glucose, and hormone imbalances in the body.[86-94] So what was meant to help our health is actually contributing to disease.

Another example of a well-intentioned lifestyle choice is starting an exercise program. A common problem is an exercise program that focuses exclusively on excessive aerobic-type exercise. This type of exercise can elicit excessive levels of cortisol with resultant acceleration of muscle and bone loss, leading to an increase in body fat! The opposite of what we would want from our exercise program.

We must control these goals to achieve healthy aging.

Student:

Is it difficult to reach these healthy aging goals? How long does it usually take?

Professor:

We talked earlier about how all of our goals are interrelated, and that when we start the process of reaching one goal, each subsequent goal becomes easier to achieve.

How long it takes to get healthy depends on your current level of health. That being said, the results come rapidly so you will begin to feel better soon after starting our program.

When you see and feel positive results, it becomes self-motivating to continue your antiaging program. It will then become a way of life.

Student:

Are there additional healthy aging goals in your Antiaging 202 course?

Professor:

Yes, there are. Pass this course and then you can find out for yourself.

What does the medical and scientific literature reveal about accelerated aging and our antiaging goals?

❖ Currently there is a dramatic increase in the number of chronic childhood conditions in the United States.

❖ Today there are more teenagers with high blood pressure, high cholesterol, and obesity, revealing cardiovascular risk factors in a young population.

❖ Men with type 2 diabetes reached moderate risk for heart disease at an average age of thirty-nine years, compared to age fifty-five for nondiabetics. Men with type 2 diabetes reached high risk for heart disease at an average age of forty-nine years, compared to age sixty-two for nondiabetics.

❖ Diabetes shortened life expectancy by eighteen years. (Accelerated aging!)

❖ Women with metabolic syndrome (from high insulin levels and insulin resistance) were three times more likely to have a recurrence of breast cancer as women without the syndrome.

❖ Women with glycosylated hemoglobin (measure of blood glucose control) of 7 percent or higher were four times more likely to develop cognitive impairment or dementia than women who tested at less than 7 percent. (Good reason to put the sweetened soda away!)

❖ Obesity increased risk of all cancers.

❖ Obesity increased all-cause mortality risk. A study found that obesity cuts lifespan by up to twenty years.

❖ A study found that high sugar consumption increased risk of pancreatic cancer. People drinking sweetened soft drinks at least twice per day almost doubled risk of pancreatic cancer. People who put sugar in coffee five times daily increased risk of pancreatic cancer by 70 percent. (Sugar is the devil!)

- ❖ A study of 4,213 men over twenty years found that a height loss of more than three centimeters from sarcopenia (muscle loss) and osteoporosis is linked to increased risk of all-cause mortality.

- ❖ A four-year study of 525 adults aged seventy-two to ninety-two years found that those who died were the ones with the highest levels of inflammatory chemicals.

- ❖ A study over twenty-five years found people with fasting insulin levels in the lowest quintile demonstrated one-third the risk of heart disease as those with insulin levels in the highest quintile.

- ❖ In a study of 2,440 nondiabetics followed for a five-year period, people with fasting glucose levels of greater than 100 but less than 125 were found to have nearly triple the risk for heart disease as those people with fasting glucose levels of less than 86.

- ❖ Inflammatory cytokines are more prominent in people with excessive stores of body fat.

- ❖ University of California study reported that inflammation is directly linked to cancer formation.

- ❖ A large European study found that increasing body mass index was associated with a significant increase in the risk of cancer for ten out of seventeen specific cancer types examined.

- ❖ Study estimated a reduction of 45 percent in the risk of breast cancer in women who lost more than nine pounds.

- ❖ Multiple studies found that the lower the blood glucose, the lower the risk of heart disease, hypertension, arthritis, and cancer.

- ❖ A study found that people with high levels of a marker for inflammation (C-reactive protein) may be twice as likely to develop colon cancer.

- *American Journal of Medicine* study of 1,293 healthy elderly people over 4.6 years found that higher levels of two blood tests of inflammation (CRP and IL-6) were associated with a twofold greater risk of death.

- *Journal of the American Medical Association* found that women who took aspirin daily (anti-inflammatory) had a nearly 30 percent lower risk of the most common type of breast cancer.

- High insulin and high glucose levels increase rate of cancer.

- Abdominal fat increases rates of inflammation and heart disease.

- High insulin levels are found to be associated with increased abdominal fat, injury to blood vessels, prostate enlargement, increased rates of cancer, lower growth hormone levels, and impotence. (Ouch!)

- A study found that high insulin levels are associated with increased risk of breast cancer and poorer survival rate after a breast cancer diagnosis.

- In a study of 7,027 women with an average age of sixty-six years, it was found that women with poor glucose control tend to have poorer mental function than those with normal blood glucose levels, and they are at a greater risk of cognitive decline over time.

- A seven-year study found that the risk of a heart attack was doubled for patients with C-reactive protein levels (measure of inflammation) in the highest quartile.

- Study found that the higher a person's body mass index (a measurement that indicates obesity), the higher his or her level of oxidative stress (higher levels of free radicals).

- A study found that men who had the highest levels of C-reactive protein at the start of the study were almost four times more likely to have a stroke ten to fifteen years after the study began than men with the lowest levels of C-reactive protein. High levels of C-reactive protein corresponded with a 60 to 70 percent increase in stroke risk.

❖ A study of overweight children found that the blood vessels of obese children show changes that can lead to heart disease later in life. Research showed that these changes can be reversed with diet and exercise. (Antiaging!)

❖ Research revealed that diabetes and obesity accelerate aging. Many of the genes recently discovered to slow the aging process when they are manipulated are genes that belong to pathways involved in the control of metabolism.

❖ A study found that the higher a person's body mass index (BMI), which is a measurement that indicates obesity, the higher his or her level of oxidative stress (higher levels of free radicals).

❖ The *Journal of the American Medical Association* study found that the vast majority of heart patients (90 percent) had heart problems because of bad health habits.

❖ Research found that among younger individuals who have increased abdominal fat, there is a greater risk of the development of diabetes, heart disease, hypertension, gallbladder disease, neurodegenerative disease, and a number of cancers, all of which are associated with aging.

❖ American Heart Association study found that women with the highest levels of inflammation were 15.7 times more likely to become diabetic.

❖ John Hopkins researchers found that the blood test hemoglobin A1C (a marker of long-term blood glucose level) is an independent predictor of heart disease risk in both diabetics and nondiabetics.

- In a study of over 400,000 men and over 500,000 women, involving a sixteen-year follow-up period, it was found that diabetes increases the risk of a number of different types of cancer.

- A mouse model of human breast cancer demonstrated that tumors are sensitive to blood glucose levels. The study found that the lower the blood glucose level, the greater the survival rate.

- An epidemiological study in twenty-one countries revealed that sugar intake is a strong risk factor that contributes to higher breast cancer rates, particularly in older women.

- A study in the *England Journal of Medicine* revealed that aggressively lowering a person's blood glucose level can cut the risk of heart attack and stroke nearly in half.

- A UCLA study found that for men with cardiovascular disease, the lower the blood sugar, the better. Their death rate over a two-year period increased from slightly more than 4 percent at a glucose level of 70 to more than 12 percent at a glucose level of 100.

- An American Diabetes Association study reported that the current diabetes epidemic costs $174 billion a year. The study reported that the incidence of diabetes has increased dramatically; there are one million new cases per year. In addition, diabetes killed over 284,000 Americans in 2007.

- Research showed that individuals who develop type 2 diabetes have a twofold increase in risk of stroke within the first five years of diagnosis compared with the general population.

- Research revealed that excessive inflammation breaks down skeletal muscle, leading to loss of lean body mass (catabolic forces.)

- A study found that higher blood levels of inflammation are associated with lower muscle mass and lower muscle strength in older men and women.

❖ A study showed that high levels of glucose deactivate the gene that controls the amount of testosterone and estrogen in the bloodstream (all of our goals are interrelated).

❖ A study from the *Journal of the American Medical Association* found that men with higher levels of insulin were more likely to develop pancreatic cancer.

❖ Recent studies have shown a close correlation between insulin resistance and a number of diseases such as cancer and Alzheimer's disease.

❖ A study published in *Annals of Internal Medicine* studied 23,000 people's adherence to four simple behaviors (not smoking, exercising 3.5 hours weekly, eating a healthy diet, and keeping a healthy weight). In those adhering to the lifestyle modifications, 93 percent of diabetes, 81 percent of heart attacks, 50 percent of strokes, and 36 percent of all cancers were prevented. (Now that's health reform!)

❖ According to analysts from the Cleveland Clinic, if lifestyle treatments were applied to all patients with cardiovascular disease, diabetes, metabolic syndrome, obesity, prostate cancer, and breast cancer, then net health expenditures could be reduced by $930 billion over five years.

And much more ...

CHAPTER 2

OPTIMAL DIET

Diet. A four-letter word. Right now you're probably thinking, *Here we go; now he is going to starve me and make me count calories.* I promise you won't have to count calories or go hungry on our program!

Healthy diet slows aging

Optimal diet is not about deprivation, sacrifice and suffering. Optimal diet is about supplying your body with the nutrients needed for optimal function. Optimal diet is the main tool to control your insulin and glucose. It also influences cortisol levels, cell function, free radicals, hormone levels, metabolism, and inflammation. All eight of our healthy goals are affected by what we eat. Imagine simply controlling what and when we eat to slow the aging process.

Of course, the opposite is what we see most commonly in medicine. That is, the wrong diet accelerating aging and contributing to multiple medical problems and subsequently multiple prescription medications. The epidemic of type 2 diabetes and obesity in this country are *huge* examples.

Optimal diet is about feeling better, having more energy, and maintaining our health. Now you are likely thinking, *This is impossible. How can a diet accomplish all of this?* Trust me, you will notice how great you feel when you eat well, and how poorly you feel when you stray.

The best advice in advance is this: eat well most of the time. You do not have to eat perfectly all the time. This makes the diet practical and doable while still getting all the benefits. This diet will directly support your healthy aging goals. Read on. I'll explain.

Eat healthy proteins, healthy fats, and healthy carbohydrates

First, let's look at the macronutrients that make up our diet. The three macronutrients are protein, carbohydrates, and fat. Many foods contain combinations of two or three of the macronutrients. For the purpose of constructing a meal, we will label food choices based on the main macronutrient ingredient. For example, proteins are meat (beef, pork, and lamb), poultry, eggs, fish, and soy. Carbohydrates are fruits, vegetables, grains, and legumes. ("Proteins move around; carbohydrates grow in the ground." Soy is an exception to the move-around protein. Soy only moves around if you throw it!) Fats include oils, nuts, avocados, and butter.

First, let's look at protein. Protein is broken down into amino acids in the body. Amino acids are then used by the body to build proteins needed to run the body (think anabolic). Many of these amino acids are classified as essential amino acids. "Essential," in diet speak, means it is an absolute requirement for health, and the body can't produce it. Therefore, it must be part of the diet. So protein, by definition, is an essential component of an optimal diet.

Next, let's look at fats. Fats are broken down in the body into fatty acids. The fatty acids are then used by the body or burned as fuels—and it's important to note that 60 percent of the brain is composed of fat. Two fatty acids are classified as essential fatty acids, which, again, means they are required for health; they can't be produced by the body and must be part of an optimal diet. Fats need to get on our wagon of optimal diet … so move over!

Finally, we have carbohydrates. All carbohydrates consumed are broken down into glucose (sugar). Since glucose can be produced in the body (by protein and fat), it is not classified as an essential nutrient. In the macronutrient world, there are *no essential carbohydrates.* The more I try to prove that chocolate-covered raisins are an essential part of my diet, the more I fail! (There are some simple sugars essential for health, and we will discuss those later.)

So does that mean carbohydrates don't get a lift on our optimal diet wagon?

No, but it does mean that if the wagon is getting heavy to pull, then carbohydrates are the first item to be thrown off. (I'll hold the beer, thank you.)

Fruits and vegetables are healthy carbohydrates, full of many nutrients and antioxidants; therefore, we encourage them in our optimal diet. But grains, breads, pasta, bagels, cookies, cake, candy, and chips are all examples of nutrient-poor carbohydrates that we will discourage in our optimal diet. There is a famous Chinese proverb: "If you eat a bagel, you will look like a bagel."

For purposes of our healthy aging diet, we consider any carbohydrate that is not a fruit or vegetable to be processed. Consumption of processed carbohydrates needs to be kept at a minimum.

In summary, proteins are broken down into amino acids, some of which are essential to the body. Fats are broken down into fatty acids, some of which are essential to the body. Carbohydrates are broken down into glucose, but since the body can produce glucose from protein and fat, none of the carbohydrates are essential to the body.

A diet so easy a caveman can do it! Eat real food. Avoid processed food.

The popular diet plans that exist today essentially recommend different combinations or amounts of the three macronutrients. There are low-fat diets (Ornish), there are high-protein diets (Atkins), there are high-carbohydrate diets (food pyramid), and there are balanced protein, fat, and carbohydrate diets (Zone).

Many diet plans exist, so how do we decide? *Mirror mirror on the wall, what is the healthiest diet of them all?*

We can address this question in a couple of ways. First of all, any healthy diet must by definition contain adequate protein and adequate fat. *Why?* Because low-protein or low-fat plans deprive our bodies of essential amino acids and essential fatty acids. Deprivation of essential nutrients leads to impaired metabolism, disease, and even death. The medical literature has many examples of problems associated with protein and fat deficiencies.

In addition, low-protein and low-fat plans usually substitute the "low" with carbohydrates, typically high-glycemic sugars that will prevent you from reaching your healthy goals. (The glycemic index is simple a measure of how rapidly specific carbohydrates are broken down into glucose in the body. High glycemic foods increase glucose and insulin levels.)

So if someone suggests you follow a low-protein, low-fat, or high-carbohydrate diet, just say no!

Another interesting way to choose a healthy diet is to go back in time and learn from the past. Let's look at the Paleolithic perspective. As humans evolved over the previous millions of years, our evolutionary forces and genetic makeup were influenced greatly by the foods consumed in our diets.[1-2] Remember "survival of the fittest"?

You may wonder why we would want to mimic a caveman diet. After all, Fred Flintstone and Barney Ruble were never portraits of good health. (Although Wilma and Betty never seemed to age!)

Anthropology data reveals that our Paleolithic ancestors were healthier than we are today. They had better bone structure, better lean body mass and strength, better dentition, and fewer degenerative diseases.

It is important for us to evaluate what these "hunter-gatherers" consumed. Clearly, they had no access to the processed, high-sugar foods that most of us consume in excess. Our ancestors ate what they could hunt, fish, or pick. There was no "shopping list" of items to pick up at the local twenty-four-hour grocery store. Most research suggests that none of the Starbucks back then even had drive-through! Imagine going all day without that Caramel Frappaccino and scone.

Their diets consisted of plenty of lean protein, natural fat, and small amounts of healthy carbohydrates when available (like berries picked in season), nuts, and seeds.

In essence, they consumed a high-protein, high-fat, high-fiber, and low-carbohydrate diet. They did not consume grains, bread, bagels, rice, pasta, sugar, candy, cakes, muffins, and so on. Remember, our "genetics" have changed less than 1 percent from the genetic blueprints of our caveman ancestors. Our genetics never evolved to consume large amounts of grains and sugars.

A high-carbohydrate diet impairs our metabolism and immune system while accelerating the risk of numerous degenerative diseases, such as diabetes, arthritis, colitis, heart disease, and obesity.[3-13]

Anthropology data shows that cultures were healthier until the introduction of grains into the diet. When cultures changed from a hunter-gatherer diet to a high-carbohydrate grain based diet, there was a marked increased incidence of degenerative diseases, as well as adverse changes to body composition and structure. (Even the incidence of road rage escalated!)

If we adopt a hunter-gatherer type diet, we have tremendous improvements in our health while simultaneously reaching our healthy goals. It is remarkably easy to eat this way, and in a short while, you will feel and look better. Simply eat real, natural food: food that you could hunt, fish, catch, or pick.

Put yourself in the mindset of a caveman (my wife indicates that the caveman mentality is not much of a stretch for me) and choose foods that you would have access to during the Paleolithic period.

Or imagine you are on a deserted island and eat foods that you would have to hunt for, fish for, pick, or grow. Eat natural foods and avoid processed foods brought to us by little elves, tigers, rabbits, or other cartoon characters.

Don't follow the food pyramid (it's a recipe for disaster).

An additional perspective in evaluating a healthy diet is to look at the hormonal response to the macronutrients. In other words, what hormones are released after we eat, and how do those hormones influence our health?

This hormone perspective is not one traditionally considered in the nutrition world. Most nutritionists and many mainstream diets recommend a diet that counts calories. The mantra of "the only way to lose weight is to eat fewer calories" has been repeated so often that virtually no one questions it.

How many times have you heard that all you have to do is eat less and exercise more? It turns out that no studies have ever proven that this "calorie theory" is the key to healthy weight loss.[14-25] That's right, no studies—zero, nada!

By decreasing calories, we usually make the mistake of limiting fat, since fat has more calories than equal amounts of protein or carbohydrates. There are two problems with limiting fat. One, fat is essential for good health. Two, by restricting fat, we usually restrict protein since fat and protein are often components of the same foods.

Thus, by choosing a diet based on the unproven and ineffective calorie theory, we migrate toward a low-fat, low-protein, high-carbohydrate diet.

This diet is similar to the diet farmers use to fatten livestock.[26-27] So if you **count** calories, you can **count** on buying a "larger" wardrobe!

Lowering calories too much often leads to a slower metabolism because our metabolism requires optimal protein and fat to run efficiently. Our hormones run our metabolism, and many of our hormones are released in response to the foods we eat, not in response to the calories consumed.[28-34]

Ironically, when we eat real, natural foods and avoid processed foods, we shift toward nutrient-dense foods instead of nutrient-poor foods and end up eating fewer calories overall. *What's easier to eat, a bag of chips or a bag of apples?* It is crucial to eat a balanced diet to obtain balanced hormone response.

Endocrinology 101

To better understand this hormone perspective, we must incorporate Endocrinology 101 into our antiaging program. Hormones are chemical messengers that interact with our trillions of cells to run the body. Hormones give cells specific instructions. Hormones tell the cells what to do and when to do it. Hormones are the drill sergeants of the body.

When we eat carbohydrates, our pancreas releases the hormone insulin.

All carbohydrates are broken down into glucose, but the *type* of carbohydrate consumed determines the rate of glucose elevation and the ultimate blood level of glucose. In other words, not all carbohydrates are created equal.

One of our healthy goals is to control insulin levels. The amount of insulin released is determined by the speed of glucose elevation, which of course is determined primarily by the type of carbohydrate consumed. If we eat high-glycemic carbohydrates, such as bread, pasta, cookies, and candy, our glucose level elevates rapidly. If we consume low-glycemic carbohydrates, such as whole fruits and non-starchy vegetables, our blood glucose levels increase gradually.

In addition to the types and amounts of carbohydrates we eat, the blood glucose rise is influenced by the amount of fiber, protein, and fat consumed.

Fat and fiber slow the rise in our blood glucose after eating. In addition to slowing our blood glucose elevation, protein also leads to the release of the hormone glucagon.

Glucagon hormone balances insulin. Glucagon's functions are the polar opposite of insulin's functions. Therefore, by eating a balanced diet of proteins, carbohydrates, and fats, we generate a balanced hormone response.[35-36] This allows us to control insulin levels while we supply the body with appropriate macronutrients to effectively run the metabolism.

So instead of worrying about calories, we focus on balanced nutrients, balanced hormones, and effective metabolism.

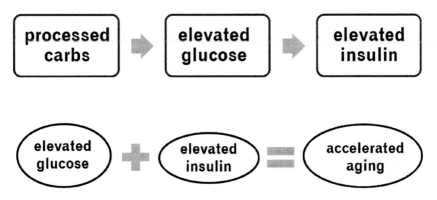

Healthy fats—all fats in a balanced diet except fried fats or trans fats—do not elevate our insulin levels. Trans fats are fatty acids that have been chemically altered in a process called hydrogenation. This commercial process is done to prevent oxidation so the fats can be utilized in processed food to extend shelf life. Unfortunately, this conversion to trans fats is damaging to the fats as well as to our health.

Since high insulin levels lead to obesity, eating healthy fat does not negatively change our hormone balance or metabolism. Just avoid chemically altered fats such as fried fats or trans fats, also called partially hydrogenated vegetable oils.

Eating fat does not make us fat! Avoiding fat makes us fat!

By eating fat, we not only supply our bodies with essential fatty acids, but we also decrease our hunger, as fat slows the absorption of food, resulting in satiety. Protein fills us up early; fat keeps us full longer.

Since it is difficult to overeat healthy protein and fat, our protein and fat intake becomes self-regulatory. Since protein, fat, and low glycemic carbohydrates are nutrient dense, we end up eating moderate amounts of calories without even counting calories!

So put your calculator away and enjoy your meal.

Pale and frail club

As we have discussed, healthy fats in our diet do not affect insulin or glucagon levels. However, fats directly influence another group of hormones called eicosanoids.

Eicosanoids are a group of hormones made directly by our cells. They are important for virtually all physiologic processes in the body. Eicosanoids influence blood flow, blood clotting, inflammation, and many other functions. The quality of our eicosanoid response is directly determined by the quality of fat in our diets.[37-47]

I can tell when someone is on a low-fat diet. *How?* Because he or she will look "pale and frail." By minimizing fat intake, eicosanoid production is adversely affected, resulting in the inevitable pale and frail body type.

By consuming balanced saturated, polyunsaturated, and monounsaturated fats, and by avoiding trans fats and fried fats, we generate balanced eicosanoids, with resulting improved health.

Eicosanoids are extremely powerful hormones. By improving our eicosanoid balance, we can dramatically improve our metabolism, decrease our risks of degenerative disease, and slow the aging process.

Fats are crucial for brain function and development. That's why I call a low-fat diet a no-brain diet!

If we eat diverse types of unprocessed food, we will by default eat a balance of different types of fats. It may help you to consider various sources for specific fats, but it is not mandatory as long as your diet has diversity.

For those who want specifics, polyunsaturated fats include omega-3 fats in fish and flaxseed, and omega-6 fats in vegetables. Monounsaturated fats are omega-9 fats found in olive oil, avocados, and nuts. Saturated fats are found primarily in animal and dairy products.

It is interesting to note that none of the naturally occurring fats and oils are made up only of all saturated or all unsaturated fats. They are mixtures of different amounts of various fatty acids.

I can't overestimate the importance of balancing different type of fats in the diet, with an emphasis on eating natural, unprocessed foods. In particular, the balance of omega-6 fats to omega-3 fats is crucial. As you will learn later in the course, a balance of omega-6 to omega-3 fats is necessary for healthy aging. Remember, the best sources of omega-6 fats are vegetables. However, processed vegetable oils are a source of excessive omega-6 fats and trans fats. This is why we discourage corn oil, for example.

Ideal sources of omega-3 fats are cold-water fish like salmon, free-range poultry, grass-fed beef, and flaxseed. Since we tend not to consume enough omega-3 fats, while simultaneously eating excessive amounts of omega-6 fats, most Americans have an unhealthy balance of omega-6 to omega-3 fats, with damaging health consequences.

In addition to balancing fat intake in the diet, we encourage organic foods when available. Organic foods are free of damaging chemical additives found in processed foods and in some nonorganic produce.

So at the risk of sounding like a broken record (should I say broken CD?), eat a variety of whole foods from nature, and you will balance the fat in your diet with improved health as the outcome.

High cortisol levels equal accelerated aging.

Yet another hormone is affected by our diets. That hormone is cortisol. Cortisol is a stress hormone; it is released from our adrenal glands to help us deal with any stress to our bodies.

Cortisol helps quickly mobilize energy and shut off non-lifesaving physiologic functions so we can get through the stressful situation. All is well if the stress response is of short duration. Unfortunately, recurrent or chronic stress—"Good news, honey. Mom is going to stay with us for a month!"—generates excessive cortisol levels.

High cortisol levels result in impaired immune function, muscle breakdown, bone loss, weight gain, and injury to the brain. Clearly, high cortisol levels are to be avoided.[48-51]

Not having optimal diets is a stress to our bodies. The brain desires a stable blood glucose level. If we eat excessive processed carbohydrates, our blood glucose levels vary from too high to too low. When our blood glucose levels spike after consuming processed carbohydrates, the subsequently elevated insulin levels drive blood glucose levels back down. These peaks and valleys are stressful to the brain and damaging to cells.

When blood glucose levels are too low, the brain is deprived of necessary energy. To deal with this stress, cortisol is released. Cortisol then breaks muscle down into amino acids. The amino acids are utilized to produce glucose to supply the brain. Over time, this recurrent stress results in loss of lean body mass (muscle) and a slower metabolism.

When we restrict calories while chasing the calorie theory for weight loss, we often go long periods without eating. This starvation response can occur by simply skipping breakfast. During this starvation period, our glucose level drops and cortisol is released to mobilize energy. We then get into a vicious cycle of low glucose, high cortisol, and impaired metabolism.

In this setting, when we finally eat, we crave high-glycemic carbohydrates to elevate our blood glucose level rapidly. This high-glycemic meal leads to the double threat of high glucose and high insulin levels.

The high insulin subsequently drops the glucose level, and the cycle is repeated. The result is poor glucose control, high insulin levels, and high cortisol levels. Three of our healthy aging goals thrown out the window because of poor diet choices! This trifecta is a perfect recipe for accelerated aging, obesity, and an increased risk of degenerative diseases.

A helpful tip to control blood glucose and insulin levels, as well as cortisol levels, is to eat every four to five hours. This improves blood glucose balance throughout the day.

If you allow blood glucose levels to drop too low, you will have low energy, irritability, and food cravings. If blood glucose gets too high, then insulin levels soar and a vicious cycle develops.

Once insulin levels go north, blood glucose levels head south and you get hungry and irritable again, leading to food cravings for high-glycemic carbohydrates. In essence, high insulin levels fuel appetite and makes you constantly hungry. No willpower in the world can battle high insulin–induced food cravings.

However, if you eat healthy foods every four to five hours during the day, you will balance glucose and insulin and end up with better energy and elimination of food cravings. I call this "proactive eating."

So don't restrict your food intake; instead, eat healthy foods frequently throughout the day. Finally, don't eat for two to three hours prior to bedtime. This will help decrease the late night junk food "pantry raid" and significantly assist fat loss efforts.

In a twenty-four hour day, you sleep approximately eight hours, leaving sixteen hours of potential eating time. If you avoid eating for a few hours prior to bedtime, you will narrow the "eating time" even further.

By eating every four hours, starting with a healthy breakfast, you will never be hungry. You will be eating four times a day at four-hour intervals, during a sixteen-hour day. *How easy is that?*

Vicious cycle: high glucose → leads to high insulin → leads to low glucose → leads to hunger → leads to food cravings → leads to eating high glycemic foods → leads to high glucose → leads to high insulin … and the cycle continues on and on.

This vicious cycle results in high body fat, accelerated aging, high medical bills, and poor quality of life.

You must avoid this vicious cycle to regain your life.

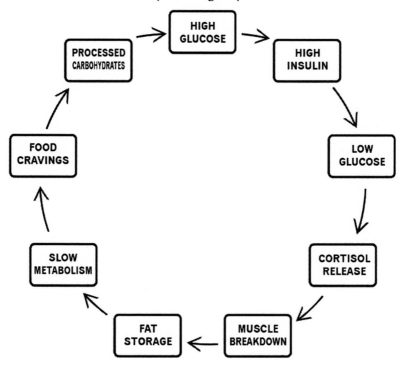

Fat burner versus sugar burner

Many of us simply want to know how to lose weight. Most people have tried various diets and exercise programs without long-term success. Because of this high failure rate, it is common for people to assume that they are destined to be overweight for their entire lifetime.

Frequently, obese patients have resigned themselves to always being heavy and never feeling their best. Others have undergone gastric bypass or other weight loss surgery because they have concluded, after multiple attempts at weight loss, that they must take drastic measures because nothing else works.

This is truly unfortunate, as we all have the ability to burn fat and lose weight. None of us need to undergo surgery simply to lose weight. It is no one's destiny to be obese. The solution is to support our biochemistry and tap into our intrinsic fat burning capabilities. Let me explain.

We discussed earlier how a Paleolithic diet is congruent with our genetics. When we eat as nature intended, we support our intrinsic physiology and biochemistry. When we support our physiology, our metabolism improves—we burn fat, lose weight, and regain our health.

An effective way to understand this is to focus on fat burning versus sugar burning. The human body has two main fuel sources: sugar and fat. Our body prefers not to burn protein unless forced to under stressful situations like starvation. Instead of burning protein, our bodies utilize protein to run metabolism and rebuild and repair under anabolic influences.

Much like a hybrid engine burns a combination of gasoline and electricity, the body burns a combination of glucose (sugar) and fat. Glucose is utilized as a fuel source for quick energy. Fat is utilized as a fuel source for sustained energy.

During our Paleolithic times, our food supply was inconsistent. We had to hunt or catch our meals. We had to endure periods of famine, especially if we were lousy hunters!

Our bodies evolved a perfect system to allow us to thrive during feast and famine. The pivotal part to this perfect system is the hormone insulin. Insulin ultimately determines whether we are primarily burning sugar or primarily burning fat.[52-56]

When we eat, our blood glucose levels, and subsequently our insulin levels, rise. The elevation of the insulin is a signal to the body that food is available. Since we historically went long periods of time when food was not available, it was critical to our survival that we eat as much as we can when opportunity allowed.

Insulin elevation stimulates appetite to ensure that we "eat when the eating is good." In addition, insulin stores much of the food we do eat as fat. This dual action of insulin is lifesaving when our food supply is inconsistent. However, when food availability is consistent, like it is today, the life saving qualities of insulin become problematic.

Our bodies are still running on our old software program, so when food is available, the message is "eat and store." If we eat foods that sabotage our glucose and insulin levels, we literally are forced to become "sugar burners" because we can't access stored body fat. Insulin locks the fat in storage and won't let it go.

When we eat foods that control our glucose and insulin levels, we become "fat burners," as the low insulin allows us to access stored body fat. This is our biochemical reality, no exceptions.[57-59]

To burn fat, we must control our insulin levels.

When we eat to control our insulin levels, we burn fat 24/7. Of course, if we don't control insulin, we store fat 24/7. This system has evolved over millions of years, so despite being old, it is very, very efficient.

We can store unlimited fat. We continue to store fat even when we have stored enough fat to fuel many lifetimes! If the "eat and store" message is sent out from insulin, guess what, we eat too much food and we store too much fat.

The only way to bypass the "sugar burn, fat store" message is to eat foods that were available during the Paleolithic times. Foods that we can hunt, catch, fish or pick, and avoid processed foods.

Just remember that when insulin levels are high, this is a one-way ticket to fat storage. Adipose, or fat cells, are meant to be a holding station for energy. When food is not available, adipose cells release stored fat in the form of triglycerides into the bloodstream. The triglycerides are transported to the trillions of cells in the body, to be burned for energy production.

When food is available, we eat, and insulin directs the storage of food energy for future use into our adipose cells. This holding station role of adipose becomes a long-term storage situation when we have predominantly elevated insulin levels.

It is critical to review which food choices will elevate insulin and which food choices help control insulin. Just keep in mind that protein will be utilized to run the metabolism, and that the body prefers not to burn protein.

In addition, protein intake does not excessively elevate insulin levels. Recall from our earlier discussion that protein elevates levels of the hormone glucagon. Glucagon has the opposite effects of insulin. Glucagon facilitates fat burning and control of blood glucose levels.

Healthy fat has no impact on your insulin levels, while simultaneously helping to slow the absorption of any carbohydrates you consume with the fat. Because of the multiple benefits of healthy fat, it is crucial to stay away from low-fat diets.

Healthy carbohydrates such as whole fruits and vegetables are, in reality, slow release sugars, so our glucose and insulin levels remain controlled.

Of course, the real culprit in glucose and insulin elevation is any processed carbohydrate. Eating processed carbohydrates will elevate glucose and insulin levels rapidly, which unfortunately leads to efficient and effective fat storage.

Fat storage will force your body into sugar-burning mode, wherein your blood glucose alternates between too high and too low. Because of your unstable blood glucose levels, you will never feel your best. You will have cravings and feel constantly hungry. While you're constantly burning sugar, the percentage of body fat grows astronomically.

When this situation develops, it usually leads to deprivation diet efforts. *Why?* Because as our body fat escalates, we become convinced, or are told, that we are "eating too much" or "not exercising enough."

Ironically, in this high-insulin state, because we are not accessing energy from stored body fat, we are actually not getting enough fuel to our cells.

When insulin is high, our bodies know times are good and focus on storage of fat for the future. While the fat storage process is going on its merry way, the nonfat storage cells of the body are starving for energy. This leads to low-energy states and malaise.

When affected people try to "eat less," their cells get even *less* fuel, and their cellular energy production plummets to lower depths. They continue on this deprivation plan until their willpower inevitably succumbs to their biochemistry. When this happens, they resume a high-carbohydrate diet, store fat at even higher rates, and become convinced, beyond any shadow of a doubt, that obesity is their destiny

It is extremely rewarding to change these patients' diets so they become fat burners, as nature intended, and watch the transformation of their body composition. When patients who felt they were destined to be obese forever finally lose the excess body fat and change their appearance and health, it is truly incredible to witness.

In conclusion, our optimal diet consists of balanced healthy protein, healthy fat, and healthy carbohydrates. This allows optimal nutrients and optimal hormone responses. The result is decreased risk of disease, improved immune function, improved brain function, and improved metabolism.

By adopting this diet, you will have renewed energy, stamina, and vitality. You will have lower body fat, better lean muscle mass and bone density. Your spouse may even think you're sexy!

Healthy proteins:

Lean meats (ideally, free-range, grass-fed beef*)
Wild game
Chicken and turkey (ideally, free range)
Eggs (from free-range chickens)
Seafood (wild, avoid farm raised)

Healthy fats:

Olive oil (extra virgin)
Coconuts/coconut oil
Avocados
Nuts (raw)
Seeds
Butter (not margarine)

Healthy carbohydrates:

Whole fruits (organic** is best)
Vegetables (organic** is best)

*Grass-fed beef has been shown to provide up to twenty-five times more omega-3 fatty acids than grain-fed beef.

**Organic foods are generally free of artificial additives, artificial sweeteners, and colorings. They are largely free of pesticides and herbicides. They have higher levels of antioxidants as well as higher levels of vitamins and minerals.

Trans fats equal slow food poisoning.

To maintain health, you must avoid trans fats like the plague that they are. Trans fats, also referred to as partially hydrogenated cooking oils, are chemically altered fats. They are chemically altered for the sole purpose of extending shelf life. This is why you can buy processed foods with an expiration date extending into the next century!

Unfortunately, they extend shelf life at the expense of shortening human life. These fake fats incorporate themselves into our cells like an unwelcome houseguest. They disrupt cell function and adversely affect health. If the only change you make in your diet after taking this course is to avoid trans fats, you will dramatically improve your health.

In our healthy diet, we minimize consumption of altered fats, such as trans fats, as well as added chemicals. Chemicals added to processed food also disrupt metabolism and are unhealthy for our cells. Common examples of chemicals added to processed food include MSG (monosodium glutamate) and artificial sweeteners, such as aspartame. Just remember to eat natural, unprocessed foods to avoid the harmful effects of chemicals and trans fats on your health.

What do trans fats do?

Raise total cholesterol

Lower HDL cholesterol

Increase risk of heart disease

Raise glucose levels

Increase body fat

Increase cancer risk

Lower testosterone levels

Shorten life

Accelerate aging

Increase the food industry's profits[60-64]

Balance of omega-3 fats with omega-6 fats

It is crucial to balance omega-3 fats with omega-6 fats to obtain good health. Most Americans have high omega-6 levels and low omega-3 levels. Omega-6 fats are prevalent in our diets, while omega-3 fats are deficient. Avoid processed vegetable oils and processed foods that raise your omega-6 levels too high. Eat cold-water fish and supplement with fish oil to raise omega-3 levels.

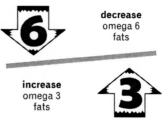

We must avoid excessive intake of the wrong kinds of fats (processed oils and trans fats) and increase intake of the right kinds of fats (unprocessed fats in grass-fed meats, wild game, wild fish, cage-free poultry and eggs, raw nuts, and extra-virgin olive oil) for optimal health and aging.

Optimal Diet Nuts and Bolts

1) Eat very well *most* of the time.

2) Base each meal and snack around a healthy protein source. Best protein sources include lean beef (organic, grass fed), chicken/turkey (free range), wild game meats, eggs (from free-range chickens) and fish (wild, not farm raised).

3) Combine your protein with low glycemic carbohydrates: whole fruits and non-starchy vegetables.

4) Add additional healthy fat to each meal. Best sources include olive oil (extra virgin), nuts (raw), avocados, butter, seeds, and coconut.

5) Encourage foods from nature in their natural state (caveman diet).

6) Don't go hungry/don't skip meals (avoid cortisol response).

7) Try to have five "feedings" daily, i.e., three meals and two healthy snacks. Plan to eat every four to five hours. Avoid eating for two to three hours prior to bedtime.

8) Avoid chemicals that disrupt metabolism: MSG, artificial sweeteners, and trans fats. Avoid processed foods. Avoid high-fructose corn syrup. Read labels to find other names for sugar: sucrose, corn syrup, dextrose, maple sugar, honey, "organic" sugar. Bottom line: *Sugar is the devil!*

9) Drink water, more water, tea, moderate coffee, and moderate alcohol (preferably red wine). No fruit drinks,

juices, sodas, or sport drinks like "sugarade," a.k.a. Gatorade.

10) Change your perspective. Optimal diet is not about deprivation and weight loss but about fueling your body for optimal function, peak performance, and healthy aging. Good health requires building your body, not breaking it down. Build the muscle and burn the fat.

11) Buy organic foods as much as possible. Shop at farmers markets and natural food stores for more diverse options. Select nature-made foods over man-made foods.

I once heard a comedian joke that "organic" meant "twice as expensive." This may be true, but it also means "twice as healthy."

I must reinforce a crucial point. When you eat, think of it as an opportunity to consume healthy foods to improve your health. Eat to build your health. You can't deny or deprive yourself of good food on your way to optimal health.

Remember, optimal diet influences all eight of our healthy aging goals!

Our antiaging diet really is the foundation for healthy aging. When we eat healthy, we control glucose and insulin levels, we control cortisol levels, we supply appropriate nutrients to support cell function, we lower free radical production, we control hormone levels, we support metabolism, and we lower inflammation.

By reaching our antiaging goals, we improve body composition, lose excess body fat, and improve energy and vitality.

Warning: you must read food labels.

Food marketing can make your food selection confusing. Watch out for statements such as "all natural" because it can contain *natural* sugar that will *naturally* lead to health problems! Avoid products labeled "low fat" or "no fat." These mean the food has been processed and usually extra sugar added to substitute for the missing fat. Also be careful with "no extra sugar added"—this simply means there already is plenty of sugar!

Instead of reading the front label, read the nutritional label on the back. Look there for artificial sweeteners, sugar content and added chemicals like MSG and high-fructose corn syrup. If you see these, be careful. They will sabotage your antiaging goals.

Remember, nature-made foods come "naturally" … without a label. The fewer ingredients listed, the better.

CHAPTER 2
QUESTIONS

Student:

On most diets, you need to count calories, fat grams, or cholesterol content. How do I know I am doing well with the healthy aging diet without counting something?

Professor:

Stay on the healthy aging diet and you can *count* on healthy aging! If you want something to monitor, simply monitor your blood glucose levels. By eating real foods and by avoiding high glycemic carbohydrates, you will stabilize your blood glucose levels at all times. This will result in fat loss as well as stable moods and energy levels, while simultaneously decreasing the risk of diabetes, heart disease, and cancer significantly. (Blood sugar ranges of 70 to 90 are optimal.)

Another easy way to monitor your progress is by paying attention to how you look and how you feel. With healthy eating, you will notice improved skin tone and color as well as resolution of chronic, recurrent rashes. You will have dramatically improved gastrointestinal health, with resolution of gas, bloating, cramps, and heartburn. You will have normal daily bowel movements (usually two per day). You will have improved energy and rarely require naps. Your moods will be stable and consistent. Your relationships could even improve (mostly because of the gas issue). You will develop a leaner body and lose excess body fat at a rate of about one pound a week. Eating this way will change your life.

Finally, you will acquire the ability to tell when you have eaten the wrong foods. When you do, your gastrointestinal symptoms will return, your mood will change, your energy will wane, and your fat loss will plateau. Your relationships may deteriorate. This allows a built-in guide to alert you to when you have strayed too far and get you back on a healthy track.

Remember, our typical American diet is making us sick. Eating well makes you feel well; eating poorly makes you feel poorly. It is that simple.

Student:

You taught us that we should "eat well most of the time." Are there any foods we should never eat?

Professor:

A goal with this diet is to allow you some flexibility in your diet to make it something you can stay on for the rest of your life. In time, you will avoid bad foods because you feel so much better when you don't eat them. However, cheating occasionally will not disrupt your ability to reach your antiaging goals. This is not about perfection.

With that in mind, here is a list of foods to avoid. These foods represent a form of food poisoning; they harm you and have no nutritional value. They are toxic to your health. Here's your list of no-no's:

Doughnuts	Fried fast foods, e.g., chicken nuggets
Candy (except for dark chocolate)	Muffins
French fries	Breakfast cereals
Bagels	Ice cream
Cake	Sugar-coated anything
Potato chips	High-fructose corn syrup
Sodas	Trans fats
Cookies	Artificial sweeteners

Student:

Are there any diet books you would recommend?

Professor:

Yes. *The Zone, Protein Power, The South Beach Diet, No-Grain Diet, Antiaging 101.*

Student:

I love french fries and potato chips. How do I live without them?

Professor:

Get over it. How old are you, two?

Student:

Everyone knows that to lose weight, you must burn off more calories than you take in, yet you teach us not to count calories. Who do we believe?

Professor:

Many physicians, nutritionists, teachers, coaches, and government agencies cling to the never-proven theory that weight loss is determined by calories in versus calories out. Everyone knows about this. Maybe this is why so many people are f-a ... *far* from their optimal weight. Metabolism and fat storage is more complicated than simply looking at calories in versus calories out. To clarify this mighty misconception further, I offer a few points to consider:

1) If you think the human body is such a simple machine that all weight loss requires is a calorie deficit ... I have some oceanfront properties in Tucson to sell you (all with plenty of beach).
2) All calories are not created equal (in the body). A calorie of fat does not equal a calorie of protein, which does not equal a calorie of carbohydrate. How we metabolize foods is important, not the number of calories.
3) The macronutrients we eat elicit a hormonal response that fuels our metabolism. The hormone response is determined by the type of food consumed, not by the number of calories consumed. For example, insulin is released when our blood sugar rises, not simply because our caloric intake increases.
4) Many studies of isocaloric diets, i.e., same number of calories but different percentage of fat, protein, and carbohydrates, have proven that it is not the calories that determine diet success but what types of foods we eat. Most compelling are studies consistently revealing that people lose more weight on a low-carbohydrate, higher-calorie diet than they do on a high-carbohydrate, low-calorie diet.[65-84] Very few people are successful with the calorie theory approach to weight loss and health.
5) The theory assumes that all overweight people, all 65 percent of us, are heavy simply because we overeat and under exercise.

Most patients I consult about a healthy diet eat too little and exercise too much.

Remember, instead of "eat less, exercise more" you should "eat less junk food and exercise more efficiently" (stay in class and I will show you how to exercise efficiently).

Student:

I had a heart attack last year. My dietician says I need to stay on a low-fat, low-cholesterol diet to avoid another heart attack in the future. You teach that fats are important to health. What should I do?

Professor:

If we look at some of the causes of heart disease, we see that this focus on cholesterol and fat is shortsighted and ineffective.

What about blood glucose, inflammation, high insulin, obesity, nutrient deficiencies, sedentary lifestyle, smoking, hormone levels, and other risk factors for heart disease? Do we just ignore them and keep you on a low fat diet?

Unfortunately, the low-fat, low-cholesterol approach ignores most of the risk factors for heart disease. In fact, a low-fat diet will raise your triglycerides, increase blood sugar levels, increase insulin levels, and increase inflammation! Ironically, by following a low-fat diet, you will actually increase your chance of having another heart attack.

Finally, not all fats are created equal so why avoid all fats or most fats?

Remember, a deficiency of omega-3 fats is a cause of blood clotting and heart disease. So don't go low fat, go healthy fat.

Student:

I have followed a low-fat diet for two years. I am elated because my cholesterol is low and my LDL cholesterol is only 90. Shouldn't I stay on the low fat diet?

Professor:

Congratulations on your low cholesterol reading. How do you feel?

Student:

I feel like hell.

Professor:

I don't doubt it son, you look a little pale and frail. I cannot emphasize enough the importance of healthy fats in the diet. Remember, balanced healthy fat intake results in balanced eicosanoid production. Eicosanoids are those cell hormones that we talked about earlier in class. Eicosanoids influence virtually all physiologic processes in the body. They greatly impact blood flow and inflammation. When people are consuming healthy fats, they have improved skin color and texture. When they are on a low-fat diet, they develop eicosanoid imbalances and have pale, dry skin. Eat balanced fats to maintain that healthy glow.

Student:

What about fiber?

Professor:

Fiber is very important. It improves colon health, immune function, and even improves your cholesterol panel. Fiber also decreases the glycemic response to foods. In other words, when fiber is part of a meal or snack, it lowers the rate of glucose elevation after eating.

If you eat healthy fruits, vegetables, seeds, and nuts, you will get plenty of beneficial fiber in your diet.

A trick for weight loss is to supplement with a dose of psyllium fiber thirty minutes before meals. This works to lower glucose levels and contribute to satiety, so you tend not to overeat. Get a brand without any sugar or artificial sweeteners added. Add the psyllium amount slowly to allow you to adjust to the extra fiber; otherwise, you may experience cramps, gas, and bloating. If you add it to your diet slowly, you should tolerate it without any problems.

Student:

You didn't mention milk; shouldn't we be drinking milk every day?

Professor:

Only if your mother is a cow (literally). In contrast to the milk mustache ads, milk is not good for you. It is a poor source of calcium; it contains lactose, a sugar that most people do not tolerate; and it is full of synthetic hormones and antibiotics.[85-87] In addition, the homogenization process results in altered, damaged fat, which can injure blood vessels. I do not encourage milk consumption.

Student:
You listed foods to avoid; do you have a list of foods you encourage?

Professor:
Great question. It is important to avoid processed foods full of trans fats, high-fructose corn syrup, sugars, and chemicals. However, it is crucial that you don't deprive your body of fuel: healthy protein, healthy fat, and healthy carbohydrates. Just remember to eat healthy for healthy aging. You can't deprive and starve your way to good health. Eat like a caveman, choosing natural foods.

Eat some of the following foods every day:

Lean meats	Vegetables
Fish	Nuts
Eggs	Seeds
Fruit	Beans

Student:
What about oils?

Professor:
Use butter, olive oil, and coconut oil. Avoid margarine and processed vegetable oils, e.g., corn oil, soy oil, canola oil, sunflower oil, and sesame oil. Although canola oil is frequently recommended for good health, it is another processed oil with excessive levels of trans fats and omega-6 fats that are damaging to health.

Butter and coconut oil are best for cooking, as they are stable fats that can endure high temperature without damage to the fats. Cooking easily damages olive oil, so only cook with olive oil at low heat. Add olive oil to salads and vegetables for optimal benefit.

Student:

How many servings of fruits and vegetables do you suggest for healthy aging?

Professor:

As many as possible. Emphasize vegetables over fruits, the more the merrier. I think it is difficult to count servings. Simply eat vegetables and whole fruits ideally with every meal and snack. They are full of phytochemicals that nourish and protect cells.

If you are not a vegetable fan, I recommend taking a "green formula" supplement daily. My favorite green supplement is called Perfect Food by Garden for Life. You can find it online or at most health food stores. It comes in powder or tablet form.

Student:

Why do you discourage grains when they make up such a large component of the food pyramid?

Professor:

Grains are not as healthy as advertised. Most grains in this country are highly processed and devoid of nutrients and fiber. Most grains simply raise your blood glucose levels with minimal if any nutrient value. Many grains are actually *anti*nutrients, which block the absorption of nutrients in food.

Many people are sensitive to gluten, a protein in grains that causes abdominal pain, bloating, diarrhea, fatigue, weight gain, and excessive inflammation. Most people are not aware of their gluten sensitivity and end up on multiple prescription medications for their symptoms, yet they continue on a high-grain diet that compounds the problem. Often, patients are given the diagnosis of irritable bowel syndrome or spastic colon, when avoiding grains would change their life (and diagnosis).[88-91]

When patients come to see me regarding weight gain, fatigue, bloating, and so forth, I have them try a no-grain diet for thirty days, often with complete resolution of their symptoms.

We should realize that we would get plenty of fiber with a diet high in whole fruits and vegetables. Psyllium, an unprocessed grain, could be added as a supplement if you would feel more in line with the government's food pyramid catastrophe ... I mean, guidelines.

Student:

What are your thoughts on portion control?

Professor:

Portion control is part of the calorie theory of weight loss. Many diet programs center around portion control with the belief that "less is better." These programs don't realize the importance of balanced macronutrients.

The logic with portion control is that if a lot of junk food is bad for you, then smaller portions of junk food are good for you. Obviously, junk food is junk food, regardless of portion size.

You must remember that you can't deprive yourself on the road to good health. You must supply the body with essential fats and essential proteins every day.

Finally, when you eat real food like a caveman, food intake becomes self-regulatory. You won't overeat healthy protein, healthy fat, or healthy carbohydrates.

Focus on your antiaging goals.

Student:

I am having trouble keeping up with all the information so far in *Antiaging 101.* Are there any foods that help my brain function better?

Professor:

In general, you will find that by supporting cell function throughout the body, as we teach in this class, every part of your body works better, including your brain. That being said, there are some foods that clearly enhance the brain and protect it from excessive oxidation and inflammation.

Here is a short but effective list of brain foods:

1) Eggs (you must eat the yolks). Egg yolks contain choline. Choline is an essential nutrient required for normal functioning of all cells. It is crucial for brain and nerve function, and it is essential for healthy cell membrane function.
2) Berries, grapes, tea, turmeric, coffee, dark chocolate, and many fruits and veggies contain antioxidants that protect and enhance brain function.

3) Omega-3 fats in fish and fish oils, flaxseed, and walnuts enhance brain function.

Student:

Do you encourage the consumption of polyphenols?

Professor:

You must have a nutrition background to ask about polyphenols. For the rest of the class, polyphenols are a class of phytochemicals found in high concentrations in tea, wine, grapes, and a wide variety of other plants. They are responsible for the colored pigments of many fruits and vegetables. They protect the plants from diseases and ultraviolet light.

When we consume polyphenols, we are also protected from disease. Polyphenols have been found to have high antioxidant activity; they have antibacterial and antiviral activity; and they have anti-inflammatory activity. They also protect and strengthen blood vessels.

Consumption of polyphenols is definitely encouraged because of the marvelous array of health benefits. They help us reach our antiaging goals.

Student:

Would you explain the difference between "glycemic index" and "glycemic load"?

Professor:

Glycemic index is essentially a measure of how much a specific quantity (fifty grams) of a food raises the blood glucose level. Glycemic load is a measure of how much a usual serving of a specific food raises the blood glucose level. The glycemic load is a more valuable tool, as it shows you the impact of a usual serving size. It is therefore more practical than the glycemic index. You can find copies of both the glycemic index and glycemic load at www.health.harvard.edu.

I believe the concept of glycemic index and glycemic load is important to understand. However, if your carbohydrate choices are primarily whole fruits and vegetables, all of which have low glycemic loads, then it becomes a moot point. In addition, when you combine protein, fat, and fiber with any carbohydrate, you lower the glycemic impact of that carbohydrate.

Student:

Why do you recommend cage-free chickens and cage-free eggs? Why do you recommend grass-fed beef? Why do you recommend wild fish over farm-raised fish?

Professor:

Why do you ask so many questions at once?

The reason for those recommendations is because the *quality* of the meat, eggs, fish, and poultry is determined primarily by what the animals eat. When the animals have access to their natural diet, they are healthier, just like humans. When they eat what nature intended, their protein and fat composition is healthier, just like humans. When we humans eat like cavemen, our body composition and health improves. When animals eat like their ancestors ate, their body composition and health improves. When poultry and eggs are free range (no cages), they have access to natural foods. When fish are wild, they have access to natural foods. When cattle have access to grass, they are healthier than if they are fed grains.

I also favor certified organic foods to avoid the addition of synthetic hormones and other chemicals currently added to our food chain. Because organic foods, cage-free poultry, grass-fed beef, and wild seafood are more expensive than other options, consume them when you can. Shop at whole food and ranch markets when you can. Remember, it doesn't have to be all the time, just most of the time. Regardless, eating meats, eggs, poultry, and fish is much, much, healthier than processed foods.

Student:

I have read that we don't need much protein on a daily basis. Why do you recommend protein at every meal and snack?

Professor:

If we simply want the *minimal* amount of protein required by the body on a daily basis, then you are correct that we will be fine with a small amount daily. However, if we approach diet with the goal of optimizing wellness and healthy aging, then more protein is required.

Protein at each meal is recommended for several reasons: Protein is used by the body all day and all night to rebuild and repair. Protein is stored primarily in our muscles. Even if we don't eat protein, our body still requires protein for "reconstruction projects." If we don't eat enough protein, then the body will break down our muscle to get it. We don't want to lose our muscle tissue!

Protein runs our metabolism. Protein at each meal is like putting another log on the fire of your metabolism. Protein keeps you in fat-burning mode. Protein consumption prompts the body to release the hormone glucagon. Glucagon helps burn fat. Glucagon also balances insulin hormone.

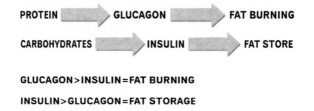

Protein promotes satiety. It keeps us content and less hungry in between meals. It helps us stay on a healthy diet forever.

Student:

How important is it to avoid artificial sweeteners and chemicals in processed foods?

Professor:

Very! People are usually surprised to learn that chemicals in their "diet" foods and "diet" drinks are detrimental to their health. Chemicals such as monosodium glutamate, aspartame, and sucralose are damaging to our health. These chemicals stimulate appetite, disrupt metabolism, and injure cells (including brain cells).[92-94] They will sabotage your antiaging efforts. Wean off them as soon as possible. Eat unprocessed foods.

Student:

It seems many people overeat processed carbohydrates and sugars because of food cravings or because they are stressed and nervous. Any suggestions to deal with this emotional component?

Professor:

By following the *Antiaging 101* program, food cravings will decrease significantly for a number of reasons. First and foremost, by stabilizing glucose and insulin, you will avoid excessive food cravings. Unstable glucose levels and high insulin levels stimulate appetite. All your brain hears is "eat sugar." This message will be silenced by following a balanced real-food diet.

Another reason for food cravings is hormone imbalances. Hormones help produce and regulate brain chemicals that affect mood. When hormones are unbalanced, brain chemicals are unbalanced, and food cravings are induced as a temporary "feel good" measure. This will be controlled with hormone balance.

Stress creates food cravings and emotional eating, again as a temporary feel good measure. Stress-reduction techniques will eliminate this component of overeating (see chapter 6).

When you start this program, it will take a few days to weeks for your cravings to be controlled. But believe me, not only will the cravings resolve, but the thought of eating junk food will literally be nauseating. You simply will not want to go back to not feeling well. Eating healthy feels too good to quit.

Student:

In your practice, what are the most common diet errors that you see with patients?

Professor:

Most common errors I find with patients' diets include not consuming enough protein in the diet. Others include counting calories instead of focusing on macronutrients, avoiding fat in the diet, consuming drinks containing high amounts of sugar, eating too many processed grains, and overeating processed foods, especially processed carbohydrates.

It is essential to realize that you deserve to be healthy. Make a commitment to yourself. Treat your body with respect. If you can't even respect yourself, how do you expect respect from others? Be a role model for your children and grandchildren.

Get out of that Accelerated Aging Club! Treat yourself well. You deserve it.

What does the medical and scientific literature reveal about diet?

❖ In a study of 4,500 adults aged sixty to eighty, higher total omega-3 fat intake deceased the risk of developing macular degeneration.

❖ A Mediterranean diet is found to be more anti-inflammatory and promotes greater weight loss than the American Heart Association "prudent diet."

❖ Older adults with diets high in omega-3 fats have higher cognitive function.

❖ Women with the highest level of folate (folic acid) intake had a 36 percent lower risk of breast cancer. Women with the highest intake of vitamin B12 had a 68 percent decreased risk of breast cancer.

❖ In a study of overweight adults, those who ate three ounces of almonds daily for six months lost 62 percent more weight than those who ate a nut-free diet with an equal number of calories.

❖ *American College of Cardiology* studied 3,000 people for one year and found the Mediterranean diet was associated with lower levels of inflammation and blood-clotting markers.

❖ Over a ten-year period, a French study of 1,640 participants, with an average age of seventy-seven, found that diets rich in antioxidant compounds could reduce the decline in mental function associated with aging.

❖ Researchers have found that people who eat a Mediterranean diet with its 40 percent fat content have a lower incidence of heart disease than people who eat a very low fat diet (10 percent fat.)

❖ A diet study that substituted carbohydrate-rich foods with protein-rich foods improved blood pressure in hypertensive patients.

❖ Study revealed that two-thirds of heart attack patients had blood glucose control problems.

❖ A ten-year follow-up study by Harvard School of Public Health found that high glycemic load increased heart disease risk.

❖ A ten-year study found blood glucose levels linked to significantly higher cancer and death risk.

❖ Multiple studies show trans fats to be associated with artery damage and a high risk of heart disease.

❖ A Harvard study compared a low-fat diet against a low-carbohydrate diet (with higher calories) and found the low-carbohydrate, higher-calorie dieter lost more weight. (It's not calories in versus calories out for weight loss.)

❖ A study of 2,000 men followed for 12.8 years found that those with the highest consumption of fruits, berries, and vegetables had a 41 percent lower risk of death from cardiovascular disease and a 44 percent lower risk of all-cause mortality.

❖ A study of 74,000 women followed for twelve years found that the women who consumed the largest amounts of fruits and vegetables had a 24 percent lower risk of obesity.

❖ Diets high in carbohydrates and omega-6 fats increase risk of blood clotting and heart attack.

❖ A large study found that one fish meal a week was associated with a 60 percent reduction in the risk of developing Alzheimer's disease.

❖ A study found that diet plus exercise reversed metabolic syndrome in three weeks. In the obese men studied, after three weeks on the program, there were significant reductions in serum lipids, insulin levels, and inflammation.

❖ A study of over 49,000 women during a sixteen-year period found that high glycemic diets increase the risk of breast cancer. Among postmenopausal women, the highest versus lowest quartile level of overall glycemic index was associated with an 87 percent increased risk of breast cancer.

❖ A diet low in total fat and saturated fat had *no* impact in reducing heart disease and stroke rates in 20,000 women studied over eight years.

❖ A 2004 Harvard University study of older women with heart disease found that the *more* saturated fat the women consumed, the *less likely* it was that their condition would worsen.

❖ A 2000 meta-analysis of the scientific literature on cholesterol-lowering diets showed that diets low in saturated fat had no significant effect on mortality or deaths due to heart attacks.

❖ A *Journal of Clinical Endocrinology and Metabolism* study found that proteins in the diet are better at suppressing an appetite-stimulating hormone (ghrelin), compared to carbohydrates and fats.

❖ *Journal of the American Medical Association* found that people eating very low-fat diets showed no improvement in body composition, blood sugar, insulin levels, or blood pressure. In fact, the study's authors called very low-fat diets "counterproductive" to health.

❖ A study reported in the *Journal of Family Practice* concluded the following: "Low-carbohydrate diets resulted in more weight loss than low-fat/low-calorie diets after six months, with no adverse impact on lipids, bone density, or blood pressure."

❖ In an eight-year study of 3,977 people, those who ate the most high-glycemic carbohydrates had a 40 percent higher risk for macular degeneration.

And much more …

CHAPTER 3

NUTRACEUTICAL SUPPLEMENTATION

Every day, our bodies are bombarded with free radicals. Every day, our brains are bombarded with conflicting information on nutraceuticals. It would be easy (and cheaper, actually) to simply throw in the towel and not bother with any dietary supplements. Resist the temptation to quit; your health and longevity depend on an effective supplement program.[1-9]

For many decades, the medical establishment has repeated the message that "supplements are worthless and only give you expensive urine!" Further, they claim that we get all the vitamins and minerals we need from your diet. (Consider all those drinks that advertise "10 percent real juice," when what they really mean is "90 percent sugar." Good luck if you think you get optimal nutrients in the "all-American diet.")

Finally, in 2002, the American Medical Association reversed their opinion. In June 2002, they stated, "All adults should take multivitamin supplements to help prevent chronic disease."[10] Maybe soon the American Dental Association will recommend flossing!

Let's give credit where credit is due. The bottom line is this: the AMA could no longer ignore numerous published medical studies revealing definite links between low-vitamin/mineral intake and disease.

These studies are found in diverse medical journals and document health benefits of supplementation on vision, skin, heart, brain, and overall health.

After reviewing this overwhelming medical literature, it becomes clear that to stay well preserved over the years, we need optimal levels of multiple nutrients in our bloodstream.

Two goals of supplementation:

- Supply cells with nutrients
- Antioxidant protection

So why should we supplement?

There are two main goals for nutrient supplementation. One goal is to provide the trillions of cells in our body with the nutrients needed for optimal function and energy production. It is difficult to fathom that every day our bodies produce millions of new cells. We must support these new cells with the raw materials they need.

Our second goal is to combat free radical damage to the cells and our DNA. Free radical damage is a major cause of disease and aging. It is a constant force that will wear you down and wear you out.

So how do we obtain appropriate levels of nutrients in our bloodstream to combat aging and provide cells with necessary raw materials? Isn't our healthy antiaging diet enough?

Well, our antiaging diet is astronomically better than the typical American diet. No study of the American diet has ever shown that we get all the nutrients we need for optimal health through food. If you live on bagels, doughnuts, french fries, and colas, then this becomes obvious.

However, what if you do eat well most of the time?

Clearly, your overall nutrient levels will be markedly improved, but they will still be under the ideal. *Why?* Primarily because of food processing, shipping, soil depletion, and a myriad of other factors that have depleted the nutrient density of our food supply.

Don't let this be a deterrent to you for following our healthy aging diet. There are still tremendous benefits, as we discussed in our last chapter. We just need a small boost in our supplement intake to reach effective levels for healthy aging and reduction of disease risk.

What about the RDA, recommended daily allowance?

Hey, I can get 10 percent of my vitamin D level by eating a bowl of Honey Nut Cheerios! In my world, the RDA equals BS. Sorry to be so blunt, but it is what it is. The RDA is the minimum level of nutrients to prevent overt disease[11-12]—for example, the amount of vitamin C you need to prevent scurvy or the amount of vitamin D needed to prevent rickets. The RDA is defined as "the average daily dietary intake level that is sufficient to meet the nutrient requirements of nearly all healthy individuals."

This RDA approach is like asking your boss to pay you the minimum wage to prevent bankruptcy! After all, you may just take the extra money and waste it on imported beer, and we know that only leads to expensive urine!

Don't confuse the RDA with optimal levels. The RDA was not established to help you achieve and maintain optimal health. It is literally the bare minimum needed to prevent vitamin deficiency disease.

Does this mean more is better?

The answer is yes … most of the time. While large doses of most nutrients are safe, we need to be careful with the doses of a few nutrients. Still, to put supplement safety in perspective, I have seen more complications from medications at prescribed doses in one week than the total complications I have seen from supplements in twenty-five years of emergency medicine.

Most vitamins are water-soluble. Essentially, this means that they dissolve in water; as a result, they do their work and are then excreted from the body in the urine. With water-soluble vitamins, the body takes what it needs and easily eliminates any excess. As a result, it is virtually impossible to overdose on water-soluble vitamins. They simply provide the blood with optimal levels and let the trillions of cells in our body choose to take in the amounts needed; any "left over" is flushed. Yes, this can mean "expensive urine"; however, the "expensive blood" has now supplied our cells with crucial nutrients for optimal function and defense. A perfect system.

On the other hand, fat-soluble vitamins are stored in body fat and can accumulate over time. This could potentially lead to problems with excessive doses. In reality, only a few nutrients are fat soluble: vitamins A, D, E, and K. In addition, it is difficult to take too much of these fat-soluble vitamins … but not impossible. Just take our suggested amounts and all will be well.

We also need to be careful with iron supplementation. Iron can act as a pro-oxidant (free radical) and can cause cell damage if excessive levels accumulate in the body. Iron is lost with monthly blood loss in menstruating women, so iron supplementation in this setting is fine, or if you are anemic and iron is prescribed by your physician. Otherwise, additional iron supplements are not usually recommended.

Biochemistry of the free radical battle

Let's look at free radical and antioxidant biochemistry. Free radicals are unstable molecules that are basically one electron short of a Happy Meal! They are products of our oxygen-based metabolism. These unstable molecules latch onto other molecules to obtain that missing electron. This process destroys the other molecule, usually our cells, our cell membranes, or our DNA.

Cell injury from free radicals contributes to accelerated aging, disease, cancer, and immune dysfunction. Antioxidants neutralize free radicals to protect cells from oxidative damage, i.e., rust. We could not live without antioxidants. We could not live very well, or for long, without optimal antioxidant levels in our blood. (When you buy your supplements, you will find that the "free" radicals are actually quite "expensive" to battle.)

We have two ways to fight this oxidant battle. One way is to decrease our production of free radicals. Although breathing increases free radical production, breath holding is not a viable option for free radical reduction!

Free radical production increases with stress, illness, toxic exposure, heavy metal exposure, and when listening to heavy metal music. Free radicals are generated during exercise. So we want to win the battle by minimizing stress, toxic exposures, illness, and by minimizing excessive exercise (I'll explain in chapter 4).

It is important to remember that the most common source of excessive free radical production is excessive calories in our diets. These excessive calories are from high-glycemic carbohydrates.

By following our optimal diet, you will be eating nutrient-dense foods and avoiding nutrient-poor foods. With this way of eating, you will avoid excessive calories from processed carbohydrates and decrease your free radical burden. A win-win diet plan.

High-glycemic carbohydrates produce excessive free radicals.

Our second method of winning the oxidant battle is by supplementation. The human body has built-in standard equipment antioxidant systems in the body; unfortunately, their activity decreases with age. What a bummer—just when we need them the most, they leave us high, dry, and rusting!

As we age and our intrinsic antioxidant systems wear down, we need to ensure protection by combining our healthy diets with an effective antiaging supplement program.

Herbs, spices, and fruits and vegetables are full of antioxidants.

Herbs, spices, and fruits and vegetables contain polyphenols and bioflavonoids that have powerful antioxidant activity. Examples include garlic, red wine, red pepper, and cinnamon. (That's cinnamon ... not cinna**bon**.)

Berries and cherries are chock-full of antioxidants. Many studies reveal that diets with higher intake of nutrient antioxidants are associated with a lower incidence of chronic degenerative diseases. So eat real food and eat it often.

In addition to our diet, we will add numerous supplements to optimize cell activity and reinforce our antioxidant defenses. We assist our cell function by supplying nutrients required for cell function and by supplying plenty of antioxidants to balance free radicals. The integrity of our cells depends on this balance of free radicals and antioxidants.

Our cellular energy production is greatly enhanced by nutrient supplementation. You will feel the difference, and your cells will thank you for it with longevity dividends in the form of healthy years.

Understanding cell function and the role of nutrients

As we look at cell function, we must emphasize that cells are constantly producing energy in the form of adenosine triphosphate (ATP), which is the chemical energy produced by our cells. Our cells convert energy from the calories we consume into this chemical energy. ATP is the form of energy that our cells use to run our metabolism. Our cells need to efficiently convert energy from the food we consume into chemical energy to make us go. The cells must constantly make ATP to meet our energy demands. The cells never get coffee breaks or time off. They are true workaholics. In upcoming lectures, you will learn how the optimal diet and supplement program greatly impacts the abilities of cells to produce ATP.

Cells produce energy in the form of ATP. Optimal energy levels require optimal ATP production.

Wake up, class—stretch and get a cup of green tea. We must now look at cell function to understand the crucial role that nutrients play in our health.

As mentioned, one of the most important functions of our cells is to produce cell energy. At the cellular level, energy is required to make new proteins, to bring nutrients into the cell, to expel cellular wastes, to repair damaged DNA, to synthesize neurotransmitters … The list of cellular activity is extensive. It ain't easy being a cell!

Everything that cells do requires energy. For the cell to carry out instructions from DNA requires energy; to produce hormones requires energy … Every cell function requires energy. No wonder you are so tired!

To look at the big picture of the body, cellular energy allows the heart to pump blood, the lungs to take in oxygen and to expel carbon dioxide, the brain to form memory, and for the kidneys to filter wastes.

The energy source the cells produce is the bio-energy molecule ATP, adenosine triphosphate. Needless to say, ATP is the energy of life. Because the metabolism of food by our cells produces ATP, and because efficient ATP production is so essential, we must consume high-quality nutrients for optimal health.

The cells utilize the macronutrients supplied in our diet—protein, carbohydrates, and fats—to produce ATP. All cells in the body take glucose from carbohydrates, the amino acids from proteins, and the fatty acids from fat to generate this cell energy.

Once inside the cell, glucose and fatty acids, and occasionally amino acids, are processed through three interlocking ATP energy production cycles. Ideally, the cells utilize glucose and fatty acids; however, under stressful conditions—e.g., starvation, deprivation diets, excessive exercise—the cells will burn amino acids (from protein) for energy. For proteins to be used in ATP production, the protein is broken down into amino acids, and then the amino acids are used to make carbohydrates or fat for cellular fuel. Clearly, we would rather have the cells burn glucose and fat instead of protein.

Not only do we benefit in appearance and health when we burn fat, but we develop more energy and feel better. This dramatic improvement is because burning fat produces over three times more ATP than does burning equal amounts of carbohydrates. Our bodies would rather be primarily fat burners than sugar burners.

Cell energy is produced in the "mighty" mitochondria.

I mentioned earlier that the cells produce ATP via three energy-producing systems. Essentially, the cells break down chemical energy bonds in glucose to produce energy. Picture a large number of people playing the game hot potato. Each time someone quickly hands off the potato to the next person, a small amount of energy is released from the potato into the room. Imagine that by handing the hot potato "down the line" of participants, we gradually release energy into the room. In this manner, the room never gets too hot to continue playing. In addition, since we can continuously release energy in small increments into the room, it never gets too cold either.

Our cells play the same hot potato game. By doing so, the cell is able to produce small amounts of ATP in a stepwise fashion. This allows cell energy production to be controlled and regulated based on the needs of the body. Unlike the hot potato game, our cell energy cycles are unique because the "potato" never cools down. This way, the cells can continuously produce energy.

The three energy production cycles are labeled glycolytic cycle, Krebs cycle, and electron transport chain. Basically, the glycolytic cycle occurs in the cytoplasm, the watery portion of the cells. This is where the hot potato game begins. Glucose, our hot potato, enters the cell, and the glycolytic cycle converts the glucose into pyruvic acid. This conversion of glucose to pyruvic acid occurs without the use of oxygen. The pyruvic acid is then "handed off" to the Krebs cycle. The Krebs cycle allows the production of ATP to occur in the presence of oxygen. This is where the majority of ATP is produced.

The Krebs cycle and electron transport chain are located inside a cell structure called the mitochondria. The mitochondria are traditionally referred to as the "powerhouse of the cell." The mitochondria are where the action is in regard to cell energy production. For the purposes of ATP production, "be in the mitochondria or be nowhere!"

In the mitochondria, our hot potato game continues in the Krebs cycle until the potato is handed off to the electron transport chain. The electron transport chain occurs in the mitochondrial membrane. In the electron transport chain, electrons are transported from one carrier to another, and energy is released during each transfer. This allows the controlled and continuous release of ATP energy.

All cells vary in the number of mitochondria they contain. It is truly miraculous to fathom that of our trillion of cells in the body, each cell contains roughly 50 to 2,500 mitochondria per cell.[13] It doesn't take a rocket scientist to realize the importance of mitochondria for cell energy production and our overall health and vitality. (You will learn in chapter 4 how the right form of exercise will increase the number of mitochondria).

A main reason we encourage you to take antioxidants is to protect and preserve mitochondrial function. In high-energy cells of the heart and brain, up to 20 percent of the cell volume is made up of mitochondria. To maintain a healthy heart and brain requires optimal cell function and optimal mitochondrial function.

Enzymes are cell spark plugs.

Let's look at how cells actually take food and produce ATP energy. The breakdown of food into energy requires "spark plugs" called enzymes. Think of enzymes as catalysts that facilitate specific chemical reactions to occur efficiently.

The chemical reactions that make up the Krebs cycle and the electron transport chain cannot occur without utilizing many enzymes. Enzymes can be enhanced or inhibited by specific compounds; from either the diet or from the supplements we take. This ability to either enhance or inhibit enzymes allows us to influence the rate and efficiency of cell energy production. If enzymes in the energy cycles are working poorly, then ATP production will suffer.

Low ATP production leads to low cell energy and poor cell function. Poor cell function leads to poor organ function. Poor organ function leads to doctor and ER visits. Doctor and ER visits lead to long waiting times. Long waiting times leads to stress. Stress leads to high cortisol levels. High cortisol levels leads to … you get the picture.

Improving enzyme function

How do we optimize enzyme function?

Glad you asked. Enzymes require two or three components. One part is a specific protein, supplied by our optimal diet. A second part of the enzyme is a coenzyme. A coenzyme is basically an active form of a vitamin.

Many of the B vitamins become coenzymes in the body. This is why the B vitamins are frequently recommended for low-energy conditions or fatigue. The third part of the enzyme complex is a coactivator. A mineral is often a coactivator. Magnesium, for example, is the coactivator for many of the enzymes of the ATP cycles. In the enzyme world, behind every good vita**man** is a mineral.

With our optimal diet, we provide plenty of protein, vitamins, and minerals to ensure adequate enzyme activity. We also supplement with vitamins, minerals, and other nutrients for ideal supply to the cells as well as antioxidant effect.

Some of the nutrients required in the ATP cycles include vitamins B1, B2, B3, B5, biotin, lipoic acid, and coenzyme Q10. In addition, vitamins B6, B12, and folic acid are required to transport various amino acids for use in the energy cycles.[14-19]

A substance called carnitine transports fatty acids into the mitochondria to be utilized for energy production. You will often see carnitine advertised as a "fat burner" because of its role in shuttling fatty acids to the mitochondrial "furnace" to be burned.

For this 101-level class, you will not need to remember the specifics, but you do need to understand the key role that vitamin coenzymes, and mineral coactivators, play in converting food into energy.

It then becomes obvious to note that complaints of malaise and low energy are common with nutrient deficiencies. It also becomes clear that the solution for fatigue is not a double espresso but a balanced diet and supplementation program. Surprisingly, the cost of our supplement program is cheaper than the daily visits to the coffee house.

To review, we want to avoid overt vitamin deficiencies to prevent vitamin deficiency diseases. But more importantly for healthy aging, we want to optimize vitamin, mineral, and nutrient levels to support cell function and energy production. Go! But go with all cylinders firing!

Because the majority of energy is produced in the mitochondria, they also become the part of the cells most at risk of oxidative stress. The activity of the mitochondria generates large amounts of free radicals that in turn can injure the mitochondria.

Where in the house are you most likely to get burned? In the kitchen … by the stove. Same with our cells. The "heat" from our mitochondrial "furnaces" can cause damage. This "heat" or "oxidative stress" can affect the activity of the mitochondrial enzymes and lead to a decline in ATP production. This mitochondrial decay accelerates the aging process. So while you are saving the whales, remember to save the mitochondria!

Save the mitochondria to save your health.

Now let's proceed with the specific components of nutrient supplementation. Remember, we are focusing on two main goals: optimizing cell function and combating free radicals.

A common mistake seen with nutrient supplementation is to supplement in an "à la carte" fashion. We will often read an article on the benefits of a specific nutrient and then take large quantities of that nutrient. Avoid this trap. It is important to realize that the body needs all the crucial nutrients all the time, not just some of the time. Our cells are working 24/7.

Another key point in nutrient supplementation is that balanced antioxidants work best. This is a team sport. All of the nutrients work together and require optimal levels of each nutrient.

In addition, different antioxidants quench different free radicals, so we must diversify our intake of antioxidants. In war, we need balanced army, navy, air force, and marines to be victorious. Likewise, in our war on free radicals, we need balanced nutrients for victory.

Antioxidants not only work as a team—they can also regenerate each other. Talk about getting your money's worth! For example, lipoic acid can significantly increase the levels of glutathione, a strong antioxidant.[20-21]

Antioxidants work best when balanced.

Finally, as we mentioned before, some nutrients are water soluble and some are fat soluble. By providing water-soluble nutrients (such as vitamin C), we protect the "watery" portions of cells, and by providing fat-soluble nutrients (such as vitamin E), we protect the fat-rich portions of cells. The fat-rich portions of our cells, such as the cell membranes and the mitochondria, are extremely vulnerable to oxidation. Because healthy cell membranes and healthy mitochondria are so instrumental to healthy aging, we must be sure to supplement with fat-soluble nutrients. In the world of supplements, balance matters.

As we proceed with specific nutrients and doses, remember that our first priority is to follow the optimal diet. Eating real, whole, and unprocessed food puts you at a major advantage in preserving health and slowing aging. A healthy diet works synergistically with our supplement program.

Let's start with the B-complex vitamins. These are, as mentioned earlier, instrumental for energy production. In addition, they support our immune systems, our nervous systems, and influence hormone balance. They are "busy *B*s." Great sources include meats, fish, poultry, nuts, and seeds. All sources are on the caveman menu.

Below is a list of specific optimal antiaging doses and a few unique properties of specific nutrients. This will be on your final exam.

Vitamin B1 (thiamine) 50 mg/day. Necessary for converting food to energy. Benefits the cardiovascular system. Enhances mental function. Food sources include legumes, meats, fish, poultry, nuts, and seeds.

Vitamin B2 (riboflavin) 50 mg/day. Regenerates glutathione, our main "built-in" antioxidant. Aids in the production of red blood cells. Needed for efficient metabolism. Food sources include green leafy vegetables, meats, dairy, seafood, nuts, seeds, and legumes. Turns our urine bright yellow (pretty cool!).

Vitamin B3 (niacin) 100mg/day. Effective cholesterol-lowering agent; increases HDL and lowers LDL. Dose for cholesterol effect is 1,000 to

1,500 mg per day. Improves metabolism. Food sources include meat, poultry, dairy, nuts, seeds, and legumes.

Niacinamide (second form of B3) 100mg/day. Improves insulin sensitivity.

Vitamin B5 (pantothenic acid) 100 to 150 mg/day. Improves energy levels. Improves wound healing and immune function. Decreases inflammation. Improves metabolism of food. Found in meat, poultry, nuts, seeds, eggs, and vegetables.

Vitamin B6 (pyridoxine) 50 mg/day. Necessary for healthy red blood cells, gums, and teeth. Helps metabolize proteins. Improves immune function. Decreases homocysteine levels, lowering the risk of heart disease. Food sources include potatoes, legumes, meats, bananas, liver, seafood, nuts, and seeds.

Vitamin B12 (methylcobalamine) 200 to 1000 mcg/day (a microgram is one-thousandth of a milligram). Important for development of red blood cells. Crucial for health of brain and nervous system. Deficiency causes depression and dementia. Lowers homocysteine levels. Helps prevent osteoporosis. Food sources include fish, meat, and liver.

Biotin (B-complex vitamin) 300 mg/day. Aids in metabolizing fats and carbohydrates. Decreases glucose levels. Improves nail strength and hair growth. Food sources include nuts, eggs, lentils, fish, vegetables, and liver.

Folic acid 400 to 800 mcg/day. Lowers homocysteine levels. Elevated homocysteine is a proven risk factor for heart disease and dementia. When combined with vitamin B-12, reduces cancer risk.

Low levels of vitamin B-12, folate, and B-6 can produce DNA damage.

Vitamin C (ascorbic acid) 1000 mg twice per day dosing. Great sources in citrus fruits, tomatoes, broccoli, and leafy greens. Essential for collagen production and immune system support. Regenerates vitamin E and glutathione. Key water-soluble antioxidant. When combined with other vitamins, it decreases risk of many cancers. Ascorbate, whether calcium ascorbate or magnesium ascorbate, is the best form of vitamin C.

Fat-soluble vitamins

Vitamin A/beta-carotene 10,000 to 20,000 IU vitamin A and 25,000 IU beta-carotene daily. Great sources of vitamin A in liver, eggs, butter, fish oils, and beta-carotene in fruits and vegetables. Essential for bone growth, immune function, skin health, and vision. Decreases risk of heart disease. Beta carotene may turn skin orange at high doses, but it is harmless (and great at Halloween!).

Carotenoids. A large group of chemicals found in leafy green and yellow vegetables and in many fruits. Many carotenoids can be converted into vitamin A as needed by the body. Only the amount of vitamin A needed is produced by carotenoids; therefore, toxicity from carotenoids is impossible. Common examples of healthy carotenoids include lycopene, alpha-, beta-, and gamma-carotene, astaxanthin, lutein, and zeaxanthin. Many of these have been found to decrease the risk of cancer.

Vitamin D 1000 to 5000 IU/day of vitamin D3 (best form). Optimal sources are eggs, butter, and fish oil. Essential for calcium absorption. People not exposed to sunlight may have low levels (UV light produces vitamin D in skin) and can become deficient in vitamin D. Low levels of vitamin D are associated with multiple sclerosis, cancer, osteoporosis, obesity, macular degeneration, and hypertension. Moderate sun exposure is crucial to obtain healthy levels of vitamin D. (Just don't burn!) During summer months, we can produce about 20,000 IU after fifteen to twenty minutes of sun exposure. Vitamin D is crucial for normal immune system function. Vitamin D is safe and well tolerated.

Vitamin E 400 to 800 IU/day. Best is "mixed tocopherols," as vitamin E is a mixture of four tocopherols and four tocotrienols. Many supplements use only d-alpha tocopherol, which is a synthetic, unbalanced form. Vitamin E is a potent fat-soluble antioxidant. Supports immune function and cardiovascular function. Vitamin E protects cell membranes; it protects arterial lining and acts like Teflon to protect LDL cholesterol from oxidation, thus rendering it harmless. Vitamin E and vitamin C work best together.

Vitamin K 70 to 140 mcg/day. Food sources include leafy greens, vegetables, and eggs. Crucial for blood clotting and bone formation.

Minerals

Calcium 500 to 1500 mg/day. Food sources dairy, broccoli, nuts, and seeds. Remember, milk is not a great source of calcium. Crucial for bone development in conjunction with other previously mentioned nutrients. Essential for blood pressure control, immune function, and nerve conduction.

Magnesium 400 to 800 mg/day. Good food sources include nuts, seeds, and seafood. A must for blood pressure control, bone formation, energy production (remember the coactivator), and immunity. Necessary for over three hundred functions in the body. Increases energy and fat burning. Enhances insulin function.

Zinc 15 to 30 mg/day. Optimal food sources include red meat, nuts, and seeds. Another important nutrient for immune function. Needed for blood glucose balance, prostate health, skin health, and brain function. Estimated to be necessary for over six hundred functions in the body. ZZZinc even works while you catch your ZZZs!

Chromium 200 mcg/day. Improves insulin sensitivity and lowers body fat; both are crucial antiaging goals.

Selenium 200 mcg/day. Found in meats and eggs (you da caveman). Excellent antioxidant and supports immune function (again). Cofactor in many enzymes.

Boron 150 mcg/day. Contains bone-building properties. Improves absorption of calcium and magnesium. Improves energy. Food sources include nuts, legumes, leafy vegetables, broccoli, apples, pears, peaches, and grapes.

Probiotics

Probiotics are beneficial bacteria found in yogurt and fermented dairy products. Examples include acidophilus, lactobacillus, and bifidus. (Feel free to use during your next Scrabble game.)

They improve digestion and the absorption of nutrients. They synthesize short-chain fatty acids that are the preferred fuel for the cells that line the colon. They biodegrade bacterial toxins, detoxify carcinogens, and help metabolize drugs and hormones. They play a remarkable role in our immune system health.

Antibiotics can destroy probiotics so supplementation is a must when you are prescribed antibiotics. Probiotics also inhibit the growth of undesirable microorganisms—for example, candida (yeast)—and keep the environment within the intestines healthy.

Please note that many nutrients are required for optimal immune function. This explains why people on healthy supplement programs get sick less often and recover quickly when ill.

Okay, class, I'm sure the list so far seems overwhelming. Relax; it won't really be on your final exam. Just know that these are all provided in most high-quality multivitamin/mineral formulas. (Find a great one at Lifestyle Spectrum).

Before making your supplement purchase, refer to the suggested doses. In addition, a capsule form or gel cap is generally much better than tablets for maximum absorption and assimilation by the body.

A twice-daily dosing format is necessary for water-soluble nutrients, and fat-soluble nutrients should be taken once a day. This provides continuous antioxidant protection and cell nutrient supply. Your cells are like that little "energy bunny" on television—they go nonstop so feed them accordingly.

Antiaging Nutrients

Now, a few more nutrients to keep you energetic, healthy, and young. Your professor encourages you to supplement with all of them so pay attention.

Coenzyme Q10 (CoQ10) is found naturally in every cell in the body. It is ubiquitous. An antioxidant, it is vital for energy metabolism. Coenzyme

Q10 unites three of the five enzyme complexes found in the electron transport chain.

It is essential for cardiac and brain function. We find that the age-related decline in coenzyme Q10 levels contributes to cancer, heart disease, and dementia risk.

Coenzyme Q10 numerous benefits include improvement of cardiovascular function and lowering blood pressure. Because of its impact on the brain, it decreases the risk of dementia, migraines, and Parkinson's disease. CoQ10 is instrumental for healthy aging.

Please note that if you take a cholesterol-lowering medication in the "statin family"—for example, Crestor or Lipitor—you must supplement with coenzyme Q10. The statins deplete the body of coenzyme Q10.

Ideal dosing is 50 to 200 mg daily. Food sources include salmon, meats, and liver. I find the small gel cap much easier to down than even a bite of liver!

Indole-3-carbinol (I3C) is a phytonutrient found in cruciferous vegetables. It assists in the healthy metabolism of estrogen and can decrease the risk of breast and prostate cancer. Truly a "his and hers" supplement.

Dose 400 mg/day.

Di-indole-methane (DIM) is also a phytonutrient found in cruciferous vegetables such as broccoli and cabbage. DIM has been found to promote healthy estrogen metabolism in both men and women. It decreases cancer risk, especially breast and prostate cancer. It has been found to improve prostate function and help increase abdominal fat loss.

Dose 50 to 200 mg/day.

Carnitine is a B vitamin–like substance made in the body from amino acids. It transports fatty acids into the mitochondria for metabolism, i.e., "fat burning." Burning fatty acids helps prevent fatty asses! Food sources include meat, fish, poultry, and dairy. Levels of carnitine, like just about everything else, decline with age.

Dose with L-carnitine at 500 to 500 mg daily.

Acetyl-L-carnitine is a form of carnitine that is able to get into the brain for optimal brain function. This supports memory and decreases risk of cognitive decline. Some interesting studies have been done in rats, with remarkable results.

Acetyl-L-carnitine should be dosed at 750 to 1000 mg daily.

Alpha lipoic acid is an essential part of ATP production. A potent antioxidant, it is unique because it has both water-soluble and fat-soluble properties.

Lipoic acid is great for improving your energy and keeping brain function at its peak. Lipoic acid improves blood flow and improves immune function. In addition, it is has strong anti-inflammatory properties.

Dose at 50 to 100 mg daily. Food sources include beef and spinach (this is why Popeye was so attractive to Olive Oil.)

Carnosine is unique in its ability to decrease the ravages of high blood glucose levels. Carnosine helps blocks glycation, the process of glucose combining with proteins and fats in cells, leading to cell injury. Best food sources of carnosine include protein-rich foods such as beef, poultry, and pork.

Dose at 1000 mg daily.

L-arginine is an amino acid made naturally in the body. Arginine increases nitric oxide (NO) production. Nitric oxide improves blood vessel health and improves the ability of blood vessels to dilate.

Arginine supplementation improves blood pressure, improves cholesterol levels, and improves blood flow. Arginine improves erectile dysfunction in men and improves blood supply to the heart in patients with angina. Since arginine is an amino acid, the best food sources include seafood, poultry, beef, pork, and nuts.

Dose is 1000 to 3000 mg daily.

Astaxanthin is a naturally occurring carotenoid with strong antioxidant properties. It is found in plants and microalgae. Crustaceans, such as shrimp and lobster, and fish, such as wild salmon, are tinted red by astaxanthin consumption. Its unique structure improves protection of cell membranes, retina, skin, and brain. Because of its powerful antioxidant capability, it has many antiaging benefits. Astaxanthin enhances immune function, heart health, skin, joint, brain, and eye health. It also has been found beneficial in exercise endurance and recovery.[22-26]

Dose is 2 to 12 mg daily.

Omega-3 fats

Now my absolute favorite healthy aging supplement: fish oil. It is truly miraculous and will affect your health in multiple ways.

In chapter 2, we covered balanced fat intake and the role fats play in eicosanoid hormone production. In the caveman times, the ratio between omega-6 fats and omega-3 fats was one to one.

A one-to-one balance leads to healthy eicosanoid balance, which has positive effects on inflammation, blood flow, blood clotting, and many other crucial physiologic functions.[27-29]

In contrast, in people eating the typical American diet, we find the omega-6 to omega-3 ratios in the twenty-to-one and even in the fifty-to-one range. With such abnormal ratios, the human body generates excessive inflammation, excessive blood clotting, decreased blood flow to major organs, and increased cancer risk.

This ratio must be restored to healthy levels immediately to reach any of our healthy aging goals. To restore the healthy ratio, eat balanced healthy protein and fats as we have discussed. Avoid processed foods and processed vegetable oils (such as corn oil), as these processed foods will produce excessive omega-6 levels. Simultaneously with the diet changes, supplement with fish oil, a rich source of omega-3 fats.

Omega-3 fats are deficient in our diet, and we require supplementation for good health. The best omega-3 source is from pharmaceutical-grade fish oil. This ensures higher potency, quality, and safety.

The two key omega-3 fats are DHA and EPA. When dosing, we want the sum total of DHA plus EPA to equal at least 1000mg.

For best results, the DHA plus EPA dose should be 3000 mg to 5000 mg daily.

Omega-3 fats are anti-inflammatory (good)
Omega-3 fats promote fat burning.

Omega-6 fats are pro-inflammatory (bad)
Omega-6 fats promote fat storage.
Goal: omega-6 to omega-3 ratio of one to one.

Concomitant with restoring our omega-6 to omega-3 ratios to a healthy range, we must reinforce the need of avoiding trans fatty acids (partially hydrogenated cooking oils). Think of trans fats as "anti-omega-3 fats." They disrupt eicosanoid balance and harm cell function, a definite no-no for our healthy longevity goals.

Please realize that fats in our diets are literally incorporated into our cell membranes. These trans fats are fake fats that are stored in our cell membranes, and they destroy cells much like termites destroy our homes.

Trans fats are cell terminators; omega-3 fats are trans fat exterminators. Our healthy aging goal of supporting cell function depends on our compliance with this essential element of our antiaging program.

Healthy fat balance in our diets produces healthy eicosanoid balance in our cells. Virtually every disease process is a result of increased inflammation and decreased blood flow. Heart disease and dementia are examples of diseases fueled by excessive inflammation. Improved eicosanoid balance profoundly decreases inflammation while improving blood flow.

As people supplement with omega-3 fats, they notice significant improvement in inflammatory conditions such as arthritis, colitis, and dermatitis.[30-36] Frequently, they can reduce and often eliminate prescription medications, such as anti-inflammatory medications or steroids that they have historically relied on for symptom reduction.

There are thousands of articles in medical journals documenting the health benefits of fish oil. The best news of all, there are minimal side effects! They may even help you swim faster.

Benefits of fish oil:

- Decreased inflammation
- Improved insulin sensitivity
- Improved metabolism
- Decreased cancer risk and metastases
- Decrease in cardiac dysrhythmias
- Decrease in plaque rupture
- Improved blood flow
- Decrease in blood clotting
- Improved mood and memory
- Decreased depression
- Improved cholesterol panel
- Improved skin tone and texture
- Help you reach all antiaging goals

Omega-3 fats = healthy cell membranes
Healthy cell membranes = better cell function
Better cell function = antiaging

Healthy fats:

Olive oil (extra virgin)
Fish oil
Flaxseed oil
Coconut oil (extra virgin)

Unhealthy fats:

Omega-6 oils (corn oil, soybean oil,
    canola oil)
Trans fatty acids (partially
    hydrogenated cooking oils)

Remember that omega-6 fats intrinsic to whole foods (e.g., fruits, vegetables, meats) are required by the body. Simply avoid processed vegetable oils, as they excessively elevate omega-6 levels in the body.

Glycoproteins

A final category of supplements is called glycoproteins. Now you are probably convinced that your professor has lost it, as "glyco" means sugar. I have spent a great deal of time warning you that sugar is the devil. Before you storm out of the classroom, let me explain.

First, our goal is control of glucose levels, not elimination of glucose. Remember, our brains require a constant supply of glucose. Second, these glycoproteins do *not* raise blood glucose levels.

So what kind of sugars are these?

They are simple sugars called "monosaccharides," which combine with proteins in the body to form glycoproteins. Glycoproteins have tremendous effect throughout the body, primarily by improving cell communication and function.[37]

It is quite extraordinary to realize that our cells communicate with each other! Cells recognize each other by identifying "tags" on the cell membranes. These tags are made up of glycoproteins.

Our ability to produce these important glycoproteins is inhibited by a poor supply in our diets, by medications, and by toxins. Six of the eight identified monosaccharides are deficient in our diets and require supplementation.

For interest sake, but not for memorization, the names of the missing monosaccharides are mannose, fucose, xylose, N-acetylglucosamine, N-acetyl galactosamine, and N-acetyl neuraminic acid.

Natural sources of these monosaccharides are plants such as aloe vera, mushrooms, fungi, certain fruits and vegetables, and unprocessed grains like psyllium.

Supplementation with glycoproteins has been shown to improve healing, decrease inflammation, inhibit tumor spread, generate antioxidants, and support immune function.[38-39]

Common supplement options are products with alpha- and beta-glucans, active hexose correlated compounds (AHCC), aloe vera, and fiber supplements. Suggested dose varies with each product.

The multiple functions of glycoproteins:

- Cellular communication
- Retain bone density and muscle mass
- Tissue resculpting
- Produce glyconutrient enzymes to generate antioxidants
- Necessary for production of cytokines
- Enhance wound healing
- Decrease inflammation
- Inhibit tumor spread
- Antibacterial and antifungal effects
- Support immune function
- Improve lipid panel
- Decrease allergy symptoms

An effective nutraceuticals supplementation program has the power to improve blood pressure, immune function, energy production, blood flow, and to slow the aging process.

Nutraceuticals can decrease your risk of many cancers (even acknowledged by the American Cancer Society) while simultaneously decreasing your risk of degenerative diseases attributed to the aging process.

You will think clearer and have better stamina and better moods. Simply stated, a healthy nutraceuticals program will keep you young longer.[40-45]

Tea

Although not a supplement in the traditional definition, the health benefits of green and white tea are too beneficial to overlook. Your antiaging program would be enhanced to a great degree by adding green or white tea to your daily program.

Green and white teas are full of antioxidants. The catechins in tea reduce risk of stroke, cancer, diabetes, and heart problems. They improve metabolism and assist with fat loss.

Tea also has tremendous anti-inflammatory benefits, and studies have shown decreased pain and inflammation in rheumatoid arthritis, colitis, and many other inflammatory conditions.[46] White tea actually contains more nutrients then green tea, but both are exceptional additions to your diet.

Resveratrol

Resveratrol is another nutrient that you should get into your daily program. Resveratrol is found in grapes, blueberries, cranberries, plums, and other plants. Its most common source is in wine, especially organic red wines.

Resveratrol is a polyphenol that has multiple benefits to health. Studies have shown resveratrol's impact on decreasing the risk of cancer, heart disease, and dementia.[13] It has powerful antioxidant activity, and it has been found to have antioxidant activity on some free radicals that other antioxidants do not touch.

It is probably best known for its cardiovascular benefits. It improves blood flow by enhancing a natural blood vessel dilator called nitric oxide. It supports healthy blood vessels throughout the body. It decreases blood clotting and protects cholesterol from oxidation. As we discussed earlier, when cholesterol isn't oxidized, it is harmless, regardless of your cholesterol level. In addition, it lowers excessive inflammation.

New research has found a unique role for resveratrol in antiaging. There is scientific evidence that we all carry a family of genes called sirtuins, which act as longevity genes. Sirtuins send out signals to all cells in the body, slowing down the aging process. The genes are activated with a nutritionally balanced but calorie-restricted diet. Resveratrol has the ability to activate sirtuins.[47-48]

Organic red wines are a good source of resveratrol. If don't drink alcohol, and even if you do, a supplement with a standardized extract of resveratrol would augment your health and decrease your risk of many age-related degenerative diseases. The recommended dose is 20 to 250 mg per day.

Curcumin

Curcumin is an extract from the spice turmeric. It has extensive antioxidant ability and powerful anti-inflammatory action. This combination of activity elicits a strong antiaging effect.

Studies have found positive influence of curcumin supplementation on arthritis, dementia, lipid profiles, and colon function. It has been found to have anti-cancer actions.[49-52]

Take at least 1000 mg daily in divided doses or add turmeric to your foods as much as you desire.

Benefits of nutraceutical supplementation:

As we learn about the many nutraceuticals available, we can appreciate the numerous and diverse benefits on our health. To reiterate the main actions, we see improved lipid panels, a decrease in inflammation, diminished oxidation, improved glucose regulation, improved insulin sensitivity, and improved cell function. Additionally, we see improved hormone balance and metabolism. Over time, we note improved blood pressure control, enhanced immunity, decreased rates of cancer, and enhanced energy and stamina.

We obtain protection of skin, teeth, and gums. There is detoxification of environmental pollutants, including heavy metals, and protection against UV light. We notice an enhanced sense of well-being, a reduction in risk of degenerative disease; an overall improved quality of life. All of the benefits of nutraceutical supplementation produce antiaging effects throughout the body.

Nutraceutical Supplementation Nuts and Bolts:

1) Choose a balanced multivitamin and mineral supplement with optimal doses.

2) Choose capsules or gel caps (when available) over tablet forms for enhanced absorption.

3) Take water-soluble supplements twice daily, fat-soluble supplements once daily.

4) Take coenzyme Q10, alpha lipoic acid, and acetyl-L-carnitine for optimal cell health and cell energy production

5) Add pharmaceutical grade omega-3 supplementation, fish oil caps or liquid, for dramatic health benefits.

6) Avoid mega dosing with specific nutrients—balance is better.

7) Combine with our healthy aging diet for optimal results

Our nutraceutical supplementation program has positive influence on all eight of our healthy aging goals.

CHAPTER 3
QUESTIONS

Student:

I always forget to take my vitamins and fish oil. Any tips for me?

Professor:

Yes ... remember. This is your health and longevity we are talking about.

Student:

My doctor says we get all the vitamins and minerals we need from food. He says if I buy vitamins, I am wasting my money. What do you think?

Professor:

Too late. I think you wasted your money when you paid your doctor. It is impossible to get optimal levels of nutrients in today's food supply. Be smart and supplement. Remember, our perspective is on health care, not on disease care.

Student:

What supplements do you recommend for "fat-burning" effects?

Professor:

You need to be careful because plenty of products are marketed as fat burners, when they are simply stimulants that rev up your metabolism. Supplements such as guarana and ephedrine are commonly utilized in these "fat burners." These are a stress to the body and increase catabolic forces (breakdown), having adverse effects on your heath.

The best way to become a fat burner is by following our healthy diet program outlined in this course. This diet will change you from a sugar burner to a fat burner.

The body prefers to burn fat for energy. However, when we overwhelm the body with high sugar and processed carbohydrates, we raise our blood glucose levels. The body wants to lower blood glucose into a safer range, as high glucose is damaging to cells. The body is forced to become a sugar burner in this setting. So instead of burning fat, it has to work on lowering blood glucose levels.

It lowers blood glucose levels by increasing insulin levels (bad) and by storing more glucose as fat (bad).

If you control blood glucose levels, the body is able to burn fat preferentially. In this setting, you burn fat all day and all night. Your energy will be higher, your body fat will by lower, and your life will be longer!

Now, in a healthy diet, there are a few supplements that assist fat burning via different mechanisms:

1) Fiber supplements such as psyllium. Lowers glucose levels and insulin levels.
2) L-carnitine. Improves fat transports to cell for fat burning.
3) Chromium. Improves insulin sensitivity.
4) Carnosine. Decreases effects of glycation.
5) Fish oil (omega-3 fats). Improves insulin sensitivity and metabolism.
6) Coenzyme Q10. Improves metabolism and fat burning.
7) Alpha lipoic acid. Improves metabolism and fat burning.
8) Pyruvate. Improves fat burning.

Student:

Recently the newspaper quoted some studies that indicated problems or lack of benefit from commonly used antioxidants. Any thoughts?

Professor:

Yes, the problems center on some misconceptions regarding antioxidants. Most commonly, the studies do not take into consideration that antioxidants are team players. Instead, they are studied individually. For example, the study uses just one vitamin or nutrient, or just a few vitamins. This creates an artificial situation.

Each of the vitamins and antioxidants utilize each other to perform their jobs. When they neutralize a free radical, they become a free radical themselves. They then require another teammate to hand off the free radical to, then that teammate becomes a weaker free radical. This process is repeated until the free radical is neutralized.

Basketball is a great analogy. We know that Steve Nash is one of the best point guards in NBA history. Steve excels in passing the ball to other teammates. He needs high-quality teammates to maximize his performance.

If we decide to play a game (or do a study) with five Steve Nash clones versus another NBA team, his team would lose. Does this study finding suggest Steve is overrated as a player? Of course not. We can't make any determinations regarding his ability by taking away his center, forwards, and other teammates. It is the same with antioxidants.

Another common problem with these studies is they often test whether a specific nutrient can be used to treat a disease that is already present. This type of study will rarely show benefits because the disease already exists. Antioxidants are for prevention or to slow progression of disease. They are not a treatment for a disease.

In addition, many studies utilize a low dose of a nutrient. We are not going to optimize results if we don't optimize the dose utilized.

Finally, there are many other conflicting variables in these studies. For example, what types of diets are the study participants eating? Are they controlling blood glucose levels? Hormone levels? Are they exercising? Are they controlling stress? Was a high-quality supplement utilized? All of these variables, and more, will impact study results.

Student:

Are there any supplements to improve results from exercise?

Professor:

Yes, here are a few supplements that can help improve your results:

Arginine is an amino acid that increases the production of nitric oxide within blood vessel walls. Nitric oxide improves blood flow and nutrient delivery to muscles. It is often found in weight lifting supplements to increase the pump felt after a weight training session.

Dose at 500 mg to 750 mg three times daily.

Creatine is another beneficial supplement. Creatine increases the muscle cells' production of ATP, increasing muscle performance and recovery. It is extremely safe to use in all ages. The only caveat is to make sure you stay hydrated to avoid cramping.

Dose 500 to 1000 mg daily.

Ribose is a natural sugar found in all of our cells. Ribose is used in the production of cellular energy, ATP. Ribose provides cells with energy; as a result, it improves stamina, endurance, and exercise recovery.

Dose is 3000 to 5000 mg daily.

Student:

I eat a lot of fish. Do I still need to supplement with fish oil?

Professor:

Yes. First, if the fish is farm raised, it contains no significant amounts of omega-3 fats. Second, a wild Alaskan salmon filet has about 700 mg to 1000 mg of the omega-3 fats, EPA and DHA. We suggest you supplement with at least 1000 mg to 5000 mg daily. Realize that you can't overdose on omega-3 fats. Some clinical studies in children dose the EPA and DHA at over 10,000 mg daily!

I encourage you to continue consuming healthy fish in your diet but still suggest you take your fish oil every day.

Student:

Can I take flaxseed oil instead of fish oil for omega-3 supplementation?

Professor:

Flaxseed contains an omega-3 called alpha-linolenic acid (ALA). The body can convert ALA to the omega-3's EPA and DHA; however, it is about a ten to one conversion. This means you have to take ten times as much flaxseed to match the EPA and DHA dose in fish oil.

Student:

What would be a good baseline supplement list to start with?

Professor:

Taking a high-quality multivitamin and mineral formula, additional vitamin D, and fish oil is a good starting point.

Student:

Is there an unbiased source of information on supplements we could access?

Professor:

I take it from your question that you consider my information biased. No offense taken, but I will remember you when I grade your final exam. *Another* source of unbiased information can be found at consumerlab.com. Consumerlab.com offers independent online evaluations about various vitamin, supplement, and nutritional products.

Student:

Recently I have read some interesting information about the multiple benefits of vitamin D. Why is this vitamin so beneficial to health?

Professor:

You are correct; vitamin D has multiple effects in the body. Vitamin D is, in reality, a hormone. A hormone is released from an organ in the body into the bloodstream and has diverse effects throughout the body. Vitamin D is released from the skin (an organ) into the bloodstream, and it has multiple effects on cells everywhere in the body. Vitamin D lowers inflammation, supports the immune system, and supports metabolism and bone density. Deficiencies of vitamin D are extremely common and are associated with obesity, cancer, osteoporosis, and many autoimmune diseases such as multiple sclerosis. It is difficult to get enough vitamin D in our diets, and since we tend to wear sunblock, we can easily become deficient. Because of the negative repercussions of low vitamin D levels, supplementation is strongly encouraged.

Student:

Do you mind telling us what supplements you take every day, and which brands you utilize?

Professor:

Sure. I hope I don't scare you when I reveal my long list of supplements, but I need all the help I can get! Here we go:

+ Multivitamin and mineral formula from LifeStyle Spectrum

- Pharmaceutical-grade fish oil, Omega Rx, from Zone Labs, Inc.

- Vitamin D-3 from Life Extension

- CoQ10 from Life Extension

- Mitochondrial Energy Optimizer from Life Extension (includes acetyl-L-carnitine, lipoic acid, and carnosine)

- Super Miraforte from Life Extension (includes chrysin and maca to support testosterone levels and lower estrogen levels in men)

- Astaxanthin from Bioastin

- Sea Health/Plus (polyphenols) from Zone Labs, Inc.

- Joint Support (includes curcumin) from Zone Labs, Inc.

- Optimized resveratrol from Life Extension

- Cruciferous vegetable extract (includes indole-3-carbinol, and DIM (di-indole-methane) from Life Extension. Women should take this as well to support healthy estrogen metabolism.

What does the medical and scientific literature reveal about supplements?

❖ Postmenopausal women taking vitamin D and calcium supplements have a 60 percent lower risk of developing cancer.

❖ Increased blood levels of the omega-3 fatty acids, EPA and DHA, correlate with decreased risk of sudden cardiac death. A 2002 study of men with sudden cardiac death found that among men with the highest levels of omega-3 fatty acids in the blood, there was a 77 percent reduction in the risk of sudden cardiac death when compared to the men with the lowest levels.

❖ Multiple studies revealed that patients on fish oil have a decreased risk of plaque rupture, improved cholesterol panels, improved body composition, less depression, and lower rates of cancer.

❖ Multiple studies have shown that low vitamin D blood levels are associated with increased risk of cancer, hypertension, diabetes, metabolic syndrome, osteoporosis, and obesity.

❖ Analysis of more than eighteen studies involving 60,000 patients found that people who took vitamin D supplements had a 7 percent reduction in mortality from all causes compared with those who did not supplement.

❖ Multiple studies have revealed cancer risk reductions of over 50 percent in people with higher vitamin D levels.

❖ American Heart Association study found that having deficient levels of vitamin D is associated with double the risk of experiencing a heart attack or stroke within a five-year period compared to individuals with normal levels.

❖ *American Journal of Clinical Nutrition* study found a positive effect of L-carnitine supplementation in individuals one hundred years of age or older. The group that received L-carnitine experienced lower total cholesterol, reduction in body fat, gains in muscle mass, a reduction in physical and mental fatigue, and better cognitive function scores compared to those not receiving L-carnitine.

❖ Numerous studies of CoQ10 supplementation have found the following: protection against skin photoaging and melanoma, decreased risk of prostate and breast cancer, decreased risk of neurodegenerative diseases, decreased risk of macular degeneration, and improved immune function.

❖ Rats supplemented with acetyl-L-carnitine and alpha lipoic acid not only avoided age-related hearing loss but also reversed hearing loss.

❖ Daily intake of vitamin C and E significantly lowers the risk of developing Alzheimer's. This study included 5,000 elderly patients over eight years.

❖ Middle-aged adults supplementing with multivitamins, B vitamins, and chromium had decrease in body fat. The supplements improved blood glucose levels and cell energy production.

❖ Analysis of existing research determined that daily intake of 1800 mg of omega-3 fatty acids by adults over the age of sixty-five could prevent nearly 400,000 hospitalizations and physician visits due to decreased heart disease over the course of five years.

❖ A study of patients with elevated triglycerides found that supplementing with fish oil decreased triglyceride levels by approximately 50 percent.

❖ A recent study of 1,059 patients admitted to the hospital with a heart attack or angina measured blood levels of omega-3 fatty acids (EPA and DHA). Compared to age-matched controls, the risk of angina or heart attack was reduced by 62 percent for every 1.24 percent increase in EPA/DHA levels.

❖ A study of more than 11,000 patients showed that fish oil supplementation resulted in a 30 percent reduction in death from heart disease and a 45 percent reduction in sudden cardiac death.

❖ A study done with healthy patients as well as those with rheumatoid disease showed that fish oil suppresses the formation of dangerous cytokines (destructive cell-signaling chemicals) by up to 90 percent.

❖ A study in *Circulation* found that supplementing mice with lipoic acid reduced arterial lesion formation, triglycerides, blood vessel inflammation, and weight gain. The supplemented mice had 40 percent less weight gain.

❖ A review of eight studies involving over 10,800 patients found that high levels of vitamin E lowered the risk of Parkinson's disease by 22 percent.

❖ *Annals of Internal Medicine* study of 13,017 adults followed over 7.5 years found that supplementation with antioxidants lowered all-cause mortality.

❖ A five-year trial involving 2,000 diabetic patients found that those supplementing with 400 IU of vitamin E daily lowered their heart attack risk by 43 percent and the risk of dying from heart disease was lowered by 55 percent.

❖ Supplementing with indole-3-carbinol suppressed a cancer-enhancing protein by almost 80 percent.

❖ Suboptimal levels of folic acid and vitamin B6 and B12 increased risk of heart disease and cancer.

❖ Study found that the lower the levels of vitamin B12 and folic acid measured, the more severe levels of hearing loss.

❖ Women who took beta-carotene for over ten years had a 69 percent lower risk of ovarian cancer than those who did not supplement.

❖ Study showed that men with a high intake of vitamin E are 65 percent less likely to develop colorectal adenomas (precursors to colon cancer.)

❖ Study found that men with the highest level of gamma-tocopherols (vitamin E) had a fivefold reduction in the risk of developing prostate cancer.

❖ A ten-year clinical study of more than 4,500 people demonstrated that people at high risk for developing advanced stages of macular degeneration (a loss of central vision that is the leading cause of blindness for those over fifty-five years old) lowered the risk by 25 percent when treated with a high-dose combination of vitamins C and E, beta-carotene, zinc, and copper.

❖ In a study of prostate cancer, the men with higher levels of omega-3 fats in their prostate tissue had lower levels of prostate cancer aggressiveness.

❖ *American Heart Journal* study found that chromium supplementation lowers blood insulin levels and lowers cardiovascular risk in type 2 diabetic patients.

❖ A study published in 2005 found that lung cancer patients who took vitamin and mineral supplements following their diagnosis had double the average survival time and better quality of life compared to those who did not use supplements.

❖ A study of 106 patients with macular degeneration reported that a combination of acetyl-L-carnitine, omega-3 fatty acids, and CoQ10 taken twice daily for twelve months significantly improved four parameters of visual function.

And much more ...

CHAPTER 4

EXERCISE

Everybody ready for recess?

Many of us have forms of exercise that we love, whether it's playing tennis, golf, hiking, swimming, or biking. I certainly encourage you to continue the types of activity you enjoy. However, in *Antiaging 101*, we will look at exercise with a different perspective.

Our perspective will be evaluating how exercise can assist in reaching our eight antiaging goals as efficiently and as effectively as possible. In other words, we want our antiaging exercise program to give us the most health benefit in the least amount of time.

Our program will be practical and doable so we can be consistent with the program for the rest of our lives. It will blend in well with our diet, supplement, and hormone therapy programs for maximal benefit. It will not require much of your time; in fact, the better you get at it, the less time you will spend exercising.

To optimize your results, I will need you to erase many of your preconceived ideas regarding exercise. Clean your slate and open up your mind to new ideas so you can use our exercise program to lower your biological age.

Antiaging exercise goal:
maximal benefit in minimal of time.

Let's list some of the amazing benefits of a consistent exercise program. Foremost, as noted above, we can lower our biological age. Now that is true antiaging. We will significantly decrease the risk of diabetes, obesity, heart disease, osteoporosis, cancer, and dementia. Imagine the benefits if we combine our diet, supplement, and hormone replacement programs with our exercise program!

With our program, you will have improved mood, improved metabolism, and improved immune function. Indeed, you will become healthier and stronger. You will look better and feel better.

Many people will acquire these benefits by spending less time on exercise than they are spending currently. Again, we want the most benefit in the least amount of time.

Finally, you will reverse the body composition changes we see with aging. By being consistent with the program, you will eliminate the accelerated aging that occurs with a sedentary lifestyle.

To understand our antiaging exercise program better, let's begin by reviewing the body composition changes that occur with aging.

As we age, we gain fat, lose muscle, and lose bone. Strike three! Remember the two main forces of our metabolism: anabolic forces and catabolic forces. Anabolic is repair and rebuild. Catabolic is breakdown and degeneration.

In our youthful years, anabolic forces exceed catabolic forces and all is well. With aging, catabolic forces exceed anabolic forces ... and we degenerate. A sedentary lifestyle will accelerate these catabolic forces and hasten the aging process.

The human body is an amazing machine. Our bodies retain the ability to repair and rejuvenate, to "go anabolic," throughout our lives, regardless of age! With the right exercise, especially with all the other components of our program, we will tap into this incredible restorative ability of the body to "become younger."

With our exercise program, we give the body appropriate stimuli to build muscle, build bone, and burn fat. By doing so, we make our bodies younger and healthier.

Our brains interpret the exercise stimuli and send out appropriate hormones and chemical signals to encourage anabolic growth. Since our brains receive youthful messages, they respond by keeping us young! You will feel the difference, and your friends will notice the difference.

Anabolic ≥ Catabolic = healthy aging

How does exercise transform our health so dramatically? Is it the extra calories we burn? Is it because we sweat off weight and toxins? Or is it because any time spent in the gym is time away from the kitchen?

You will be surprised to learn that many of the benefits of exercise are a direct result of the hormone response to exercise.[1-17] We don't usually think of exercise and hormones as being interrelated, but indeed they are. Understanding this allows us to plan our antiaging exercise program more effectively.

With exercise, we lower our insulin levels and improve insulin sensitivity. We increase our glucagon levels. Glucagon is the balancing hormone to insulin. We increase our levels of HGH (human growth hormone), DHEA (dehydroepiandosterone) and testosterone, all of which are anabolic hormones. HGH is produced by the anterior pituitary gland in the brain, while DHEA is produced by the adrenal glands. Testosterone is produced by the testicles in men and in the ovaries and adrenal glands in women. Testosterone, HGH, and DHEA improve fat burning, muscle strength, and bone density. These hormones improve anabolic metabolism and helps us build better bodies.

Exercise balances our cortisol stress hormone (unless we exercise excessively), and exercise increases endorphins that affect mood and pain relief. Exercise also impacts leptin hormone. Leptin is a hormone released from our fat cells. When we are sensitive to leptin, the brain receives the message from fat cells to decrease appetite. When we have leptin resistance, which is similar to insulin resistance, the brain ignores the leptin message and we stay hungry. Exercise helps restore leptin sensitivity, with the net effect of decreased appetite and decreased fat storage.

This combined hormone response to exercise results in lower body fat, increased muscle mass, increased bone density, improved metabolism, decreased stress, improved mood and sleep, and improved immune function.

The resulting hormone response to exercise allows us to reach our healthy aging goals and significantly decrease our risk for multiple degenerative diseases.

Quite a remarkable array of benefits. So lace up your sneakers and get going!

Hormone changes with exercise:

Lower insulin levels
Increased glucagon levels
Increased HGH levels
Increased DHEA levels
Increased testosterone levels
Balanced cortisol levels
Improved leptin function

Muscles matter!

At the 101-course level, I find it helpful to simplify our exercise goals to improve your understanding as well as your compliance with the program. I simplify our exercise program by giving you one specific target. That target is your muscle strength.

We will focus entirely on the muscular system because every benefit of exercise will come to fruition by simply strengthening our muscles. When you add muscle and get stronger, your heart works better, your immune system works better, your metabolism improves dramatically, and you burn fat more effectively.

By exercising our muscles and getting stronger, we literally send a signal to the brain that we are young and active. In response, the brain will take care of the rest to ensure we grow biologically younger. Now how cool is that?

Unfortunately, the opposite is true. A sedentary lifestyle signals our brain that we are old and lazy. In response, the brain facilitates the catabolic processes, and we begin our "breakdown."

Without the stimulus that exercise provides, we lose muscle. We can lose two to six pounds of muscle every decade!

Consider your muscle as your most valuable real estate. You worked hard over the years with exercise and nutrition to stay strong and to build and maintain muscle. Simply by becoming inactive, you give away that expensive real estate for free. Don't allow nature to take away this valuable component of your health portfolio!

If we combine a deprivation diet with a sedentary lifestyle, the speed of muscle loss accelerates. Ironically, excessive exercise, such as running marathons, will result in accelerated muscle loss, compounding the problem further. Allowing this muscle loss to occur can ultimately affect your ability to live independently.

With muscle loss, people become too weak to lift groceries and to get up if they fall, and they are unable to stay mobile. Many people end up in an assisted living or nursing home residences simply because they lack the muscle strength to live independently. This is tragic and completely avoidable.

With your muscles, it is certainly "use it or lose it."

Main goal of antiaging exercise: muscle strength and definition.

Okay, class, now let's turn our attention to our muscles. A little muscle physiology is needed to appreciate the goals of our program.

Muscles are made up of different muscle fibers. The muscle fibers differ in size, speed, and their use in the human body.

There are three main types of muscle fibers. We have slow twitch, intermediate twitch, and fast twitch. The slow twitch fibers are the smallest fibers. They are activated first as we start exercising, and they are used for endurance activity. Intermediate twitch fibers are a combination of slow and fast twitch muscle fibers.

At the other end of the fiber spectrum are fast twitch muscle fibers. These quick dudes are the biggest fibers, and they are activated later as the muscle is stimulated. Fast twitch fibers are for power and are used only for short durations.

Another difference in the fibers relates to their primary energy source. Slow twitch fibers burn mostly fat for energy, intermediate fibers burn fat and glucose, and fast twitch fibers burn glucose for energy.

As we gradually increase our intensity of exercise, our "fuel" mixture changes from predominantly fat to a mixture of fat and glucose, and ultimately, it's predominantly glucose.

Essentially, glucose is used when we need quick energy; fat is used when we need sustained energy.

At low intensity, such as with walking, we use slow twitch muscle fibers and burn mostly fat. During high-intensity exercise, such as weight lifting, we use fast twitch fibers as well as intermediate twitch fibers, thereby burning mostly glucose. (Later on, we will review why the energy source burned *after* an exercise session is crucial for antiaging.)

So how do our muscles grow? Basically, exercise results in microscopic tears to our muscle fibers. The anabolic repair process results in increased muscle protein synthesis to repair and reinforce the injured muscle fibers. The result is stronger and larger muscles.

With this repair process, muscle fibers increase in density and number. Muscles also respond to exercise by increasing the number of mitochondria "furnaces." With additional mitochondria, the muscle can burn fuel more efficiently and effectively. Increased mitochondria mean enhanced energy production and better stamina. The improved burning of fuel helps in the fat loss department. We become stronger and leaner!

Concomitant with the improved muscle fiber strength and the escalating number of mitochondria is the enhancement of enzymes in the body. This increase in enzymes, or "up regulation," results in superior fat burning and glucose transport. (Remember the energy cycles.) This translates into a stronger, leaner, and healthier you.

You will "retool" your metabolism with an effective exercise program.

Exercise increases:

Muscle strength
Mitochondria
Enzymes

When we improve our muscular systems with exercise, we simultaneously improve our cardiovascular systems. Most people have this backward. They focus on improving their "cardio" but neglect their muscular real estate. They frequently choose exercise with the focus of raising their heart rates or burning the most calories. This approach will actually produce muscle loss and have minimal effect on cardiovascular health.[18-25] Remember to focus on your muscle strength.

It may seem counterintuitive that adding muscle strength results in better heart health, so let's evaluate this concept further. Remember that the heart is a muscle. Improving this muscular pump is crucial for cardiovascular optimization.

In addition, when we exercise our muscles to get stronger, two things happen. First, our muscles improve their ability to take up oxygen from the blood via enzyme upregulation. Second, stronger muscles result in increased blood flow to the muscles.

Stronger muscles result in both dilated blood vessels as well as increased number of blood vessels to supply the muscle with blood. These changes in the muscular system lower blood pressure while simultaneously improving nutrient delivery to the cells.

Combined, these changes mean the heart pumps more efficiently and effectively. Enhanced oxygen and nutrient delivery to the muscles occurs, resulting in improved stamina.

When your strength increases, you improve your cardiovascular health immensely. We turn you into a strong "muscle head," but you develop a strong "muscle heart."

With exercise, muscles increase glucose uptake thirtyfold. Consequently, muscle strength lowers blood glucose levels and improves insulin sensitivity dramatically.

Combining the improvements in glucose metabolism with the hormone response to exercise works synergistically to improve health. It is easy to appreciate how a consistent exercise program facilitates reaching all of our healthy aging goals.

Come on, Professor; tell me what to do at the gym.

Let's set up an exercise program. For teaching purposes, we will break exercise options down into two categories: aerobic (a.k.a. "cardio") and resistance training (a.k.a. weight lifting).

Aerobic exercise is what most people think about when discussing exercise. Aerobic simply means "with oxygen." I can't imagine exercising without oxygen!

Basically, aerobic means exercising at an intensity that allows sufficient oxygen to be delivered to the muscle cells. Walking, jogging, biking, and swimming are examples of aerobic exercise.

At lower levels of intensity, the muscle cells get plenty of oxygen to burn fat and glucose efficiently. The slow twitch fibers are utilized to allow the endurance activity to continue.

If the intensity is increased—for example, when picking up the pace or sprinting—the muscle cells reach a point where they don't get sufficient oxygen. When glucose is burned without sufficient oxygen, lactic acid is produced. The lactic acid released causes the "burn" sensation that is felt in the exercising muscles.

At high intensity, we utilize the fast twitch fibers; we burn glucose first with oxygen, then glucose without oxygen until we feel the burn. When we feel the burn sensation, we must stop or slow down so we can utilize slow twitch fibers to continue our activity.

If we maintain a relatively slow, stable pace, typical of jogging, for example, we can exercise much longer, as we don't reach the "burn" phase.

Aerobic exercise has many benefits. It lowers glucose levels, it lowers insulin levels, it lowers cortisol levels, it stimulates endorphins, it improves mood, and it helps with fat loss. It is also a type of exercise that everyone is comfortable and familiar with.

Despite its many health benefits, aerobic exercise has some limitations that we need to be aware of. This knowledge allows us to utilize aerobic exercise to reach our healthy aging goals.

The first limitation of aerobic exercise is that it does not build muscle. The reliance on slow twitch muscle fibers exclusively precludes us from stimulating muscle fibers required for growth.

In addition, prolonged excessive aerobics, like running a long marathon, actually lead to muscle loss. With excessive aerobics, muscle loss occurs for a couple of reasons. First, prolonged exercise is a stressor that results in increased release of cortisol. Cortisol is catabolic and will cause muscle and bone loss at high levels.

Second, after roughly forty to sixty minutes of exercise, our bodies start breaking down muscle to supply energy to the exercising muscles. This catabolic response is why marathon runners often look frail, especially in the face and upper body. The muscles from their upper bodies are broken down to fuel the exercising leg muscles.[26-30]

Since the main focus for our antiaging exercise program is muscle strength, excessive aerobics will not be part of our plan. I don't know about you, but I don't want to run miles burning calories so I can end up weaker!

Another limitation of aerobics is that it will not produce significant body composition changes. If your body type is an apple, aerobics will make you a smaller apple, but you will still be the shape of an apple. If you are built like a pear, aerobics will only make you a smaller pear.

Finally, many forms of aerobic exercise result in repetitive trauma on our joints and contribute to chronic knee pain and chronic foot pain from conditions such as tendonitis and plantar fasciitis.

Benefits of aerobic exercise:

Lowers glucose levels
Lowers insulin levels
Lowers cortisol levels
Lowers body fat
Improves mood
Improves metabolism

We will design our exercise program to glean the many benefits of aerobic exercise without the negative influences of its limitations. This is accomplished two ways.

One, simply limit the time spent on your aerobic activity. For most people, this translates into sessions less than thirty minutes. Of course, this does not mean you can't take a long hike or long bike ride occasionally. It simply means don't plan on frequent, prolonged aerobic sessions. To do so means wasting large blocks of time with minimal antiaging benefits.

Interval training

The second way is by utilizing interval training. Interval training can be done with any type of aerobic exercise—by alternating short bursts of higher intensity aerobics with short periods of lower intensity aerobics.

For example, walk at your usual pace for a few minutes, then walk faster for thirty seconds to a minute, then slow down to your baseline pace. Repeat this cycle every few minutes. This can be applied to jogging, biking, jumping rope, or any form of aerobic exercise. Most newer exercise bikes, treadmills, and elliptical trainers have built-in computer programs for interval training.

The interval training session should be limited to twenty or thirty minutes. Gradually, as you get in better shape, you will increase your intensity, but you will never have to increase time spent exercising!

Interval training has multiple advantages over traditional aerobics. By alternating intensity, we incorporate all of our different muscle fibers, optimizing the stimulus to our muscular systems. Doing so maximizes fat burning during and after exercise.[31]

In addition, interval training optimizes the anabolic hormone response, allowing us to tap into the restorative power of our hormones.

Another benefit of interval training is we avoid the body "adapting" to the same exercise repeatedly. When the body adapts, there is a significant decrease in the positive effects of the exercise program.

Finally, by capping the amount of time spent on interval training, we avoid repetitive trauma-related injuries. This allows you to get more benefit, spend less time exercising, and decrease the risk of injury. That's why we call it smart exercise!

Interval training is effective regardless of your current level of fitness. In essence, with interval training you are performing aerobic exercise, "cardio," simultaneously with anaerobic exercise, "resistance training," making it an efficient exercise routine. We don't want to waste your precious time.

Off the treadmill; let's move on to resistance training. (That's resistance training, not resistance to training!)

Resistance training can be done with free weights, machines, rubber tubing, and even with your own body weight. For this class, the main focus will be on weight training, but the principles discussed apply to all forms of resistance training.

Most people are surprised and skeptical that weight training is advocated for an age management program. However, you will soon understand why it is such a crucial element of the program. You will realize that resistance training can benefit people of all ages, regardless of fitness level.

Most importantly, the impact of resistance training on our healthy aging goals is immense. We will cover why resistance training is the single best form of exercise for improved health. If we are going to shift the tide of the catabolic forces of aging, then resistance training is necessary.

Weight training is often referred to as anaerobic exercise. Again, this simply means exercising at an intensity that causes insufficient oxygen delivery to the muscle cells. The resultant production of lactic acid elicits the "burn" felt in exercising muscles.

Clearly, resistance training involves both aerobic and anaerobic components. One of the reasons weight training is so beneficial is this dual component. This is also why weight training is so time efficient, as you are participating in aerobic exercise simultaneously with anaerobic exercise.

Remember, our main goal of exercise is to improve our muscular systems—and nothing strengthens muscle more than weight training!

The beauty of a weight training program is the ability to get stronger and leaner at the same time. In addition, no other form of exercise can change your body composition to the degree that occurs with weight training. Even if you have the typical apple or pear body shape, weight training will help alter and improve your body shape. You can finally lose that apple or pear appearance!

Weight training alters your body composition by lowering body fat while building muscle. One pound of muscle takes up one fifth of the space occupied by one pound of fat. This leads to a leaner, firmer body type.

Weight training also produces a better hormone response, all in line with our healthy goals. Insulin is lowered; testosterone release and HGH release are enhanced. Cortisol production is diminished. Again, these multiple hormonal benefits allow the body composition changes to take place.

Our shift from catabolic metabolism to anabolic metabolism will be dramatically impacted by this hormone response.

Additional benefits of weight training include improved joint strength and flexibility. Many people assume the best exercise for joint health is cardio. Interestingly, by strengthening the muscles and tendons that move the joints, we improve the joint function.

Indeed, most orthopedic rehabilitation exercise involves resistance training. After knee surgery, for example, we don't have you pounding the pavement running. On the contrary, we have you participate in a resistance program that gradually increases the intensity to strengthen your knee joint.

Another benefit of weight training is the cross-training benefit toward other sports. Most sports require short bursts of high intensity alternating with low intensity. This, of course, is exactly what happens with weight training and interval training.

We previously reviewed the cardiovascular benefits of weight training. The heart benefits combined with improved strength, improved flexibility, and joint health translates into better athletic performance regardless of the sport.

Many examples of the cross-training benefit of weight lifting occur in the athletic world. Andre Agassi added years to his tennis career simply by lifting weights. Tiger Woods remains a world-leading golfer while continuing a year-round weight lifting program.

Most professional and college athletes participate in a weight training program throughout the year because of the cross-training benefits toward their different sports.

Benefits of weight training:

Improved muscle strength
Lower body fat
Increased bone density
Lower glucose and insulin
Improved metabolism
Anabolic hormone response
Lowered inflammation
Improved cardiovascular function
Improved joint strength
Cross-training benefits
Improved appearance/body composition
No need to purchase jogging shoes

Even when we are beyond our high school and college athletic careers, we can still capture the age management benefits of resistance training. Many excellent studies in the medical literature have documented the multiple health benefits of weight training, regardless of age and prior fitness level. The human body has a remarkable ability to build muscle and to get stronger regardless of age.

Weight training programs in elderly patients, even with no prior weight training experience, have resulted in improved body composition, improved balance, and improved flexibility. The ramifications of these changes in their health were miraculous, leading to less dependence and even elimination of walkers and canes. Now we're talking antiaging!

Let's discuss some principals of effective weight lifting programs. Many people who have never lifted weights may feel intimidated walking into a gym and starting a program. Rest assured that we have many different options and opportunities.

Private exercise studios with personal trainers are a great way to start a program in a comfortable setting with individual attention. SWAT Fitness is a perfect example.

There are also great and affordable home gym opportunities and even trainers who come to your house or workplace. You're going to "run" out of excuses! (And you don't even have to run to exercise!)

The primary goal of a weight training program is to exercise your muscles to induce microscopic injury to the muscle to allow the muscle to rebuild and strengthen. You may wonder how we know we have reached the point of microscopic injury without a microscope.

Fortunately, it is quite easy. We simply perform an exercise until we reach muscular fatigue and feel that 'burn" of lactic acid production. This "burn" alerts the body to begin the repair process.

Muscular fatigue is the point where you can't lift the weight even one more time. With this in mind, we pick different exercises for each of our major muscle groups—chest, back, legs, shoulders, abdomen, and arms. We then perform each exercise until we reach muscle fatigue.

Ideally, the amount of weight selected should allow you to lift and lower the weight about six to fifteen times. If you can't lift the weight six times, then chose a lighter weight. If you perform fifteen repetitions, or "reps," without reaching muscular fatigue, then simply choose a heavier weight.

After you have completed an appropriate number of reps and have reached muscular fatigue, you are done with that major muscle group. You have just completed a "set." You now rest for about one minute and catch your breath, then move on to the next major muscle group and repeat, again aiming for six to fifteen reps.

Repeat this routine until you have exercised every major muscle group. To hit every major muscle group and lift until fatigue only means you will be doing about six to eight different exercises for a total body workout. With about a minute rest between sets, the whole routine only takes approximately thirty minutes.

As you progress, you will get stronger and more efficient. Your workout will take even less of your time. You will also be able to do additional sets of each exercise as you become more proficient. In addition, you will shorten the rest interval as you progress.

A goal with your weight training program is to keep the workout session under thirty minutes. This will make it more practical and keep you on the program forever, while making sure you tap into all the benefits of a weight training program.

> Cap weight training session at thirty minutes.
> Cap interval training session at twenty minutes.

Focus on intensity without extending duration.

This program can be utilized with free weights, machines, or a combination of both. A sample workout sequence follows.

Warm-up only requires doing a few sets of squats at low weight and/or a few sets of bench presses at low weight.

Do the following workout three days a week, i.e., Monday, Wednesday, and Friday, or Tuesday, Thursday, Saturday:

1. **Squats** (legs) 6–15 reps
   Rest 30 to 60 seconds (or until you can speak comfortably)
2. **Bench press** (chest) 6–15 reps
   Rest 30 to 60 seconds (or until you can speak comfortably)
3. **Row** (back) 6–15 reps
   Rest 30 to 60 seconds (or until you can speak comfortably)
4. **Reverse crunches** (abdomen) until fatigue
   Rest 30 to 60 seconds (or until you can speak comfortably)
5. **Military press** (shoulders) 6–15 reps
   Rest 30 to 60 seconds (or until you can speak comfortably)
6. **Curls** (arms/biceps) 6–15 reps
   Rest 30 to 60 seconds (or until you can speak comfortably)
7. **Arm extensions** (arms/triceps) 6–15 reps

Hit the shower. Eat a healthy meal. Ball game over.

In time, you can add a second or third set, each to fatigue, to all of the different exercises. You will become more efficient, and the extra sets will not add much time to your workout. In fact, as you get more proficient with experience, eventually you will get a great workout in twenty minutes.

There are a few principles to be aware of with resistance training. First we choose a primary muscle group(s) to exercise; we strain that muscle group(s) until fatigue; then we rest and go to the next muscle group(s). Our end goal is muscle fatigue instead of a specific number of repetitions.

When you can no longer lift one more rep and you feel the burn, know that the appropriate stimulus has been released. The body will then initiate the repair process sequence for the exercised muscle group(s). Then move on to the next muscle group(s).

It is crucial to be consistent with the program and to increase the intensity progressively—but not the duration of your exercise. There are a number of ways to progressively increase the intensity. One is to simply increase the amount of weight lifted. Another technique is to slow down the speed of motion, lift the weight slowly, and lower the weight slowly with controlled motion. A third option is to lift the weight rapidly but lower the weight slowly. A final technique is to change the position of the specific exercise—for example, incline the bench during chest exercise or stand during arm curls.

Subtle changes increase the muscle fiber recruitment to incorporate more muscle fibers into the exercise for additional benefit. Additional options include lifting to add more power, or lifting to enhance endurance. For power, select heavier weights that allow fewer repetitions until reaching muscle fatigue. For endurance, select lighter weights that you can lift a higher number of repetitions until reaching muscle fatigue.

Switch around the program periodically—for example, choose different workouts every other week, or you can do one specific sequence for four to six weeks, then change for another four to six weeks. You get the picture. The options are endless, but as long as the basic principals are adhered to, there will be tremendous benefits.

Do weight lifting and cardio on different days.

For maximal exercise results, do your cardio and weight training on different days, or do your weight training first, followed by your cardio training.

With weight training, never exercise the same muscle group(s) two days in a row. Remember, muscle grows while you rest it. After a weight training session, the body takes roughly forty-eight hours to recover.

The recovery process requires proper nutrition and hormone balance. It also requires a tremendous amount of energy, which explains why you are burning fat even on your rest days. After a cardio session, metabolism is increased for a few hours. After a weight training session, metabolism is increased for two days.[32-33]

I liken this metabolic difference between cardio and weight training to renting property versus owning property. With renting, you do not build equity, and with cardio you don't build long-term metabolic gains. With ownership, you build equity over time, and with weight training, you have long-term metabolic gains. With weight training, equity equals increased muscle mass and enhanced metabolism.

On your rest days, in between resistance training sessions, you could do an interval training session or a thirty-minute walk or bike ride. Or you could simply rest and let your body repair from the previous day's workout.

You will receive multiple benefits from this exercise program. Be consistent with the program for best results.

Overall, you will end up spending less time exercising yet attain better results over the upcoming years. Since you will see and feel the difference in your health and energy, you will not want to live without making exercise a part of your life.

Exercise your right to be healthy!

Benefits of exercise program:

Lower biological age

Decreased risk of degenerative disease

Improved bone density

Improved strength

Improved mood

Improved metabolism

Lower body fat

Improved immune function

Slow aging process

Improved glucose control

Improved insulin control

Lower cortisol levels

Improved hormone levels

Decreased inflammation

Optimized cell function and cell
  energy production

Exercise Nuts and Bolts:

1) Be consistent. Benefits accrue over time. Consistency is more important than duration.

2) Schedule workout times. Make it a priority in your life for healthy aging.

3) Start with realistic goals, e.g., weight training thirty minutes, two to three times per week; cardio twenty minutes, two to three times per week. Remember your rest days.

4) Quality of exercise is better than quantity; intensity is more important than duration. Think brief exercise sessions.

5) Remember the main goal of your exercise program: improving the muscular system.

6) Lift weights or do another form of resistance training to optimize body composition and metabolism. Resistance training is necessary for muscle preservation.

7) Brief cardio or interval training sessions avoid excessive cortisol response.

8) If you have time for only one type of exercise, choose weight training.

All of our healthy aging goals will be positively impacted with an effective exercise program.

Exercise is a perfect antiaging modality. When we make a commitment and exercise intelligently, we find it becomes more efficient yet less time consuming.

Exercise has a tremendous impact on glucose, insulin, and cortisol control. Exercise improves cell function and metabolism.

Intelligent exercise avoids excessive free radical production and, remarkably, decreases inflammation. The anabolic stimulus of our exercise program balances hormone levels.

Together, by reaching all of our antiaging goals, we become leaner, stronger, energetic, and youthful.

CHAPTER 4
QUESTIONS

Student:

Since heart disease is such a common cause of death in Americans, shouldn't we focus most of our exercise time on aerobics and cardiovascular health instead of resistance training?

Professor:

Focus on muscle strength. By getting stronger and improving your muscular system, you will vastly improve your cardiovascular function. Simply getting your heart rate in an aerobic zone does not come close to the cardiovascular benefits of a resistance training program.

Student:

My physical education teacher said that lifting weights would decrease my flexibility and make me "muscle bound." Is that true?

Professor:

No. Contrary to popular myth, weight lifting will not restrict your flexibility or limit your movements. In fact, with resistance training, you will have better joint health, better balance, and improved flexibility. Watch Tiger Woods hit the golf ball if you have any doubts (he lifts weights throughout the golf season). Or watch video of Andre Agassi (another weight lifter) playing tennis; his speed and quickness should convince you. Most, if not all, of the elite college basketball programs have year-round weight lifting programs. Do those athletes look stiff and muscle-bound to you?

Student:

I bought my wife a heart monitor for her birthday next week. You didn't mention heart rate monitors in your lectures. Should I return it?

Professor:

I'm glad to see that I'm not the only idiot who gives exercise equipment gifts to his wife. I will give you two reasons to return the heart monitor: (1) she won't like it; and (2) she doesn't need it.

During rest periods, tell her to focus on her breathing, once her breathing rate slows and she can talk comfortably, it is time to start exercising again. No need for watches, clocks, or monitors.

Student:

Do you have a favorite weight lifting routine?

Professor:

I aim for a twenty- to thirty-minute session three times a week. I choose five to eight exercises to hit all major muscle groups. I like to vary my routine to avoid monotony, but my most common workout is one of the following:

For each exercise, I do one set at a weight I can lift about fifteen times—but lift until fatigue. Rest briefly. Then I do a second set at a higher weight, aiming for about ten reps, again lifting until fatigue. Rest briefly. Finally, I do a third set with a heavier weight, aiming for six reps, again lifting until fatigue. Rest briefly and go to the next exercise. This sequence is repeated until all exercises are done or my thirty minutes is up.

Or, when I really want to make my workout brief yet maximize my fat burning, I do a version of the following:

Pick five to eight exercises to hit all major muscle groups. Pick a weight for each exercise, one that you can lift for between eight to twelve repetitions. Do the exercise until muscle fatigue, i.e., can't lift even one more time. Rest for six seconds (yes, six seconds!), then do the same exercise with the same weight until muscle fatigue. Rest another six seconds and repeat the exercise until fatigue. Repeat the cycle until you can only lift once or twice until fatigue.

Rest as briefly as possible, about five to thirty seconds, and go immediately to your next exercise, doing the same sequence until you have completely fatigued another muscle group. Repeat the cycle until all exercises are completed. In time, you will become faster and will be able to recycle through the workout again (if you want to) and still finish within thirty minutes.

I love this approach because it is fast and effective. Keep in mind that shorter rest periods mean you are burning fat and building muscle.

To avoid monotony, I will change it up even further. Sometimes I will alternate exercises that involve opposing muscle groups. For example, a "push" exercise followed by a "pull" exercise. Opposing muscle group examples would include a chest exercise followed by an upper back exercise … or a biceps exercise followed by a triceps exercise.

When I alternate opposing muscle groups, I try to alternate back and forth with minimal, if any, rest periods. In other words, complete one exercise and then go to an exercise for an opposing muscle group in rapid succession. This increases the intensity while simultaneously decreasing the total workout session. With every workout, the goal is increasing intensity but never increasing time spent in the gym.

Keep a journal and write down weights and reps for each exercise; this will facilitate future workouts. Always try to do a little better with each workout.

In time, you will become efficient with the workouts, yet they will continue to challenge you and provide the stimulation needed for great results.

Student:

How long should I rest between sets?

Professor:

The best way is to pay attention to how you are breathing. After a set, you will feel short of breath and notice that your breathing rate and heart rate have escalated. This is because your body is trying to increase the oxygen to the muscles.

Simply wait until your breathing rate has slowed enough to allow you to speak comfortably. When that occurs, you are able to start exercising again.

Initially, this rest period may be a few minutes; however, in time you will notice that the average rest period will be between thirty and sixty seconds.

As you get stronger, you will be able to do some sets sequentially, without a rest period. This will shorten your exercise session even further! Listen to your body instead of watching the clock.

Moreover, when you first start your weight training program, I suggest turning off the music or television and paying attention to how you feel while exercising and during your rest periods.

After each weight lifting set, you should notice a few things to make sure you are performing the exercise well. First, you will be short of breath. Second, you will notice that your heart is beating rapidly (high pulse rate). Third, you will notice a burning sensation in the muscle groups that you just exercised. And finally, you will notice that you are sweating. (You will also notice the desire to quit!)

If you notice all of these, you will know you are exercising well. It's simple and it doesn't require a fancy monitor or clock. Just remember the five Bs of effective weight lifting exercises:

Beating heart
Burning muscle
Breathing fast
Beads of sweat
Desire to make a **"B" line** to the exit

If you notice the **B**s, you can **b**et you are **b**uilding a **b**etter **b**ody and **b**urning fat!

Student:

I have read that compound exercises, incorporating multiple muscle groups into one exercise, and functional training are effective. What is your opinion?

Professor:

Absolutely, and I'll tell you why, but first let me briefly explain the terms "compound exercise" and "functional training" for students who are unfamiliar with the concepts. Compound exercises involve motion in multiple joints, thereby simultaneously training more than one major muscle group at a time. A squat is an example of a compound exercise, as it involves several joints—hips, knees, and ankles—while targeting muscle groups: buttocks and upper and lower legs. Functional training involves specifically training the body for an individual sport or for real-life activities. Compound exercises and functional training are great ways to maximize results while simultaneously decreasing exercise time. I would suggest working with a certified personal trainer for guidance. If you live in Tucson, then see Ron Holland at SWAT Fitness. He is a master at functional training programs.

Student:

Doesn't weight training increase the risk of injury?

Professor:

No. In fact, the opposite is true. Weight training is safe and effective regardless of your current fitness level. In addition, the anabolic stimulus generated by the body with resistance training is anti-inflammatory and allows the body to build and repair.

Student:

Isn't weight lifting more difficult for older people?

Professor:

Weight training is effective and appropriate for people of all ages, even the elderly. Studies have proven that an elderly population reaps enormous benefits from a weight-training program, regardless of whether they have ever lifted weights before!

Most people find prolonged aerobics increasingly more difficult to do as they age. This is usually because of repetitive trauma to their joints and the fact that aerobics are often boring as hell.

Student:

Do you ever have days where you just don't feel like exercising?

Professor:

For sure, but only on days that end in *y*! Joking aside, we all have days when we aren't motivated to exercise. My suggestion on those days is to try the "ten-minute rule."

On the days you don't feel motivated to exercise, start your exercise session and plan on working out for only ten minutes. Anyone can work out for ten minutes.

After ten minutes, reassess how you feel. Usually, you will feel so much better that you decide to finish your workout session. If you don't feel better, then stop your workout. Your body may simply need a break.

Another effective trick for motivation is called the "mirror test." I use this frequently. On the days I don't want to work out, I take off my shirt and look in the mirror. One glance at my gut and I'm back in the gym!

Student:

You recommend interval training over traditional aerobics. Please describe interval training again, explaining how intense the intervals need to be for optimal benefit.

Professor:

The intensity of the intervals depends on your level of fitness. If you are a novice, then walk at a comfortable pace for a few minutes, walk faster for thirty to sixty seconds, and then go back to your baseline pace. Repeat the sequence about five to ten times.

If you are experienced with exercise, you could jog at a comfortable pace for a few minutes, then sprint for thirty to sixty seconds, and then go back to your baseline pace. Repeat the sequence about five to ten times.

You can apply this to biking, swimming, jumping rope, elliptical trainers, or whatever form of exercise you like.

Just limit the total time to about twenty minutes. No matter what your baseline level of health, you will notice incredible benefits of interval training.

The goal with interval training is to create an oxygen debt. An oxygen debt is reached by briefly raising the intensity of the exercise until you can't continue that pace any longer, then slowing back down to a comfortable pace.

After slowing down, you will be short of breath, and your pulse and breathing rates will have accelerated. Your rapid breathing and heart rate is your body's way of working to get more oxygen to "pay back" the oxygen debt.

When your breathing slows again, repeat the higher-intensity interval.

This oxygen debt is the stimulus you are striving for to tap into the fat burning benefits.

> Goal of interval training: oxygen debt
> Pay the debt back with fat currency!
> Dividend is better health.

Student:

What type of snack do you recommend prior to and after an exercise session?

Professor:

Eating as we discussed in chapter 2 will augment your exercise program nicely. While some people prefer to exercise on an empty stomach, most feel better and get better results by consuming a healthy snack an hour or so before the exercise session.

Ideally, this snack should consist of both a healthy protein and a healthy carbohydrate. A balanced snack helps fuel your muscles for your workout while simultaneously supporting a balanced hormone environment.

Most important is to eat a healthy meal or snack within a few hours of completing your workout. This is crucial to provide needed nutrients for the recovery process. This post workout meal should provide healthy protein, carbohydrates, and fat.

Student:

While lifting weights, what is the best way to breathe? What pace do you recommend while lifting and lowering the weights?

Professor:

While lifting weights, breathe comfortably and don't hold your breath. Inhale while you lower the weight and exhale while you raise the weight.

For lifting pace, think of your muscle as a spring or coil. Lower the weight slowly to contract the coil and then lift the weight quickly as if the coil has sprung lose. When you lower the weight slowly and then raise the weight quickly, you maximize utilization of your different muscle fibers. This helps optimize your results.

Student:

When is the best time to exercise?

Professor:

As Ron Holland from SWAT Fitness says, "The best time to exercise is the time that works for you and your schedule." One simple trick is to set your alarm and wake up earlier than usual to exercise. After a while, it will seem as if you have added more time to your day.

Student:

What are your thoughts on "carb loading"?

Professor:

Carbohydrate loading is ineffective. For students who are not familiar with the term, let me briefly explain what carbohydrate loading is before I answer your question. Carbohydrate loading is often used by endurance athletes. "Carb loading" is a diet high in processed carbohydrates, such as bread, pasta, and potatoes, consumed for several consecutive days prior to a competition. The athlete will eat this way in an attempt to maximize carbohydrate storage in muscle. The goal of carbohydrate loading is to load your muscles with glucose, in the form of glycogen, so you can exercise for prolonged periods. The thought is that with carb loading, you optimize the storage of glucose so you have a steady flow of energy for the duration of the athletic event. While it certainly sounds good, it doesn't work because of our physiology and biochemistry. Here's why.

First, there is a limit of how much glucose the body can store. Glucose is stored in the form of "glycogen," primarily in muscle and the liver. Once the glycogen stores are full, any excess glucose can only be stored as fat. Unlike glucose, there is no limit to the amount of fat we can store.

Second, carbohydrate loading or excess leads to high levels of insulin, which initiates a whole host of problems, as discussed in this course. High insulin levels prevent the release of stored body fat as well as the breakdown of glycogen into glucose, which deprives the athlete of two major fuel sources.

Ironically, when insulin is elevated, the goal of carbohydrate loading is impossible. What the carbohydrate loader wants to accomplish is supplying his cells with a stable and consistent blood glucose level so he can continue his exercise for long periods.

When you load with carbohydrates, your blood glucose is elevated briefly before your insulin levels soars. The elevated insulin level then lowers your blood glucose level. When the glucose level drops, your body releases stress hormones like cortisol and epinephrine.

The stress hormones break down fat and muscle to burn in an attempt to raise the glucose level into a better range to propel the exercise activity. High-stress hormones result in catabolic metabolism. Catabolic metabolism leads to muscle breakdown. If athletes realized that carbohydrate loading promotes muscle breakdown, they would be horrified.

So instead of carbohydrate loading, eat protein, fat, and low glycemic carbohydrates. Eating this way will prevent the overstimulation of insulin and allow stable blood glucose levels for exercise, thus preventing the catabolic hormone release. Eating in this manner optimizes the release of body fat to supply our cells with a virtually endless source of fuel.

Student:

What are the most common exercise errors you see with patients in your practice?

Professor:

The most common exercise errors I see are the following: (1) excessive aerobics; (2) infrequent use or lack of resistance training; and (3) daily excessive exercise without time off for effective recuperation.

What does the medical and scientific literature reveal about exercise?

❖ Resistance training improved age-related loss of muscle mitochondrial function in older adults.

❖ Over an eight-year period, a Harvard study of 72,000 female nurses, aged forty to sixty-five years, found that sedentary women had substantially higher rates of heart attacks and death. Walking three to four hours a week reduced the risk of coronary events by 30 to 40 percent.

❖ A study comparing a group on a diabetic medication to a group participating in a walking and diet program found that those who participated in the lifestyle changes reduced their risk of becoming type 2 diabetics by 58 percent over 2.8 years.

❖ A 2001 study over eight years found less cognitive decline in elderly women who participate in walking program.

❖ Benefits of resistance training for women over sixty years included improvements in muscle strength and body composition.

❖ Aerobic exercise resulted in reduction in abdominal fat and improved insulin sensitivity in middle-aged and older men.

❖ Men who do endurance training for more than eight hours a week have a significant reduction in testosterone level (excessive exercise becomes catabolic; do interval session instead).

❖ Interval training increases levels of HGH and testosterone.

❖ Studies involving regular exercise have found improved lipid panels, decreased body fat, increased lean body mass, and reduced blood pressure. In addition, the studies found a reduction in cancer rates, improved insulin sensitivity, less depression, and improved coronary blood flow.

❖ Studies involving resistance training have found an increase in muscle mass, enhanced basal metabolic rate, and increased bone density. The studies revealed improved walking gait and fewer falls, a decrease in chronic low back pain, and improved immune function in the elderly.

❖ Studies of sedentary lifestyle have found an increased rate of chronic disease, including type 2 diabetes, heart disease, and metabolic syndrome. The sedentary group had increased rates of obesity and increased rates of all-cause mortality.

❖ A study of ninety-year-old nursing home residents found that after eight weeks of a weight lifting exercise program, the elderly residents increased their leg muscle strength by 174 percent and their muscle size by 9 percent. (Weight training slows aging!)

❖ A study published by the American Heart Association reported superior benefits of interval training compared to moderate continuous training in elderly patients with stable prior heart failure. The interval-training group had a greater improvement in their aerobic capacity as compared to those in the moderate training group (46 percent versus 14 percent).

❖ Study found that resistance training reverses aging in human skeletal muscle. After six months of resistance training, participants showed a *reversal* of most of the genes affected by age in muscle tissue. (Wow!)

❖ Study found that increased fitness is associated with a 50 to 70 percent reduction in all-cause mortality. (Read that again!)

❖ A 2001 study compared two groups of women; one group exercised using standard aerobic training, and the second group used interval training. Despite exercising longer and burning the same number of calories, the aerobic group lost less body fat at the end of the study compared to the interval group. In addition, fitness in the interval group was substantially greater than in the aerobic group. (Intelligent exercise.)

❖ A 1996 study showed that interval training burned more fat than aerobic training. Not only did the interval group burn more fat during exercise, but they also had increased fat-burning effects that persisted for twenty-four hours after exercise. In addition, the interval group sessions were fifteen minutes shorter than those of the aerobic group. (Short and sweet exercise sessions!)

❖ A study in *Diabetes Care* found that resistance training improves muscle strength and the ability to perform activities of daily living, while improving quality of life, in patients with metabolic risk factors.

❖ An *Archives of Internal Medicine* study involving a group of 2,401 twins took blood samples to measure telomere length (telomeres are at the end of each chromosome and serve as a biological measure of age, as they progressively shorten over time). Less physically active men and women displayed shorter telomeres than those who were more active. The most active subjects had telomeres the same length as sedentary individuals up to ten years younger, on average (proving that inactive lifestyles accelerate aging!).

❖ In a study comparing long-duration training (forty-five minutes without interruption) and short interval training (duration of fifteen to ninety seconds with resting in between), the researchers found that the short-interval-training group lost nine times more fat than the endurance group. (Short and sweet exercise sessions means being leaner too!)

And much more …

CHAPTER 5

HORMONE REPLACEMENT THERAPY

Hormones for health

Our healthy aging goal #6, control hormone levels, is critical in attaining and maximizing your good health and slowing the aging process. In this course, we will discuss why these hormones are so pivotal to our health and vitality.

People from across the country and throughout the world have experienced the life-enhancing benefits of hormone therapy. Despite this clinical success, and despite large quantities of high-quality research supporting hormone therapy benefits, the topic of hormone supplementation remains controversial in medical circles in this country. In fact, many within our current medical system will criticize much of what we cover in this section of the course.

The warning that we will be scrutinized by traditional medicine is not meant to scare or intimidate; it is mentioned so we can bring the topic out in the open for objective discussion. It is okay that your physician may not endorse hormone therapy or may recommend traditional synthetic hormone therapy for you instead of bioidentical hormones. It is important to consider his or her perspective on hormone programs. It is imperative that you learn as much as you can regarding hormone therapy in order to allow an informed decision.

Once we review the science and clinical benefits of restoring your physiology with hormone therapy, you will be comfortable making the personal decision that is best for you.

Yes, there is disagreement among physicians regarding hormone therapy, but you must learn all sides and consider all perspectives prior to choosing whether to begin a hormone program. Patients often ask me why there is so much controversy regarding hormone therapy, and why physicians can't reach a compromise. I believe the main reason there is disagreement is differences in perspective.

The focus of our current medial system is on disease care; in contrast, the antiaging focus is on prevention and wellness. In traditional medicine, "If it ain't broke, don't fix it." In age-management medicine, we try to fix it before it breaks. If you are having chest pain, I will send you to the hospital emergency department, not to my antiaging clinic! If you want to optimize your health and vitality, I won't send you to the hospital; instead, I will see you in my clinic.

Because of this different focus, our mainstream medical system is not current on hormone therapy, tending to follow outdated protocols or, more commonly, not advise hormone therapy at all. But that does not mean you don't have options. Many patients tell me that being on bioidentical hormone therapy has changed their lives. Even if you don't get an endorsement from your physician, it does not mean that you can't or shouldn't consider hormone supplementation. Again, learn and make a decision you are comfortable with.

Hormone therapy may not be for you—it certainly may not be for everyone—but the benefits are so vast that you owe it to yourself to at least consider it with an open mind. Even if you elect not to start hormones, you can always revisit you decision in the future. If you do decide to begin a hormone therapy program, just be aware that you are likely to hear **moans** about hor**mones.**

The beauty of this course is that we will review the topic, give you the essentials, and empower you to make healthy choices for yourself. You would be wise to take a proactive stance on your health and lifestyle choices. The more you learn in this course, the better your choices will become.

To repeat, we have a great medical system is this country. Without a doubt, when you need acute medical care, enter our medical system with confidence that you will receive the best treatments available. However, for prevention and healthy aging, our antiaging approach veers away from what traditional medicine currently offers.

I practice medicine in both traditional and nontraditional settings. I would never want to live without having the benefits and choices from both mainstream medicine and age-management medicine. I want the same access and choice for my patients. After completing this course, we want you to eat like a caveman, but you won't be thinking like a caveman! You will be educated to make healthy decisions for your entire lifetime.

Unbalanced hormones accelerate aging. Hormone deficiencies accelerate aging.

So what is bioidentical hormone replacement and why is it so beneficial for health?

As we age, certain hormone levels decline, creating hormone imbalances that increase our risk for many degenerative diseases. These hormone imbalances and deficiencies will accelerate the aging process.

Supplementing with bioidentical hormones can raise hormones to youthful levels and restore energy and vitality, greatly enhancing the quality of your life.

To appreciate the potential for bioidentical hormone replacement, it is necessary to review what hormones do in the body and to understand the diverse role they play in health and well-being. Remember, hormones are chemical messengers that control all the body's functions. Let me repeat, for emphasis, *all the body's functions.*

Hormones control our metabolism, energy production, mood, and memory, and they contribute greatly to our libido and sexual performance. (Okay, sign me up.) Hormones direct cells throughout the human body by giving cells chemical messages, or "instructions," to carry out cellular function. These instructions are like honey-do lists that I receive periodically from my wife. Without these instructions, I am inefficient, and without these instructions, cells become inefficient.

Every cell in the body requires interactions with hormones for optimal cell function and optimal health. If hormone levels are deficient, cell function and, subsequently, organ function will suffer. To maintain our health, we must maintain youthful hormone levels with bioidentical hormones.

So why are people receiving advice against hormones when they are so important to all facets of the body? It boils down to misunderstanding and misinformation. So let's clear up the issue.

Understanding the wellness benefits of bioidentical hormones requires differentiating bioidentical hormones from traditional synthetic hormones. Bioidentical means that the hormones used are exact replicas of hormones produced naturally in our bodies. Same shape, same structure, same effects. Traditional synthetic hormones are not the same as our own hormones. They are chemical substitutes for our hormones—different shape, different structure, different effects.

Hormones interact with cells throughout the body by binding on to cell receptors. Cell receptors "recognize" different hormones based on shape and structure of the hormone. If we want a specific hormone effect in the body, we must use a hormone that is biologically identical to that hormone, not a synthetic mismatch.

By supplementing deficient hormones with the exact hormone, we allow the body to utilize the hormone naturally and with minimal side effects. Our bodies have been utilizing natural bioidentical hormones since puberty. The body knows what to do with them and how to metabolize them efficiently.

We want hormones to do their job" and then be metabolized away. This natural hormone metabolism means we don't give excessive cell instructions that could be problematic by creating an imbalanced hormone response.

Unfortunately, synthetic hormones are not metabolized appropriately. For example, one dose of Premarin, which is a commonly used synthetic estrogen, stays in the body for two weeks. It hangs around like an uninvited houseguest. (Oh, hi, Mom. I didn't realize you were still here!) In contrast, bioidentical hormones are metabolized away within twenty-four hours and utilize normal metabolic pathways.[1]

If that isn't convincing enough, then please realize that Premarin comes from **pregnant mares'** urine. Sure, urine is natural, but come on! The fact that we equate horse-derived estrogen with human estrogen reveals the power of pharmaceutical companies' marketing. Since pharmaceutical companies can't patent a natural substance, they make a different chemical and then advertise that it is better than natural hormones. (Yet bioidentical hormones are controversial?) Remember, don't think like a caveman.

Bioidentical hormones are identical replicas of human hormones.

Let's move on to the specifics of bioidentical hormone therapy. As women age, they produce less estrogen, progesterone, and testosterone hormones. Estrogen and testosterone have the most impact on overall health.

Estrogen is a broad term for three main hormones called estriol, estradiol, and estrone. Estradiol is the main estrogen that we want to optimize. Estradiol has the most benefit on brain and heart health. Estradiol plays a huge role in improving and maintaining bone density.

Estriol is a weaker estrogen. Estrone is a more aggressive estrogen. With bioidentical hormone replacement therapy, we restore a healthy ratio of estradiol to estriol and to estrone.

Prior to menopause and perimenopause, a women's estradiol to estrone ratio is approximately two to one. This two to one ratio means that prior to any hormone imbalances or hormone deficiency states, a woman has twice as much estradiol as estrone. Maintaining this estradiol to estrone ratio of two to one creates a healthier estrogen balance. Remember, this is the ratio in the body when women are at their hormonal prime.

If we elect not to utilize bioidentical hormone therapy, then women will lose this healthy estradiol to estrone balance. Losing this balance is felt to contribute to some of the problems related to estrogen. This is why not utilizing bioidentical hormones during perimenopause and menopause may put patients at more risk than utilizing bioidentical hormone therapy.

Ironically, synthetic hormones not only do not restore this estradiol to estrone balance, but they also reverse this balance. With synthetic hormones such as Premarin, we subsequently can measure twice as much estrone in the body than estradiol.[2] This is literally the opposite effect that we want to maintain with hormone therapy. Birth control pills also have a negative impact on the normal estradiol to estrone ratio.

Could this be why we see an increased risk of breast cancer with synthetic hormones and an increased risk of breast cancer with birth control pills?

The more we replicate nature, the better.

Testosterone hormone is immensely beneficial to woman's health. Testosterone improves energy levels, libido, metabolism, and body composition. Women report enhanced focus and concentration when testosterone levels are optimized. Testosterone levels often drop in the fourth decade of a women's life. We frequently see low energy levels, low libido, poor focus, and weight gain at this stage of a women's life.

Another hormone that we measure and monitor is called follicle-stimulating hormone, or FSH. FSH is released from the pituitary gland in the brain. The pituitary gland is the command center for hormone regulation in the body. The brain is constantly monitoring our hormone levels in the blood. When our hormone levels drop, the pituitary gland sends out stimulatory hormones, such as FSH, to increase the production of specific hormones.

For example, if estradiol levels are low in women or testosterone levels are low in men, the pituitary gland will release more FSH to stimulate the ovaries and the testicles to produce more estradiol and more testosterone, respectively.

If there are optimal levels of estradiol and testosterone in the bloodstream, then the pituitary gland will lower the release of FSH. This inverse relationship between FSH levels and estradiol and testosterone levels is part of a "feedback system."

The feedback system is a perfect example of how the body works its wonders to maintain hormone balance. The brain wants optimal hormone balance. If the balance is lost, the pituitary gland amplifies its commands to ramp up hormone production in the body.

When women have low estradiol levels, as in menopause, or men have low testosterone levels, as in andropause, the pituitary gland secretes more FSH. Of course, the goal of higher FSH levels is to raise the level of bioidentical estradiol and testosterone in the body.

If the levels of estrogen and testosterone do not increase, as in menopause or andropause, the pituitary gland will continue to release FSH in an attempt to restore hormonal balance. Many symptoms of hormone deficiencies, such as night sweats and hot flashes, are related to the high levels of FSH.

When we correct hormone deficiencies with bioidentical hormones, the FSH level improves and symptoms resolve. We measure this improvement of the hormone levels in the body to help us monitor and adjust hormone doses for optimal health.

Not surprisingly, synthetic hormones do not re-create balance and don't correct elevated FSH levels. As a result, patients don't obtain relief of all symptoms when synthetic hormones are utilized. Interestingly, many physicians never measure the blood levels of estrogen, testosterone, or FSH.

We can't reproduce optimal hormone levels if they are not measured and monitored with ongoing hormone therapy.

As men age, they produce less testosterone and gradually produce more estrogen. Men are usually quite surprised to find out they make estrogen. Paradoxically, with aging, some men can actually have higher estrogen levels than women of the same age.

With bioidentical hormone therapy, we measure and monitor both the testosterone level and estrogen level. When men are in their prime, they have high levels of testosterone and low levels of estrogen. A high ratio of testosterone to estrogen is the rule in healthy men.

When we correct hormone deficiencies in men, our goal is to re-create this healthy testosterone to estradiol ratio. If this healthy ratio is not maintained, then we will not optimize the impact of the bioidentical hormone therapy. We will discuss this testosterone and estrogen balance in men later on in this lecture. We have many therapeutic options to utilize when men have low testosterone and high estrogen levels.

As estradiol is the pivotal hormone in women, testosterone is the pivotal hormone in men. Testosterone is essential for metabolism, body composition, cardiovascular health, brain health, energy, and libido. One of the most important healthy lifestyle decisions men can make is to restore testosterone levels in the body.

With aging, both men and women release less HGH and less DHEA. It is crucial to acknowledge that insufficient levels of some or all of these hormones result in hormone deficiency states that will adversely influence health and aging. Both DHEA and HGH have multiple effects throughout the body.

Low hormone levels will mean suboptimal metabolism, leading to:
- Higher body fat
- Less muscle
- Less bone density

Remember, these hormones interact with every cell in the body.

Suboptimal cell function leads to:

- Accelerated skin aging
- Increased risk of heart disease, dementia, and stroke
- Increased risk of osteoporosis

With deficient hormone levels, our immune systems are adversely affected so we are less resistant to bacterial and viral illness as well as cancer. To add insult to injury, mood and libido will suffer from low hormone levels. As hormone levels drop, symptoms of night sweats, hot flashes, fatigue, depression, dry skin, and insomnia can develop. The result of hormone deficiencies is a decreased quality of life.

So if you receive advice against hormone therapy, review the list of advantages of maintaining deficient hormone levels (none) and then compare that list to the advantages of hormone replacement discussed above. Then make an informed decision for your health.

Many patients hear negative comments about hormone therapy because of some common misconceptions. One misconception propagated is that hormone therapy increases your risk of cancer. It is commonly assumed that testosterone replacement increases the risk of prostate cancer in men, and estrogen replacement increases the risk of breast cancer in women. These erroneous assumptions are a tremendous disservice to people interested in healthy aging.

An extensive review of the medical literature does not support these assumptions. After a review of the medical literature on testosterone replacement, Morley is quoted in the Mayo Clinic proceedings: "There is no evidence that the risk of either prostate cancer or prostate hypertrophy increases with testosterone replacement therapy."

Dr. A. Morgentaler, a urologist from Harvard Medical School wrote the following:

> There is an absence of scientific data supporting the concept that higher testosterone levels are associated with an increased risk of prostate cancer. Specifically, no increased risk of prostate cancer was noted in (1) clinical trials of testosterone supplementation, (2) longitudinal population-based studies, or (3) a high-risk population of men with low testosterone levels receiving testosterone treatment.
>
> Moreover, hypogonadal men (men with low testosterone levels) have a substantial rate of biopsy-detectable prostate

cancer, suggesting that low testosterone has no protective effect against development of prostate cancer. These results argue against an increased risk of prostate cancer with testosterone replacement therapy.

Another study looked at testosterone levels in 708 men diagnosed with prostate cancer and in 2,242 men without prostate cancer. Findings revealed that the risk of prostate cancer was lower in men with higher blood levels of testosterone.

In addition, prostate disease increases as natural testosterone levels decline. The decreasing testosterone levels and increasing estrogen levels in aging men create an imbalance that produces a hormone environment that supports the development of prostate disease. By following a hormone therapy program, men can avoid this abnormal hormone environment and decrease the risk of prostate issues.

The voices against female hormone therapy are much louder than those against male hormone therapy. The assumptions are fueled by data from the Woman's Health Initiative (WHI). This study revealed an increased risk of breast cancer, blood clots, and strokes in women on *synthetic* hormone replacement.

So why am I still advocating hormone therapy for women?

Well, for many reasons. First, the WHI study uses Premarin (horse urine–derived estrogen) and Provera (chemically altered progesterone). These are not bioidentical hormones and never will be. Any conclusions from this study cannot be applied to bioidentical hormones.

Second, other studies have proven that Provera increases the risk of breast cancer and blood clotting, while natural progesterone has the *opposite* effects. (It is essential to acknowledge that Provera does not equal progesterone. The only similarity is that they both begin with the letter *p*!)

As discussed earlier, Premarin does not equal bioidentical estrogens. So none of the hormones used in the WHI were bioidentical.

Finally, the WHI study has other major flaws. For starters, the average age of the participants was sixty-two years old, and none of them had any prior hormone therapy. This means an average of twelve years from menopause without the benefits of hormone supplementation. This group of women will have a higher risk of medical problems because of untreated hormone deficiency states.

In addition, none of the women in the study had hormone blood levels obtained either prior to, during, or after the study. Imagine the value of any type of hormone study that not only uses the wrong hormones but also never measures the hormone levels in the body! Hell, I should be moaning!

In the medical literature, we do not expect identical results from different studies. We do, however, look for a trend in the literature to make informed decisions. With that in mind, please realize that no data in the medical literature clearly and consistently reveals an increased risk of breast cancer with hormone therapy.

Some literature reveals a *decreased* risk of breast cancer with hormone therapy. Some literature reveals a neutral effect on breast cancer with hormone therapy. A few studies (with the wrong hormones) show a slight increase risk of breast cancer with hormone therapy.

Even in the WHI study, the absolute risk was small. Of the women on the wrong (synthetic) hormones, 1.9 percent were diagnosed with breast cancer. Of the women not on any hormones, 1.5 percent were diagnosed with breast cancer. Thus, the actual risk was 0.4 percent! Hardly a huge vote against hormone therapy, especially considering all the flaws of the study, including the fact that synthetic hormones were used.

The last nail in the coffin against the WHI is that there was no consideration of other risks of breast cancer. In other words, some of these women were obese, some smoked, and some had family history of breast cancer. Many of these women were at risk regardless of the hormones used.

Remember, breast cancer was present in both the hormone group and the non-hormone group. In fact, we find that the longer a woman is in menopause without hormone therapy, the higher the rates of breast cancer.[3-4]

In addition, the majority of breast cancer patients have not ever been on hormone therapy—90 percent of them. Also, having a low or deficient blood level of estradiol does not protect you from getting breast cancer. In fact, there is no physiologic advantage to living with low estrogen or low testosterone levels in the body.

With this knowledge, make your decision regarding hormones with an open mind and with consideration of all the information that is available to you. Don't make your choice based only on the erroneous assumptions repeated over and over again in the media and by medical professionals.

A recent review of two hundred published medical studies reinforces the key differences between synthetic hormones and bioidentical hormones. The review compared synthetic hormones to bioidentical hormones and found that synthetic hormones increased the risk of breast cancer and heart disease while bioidentical hormones *decreased* the risk of breast cancer and heart disease. The findings of this study indicate that not utilizing bioidentical hormone therapy is detrimental to your health. Remember, sometimes the risk of no action is greater than the risk of taking action.

Another reason for misinterpretations about hormone therapy is steroid abuse seen in athletics. When athletes abuse steroid hormones with goals of performance enhancement, they use high doses of synthetic hormones. This results in "supraphysiologic" levels of hormones. These abnormally high levels of hormones increase risk of side effects and are clearly not advocated with our antiaging goals of optimizing hormone levels.

Unfortunately, when we see negative results of testosterone or HGH abuse, we apply it to all hormone replacement. With this logic, if a capsule of an antihypertensive agent improves your blood pressure, then taking the whole bottle at one time would really help your blood pressure! *If we see side effects from an overdose of medications, does it mean all medications are bad?* Obviously, class, you're smarter than that!

Yes, we believe deficient levels of hormones are to be corrected, but we don't want to correct deficiencies with excessive levels of hormones. Our ultimate goal with bioidentical hormone therapy is to restore your physiology. We emphasize correction of deficiencies, not utilizing excess dosages.

This restoration requires us to utilize the identical hormones that are deficient to maintain optimal blood levels and cellular effects. It is impossible to restore your physiology with chemical hormone substitutes.

Hormone balance is the key.

This discussion leads us into another essential component of safe hormone therapy. A key goal in bioidentical hormone therapy is "balance." Balance means we correct all deficient hormone levels instead of focusing only on estrogen supplementation in women or focusing only on testosterone supplementation in men. Unfortunately, isolated hormone therapy with synthetic hormones has been the norm with traditional hormone programs.

All the hormones work together for optimal effect and safety in the body. If we focus on only a few deficient hormones, then we will never restore hormonal balance and never reach optimal health. Analogous to nutraceutical supplementation, hormone therapy is a team sport.

Arguments against hormones focus on potential negatives of hormones but never seem to look at potential positives of hormone therapy. Any risk versus benefit analysis requires looking at both sides of the issue.

One major benefit of hormones is our cardiovascular health. The risk of dying from heart disease is many times greater than the risk of dying from breast cancer or from prostate cancer. Heart disease is a leading cause of death. Bioidentical hormones play a tremendous role in decreasing many cardiac risk factors.

For example, both estrogen and testosterone improve cholesterol panels, improve blood flow to the heart, improve blood pressure, improve blood glucose and insulin levels, and decrease the risk of blood clotting.

Our natural hormones also benefit the cardiovascular system with anti-inflammatory and antioxidant effects. In addition, balanced hormone levels decrease the stress response, also immensely beneficial to our cardiovascular systems.

The impact of hormone balance offsets the weight gain and obesity that occur with hormone deficiency states such as menopause and andropause. This improvement in our body weight is an additional cardiovascular benefit.

Many of the benefits of bioidentical hormones on heart function also apply to brain function, with improved memory, mood, and decreased risk of dementia and stroke.

The brain requires estrogen and testosterone to produce neurotransmitters (brain chemicals) that are required to formulate memory, and influence mood, focus, concentration, and cravings. A deficiency in our bioidentical hormones results in a deficiency of neurotransmitters.

The lowering of inflammation, oxidation, and glycation that we obtain with hormone balance plays a critical role in the brain benefits of bioidentical hormone replacement therapy.

With traditional hormone therapy, we tend to focus only on symptom reduction—for example, night sweats and hot flashes—while ignoring the huge impact of hormones on heart and brain health.

When patients live without the benefits of bioidentical hormones, then we are forced to treat their symptoms of hormone deficiencies with prescription medications. You have insomnia—here is a sleeping pill. Mood issues—here is an antidepressant and/or antianxiety medication. Libido issues—here's some Viagra. Your cholesterol is high—take this Lipitor. Your bone loss is accelerating—take this Fosomax. A prescription drug for all your needs. None of those prescriptions will help you reach any of your healthy aging goals.

With the current medical paradigm, prescription medications are frequently the treatment for hormone deficiencies. Now, I have not won the Nobel Prize in medicine, but why are we not treating hormone deficiencies with the deficient hormones?

If your thyroid is low, should we prescribe an energy stimulant instead of natural thyroid?

Can you imagine treating insulin-dependent diabetes (an insulin hormone deficiency) with anything other than human insulin?

Why does anyone believe that prescription medications are a safer alternative than our bioidentical hormones when treating hormone deficiencies?

A more sensible approach would be to utilize hormones first and then try medications only when absolutely needed. Without a doubt, prescription medications are crucial to treat infections, control pain, and to save lives in the acute care medical setting. Many pharmaceuticals are of tremendous benefits to millions of people. But we should not use pharmaceuticals instead of bioidentical hormones to correct hormone deficiencies. We should also not utilize pharmaceuticals simply to control symptoms of low hormones.

Symptoms are the body's way of alerting us that something is wrong or out of balance. It is not enough to suppress symptoms. We need to elucidate the cause of the symptoms and then *treat* the cause of the symptoms.

With this approach, symptoms resolve as we restore hormone balance. If symptoms don't resolve or if someone doesn't tolerate hormone therapy, then at that time we can consider medications. Again, please keep these issues in mind when making decisions regarding your own hormone therapy program.

Remember, do your own risk-versus-benefit analysis. Any medical decision must include an analysis of risk versus benefit. Not going on hormones has risk. In fact, not going on hormones has a long list of risks. Yes, a hormone therapy program may have risks in certain patients, but for the vast majority of people, there is minimal to no risk at all to receiving the benefits of hormone therapy.

Even if going on hormones has a short list of risks, they should still be entered into your analysis of hormone therapy. I frequently see patients that have previously made the decision not to try hormone therapy without ever considering that there is clearly more risk in not using hormones than there is risk in using hormones. In many areas of life, and certainly in medicine, inaction can be more detrimental than taking action. Be empowered.

Thyroid replacement

With bioidentical hormone therapy, we also take a slightly different approach to thyroid replacement than what is done historically in conventional medicine. Thyroid is a vastly important hormone that influences mood, metabolism, energy levels, and overall health.

Traditional medicine screens for a thyroid hormone deficiency with a blood test called TSH (thyroid stimulatory hormone). TSH is inversely related to the blood thyroid levels. If blood thyroid levels are low, TSH levels are high. If the TSH comes back very low, your thyroid levels may be too high.

If your TSH comes back elevated, you will be diagnosed with low thyroid, "hypothyroidism." The current treatment for hypothyroidism is usually a prescription of a synthetic thyroid replacement.

Despite this common approach to thyroid deficiencies, it has some significant limitations. For one, TSH "normal ranges" are broad, so you could be hypothyroid yet have a "high but normal TSH value." With the current medial paradigm, you would not be given a prescription for thyroid hormone replacement.

This is unfortunate because medical literature has shown that an elevated TSH, even if in "normal range," is not an optimal TSH. When TSH is on the high side of "normal," it suggests suboptimal thyroid function. When suboptimal thyroid function is ignored, patients suffer unnecessarily.

When thyroid function is not optimized, patients often have weight gain, fatigue, depression, cold intolerance, and many other symptoms. We also frequently find elevated cholesterol levels in these patients.

With bioidentical therapy, if your TSH is elevated yet "normal," and you have symptoms consistent with hypothyroidism (again, fatigue, weight gain, depression), then we will initiate thyroid supplementation, usually with tremendous benefit. We monitor your progress as well as follow-up blood tests to maintain optimal but safe thyroid levels in the body.

Another deviation from the traditional medicine approach is that with bioidentical programs, we also measure two additional blood tests for thyroid: free T4, thyroxine and free T3, triiodothyronine. These tests give us a better look at your overall thyroid function.

T4 is a measure of the thyroid hormone released from the thyroid gland. T4 is then converted in the body to T3. T3 is the active thyroid hormone. Because T3 represents thyroid activity, it is important that it be measured in addition to the TSH test. This is crucial because we have discovered that many patients have decent TSH levels yet can have low T4 or T3 levels; they often benefit greatly from thyroid replacement.

The final difference from traditional medicine is the actual thyroid prescription used. In traditional medicine, we usually prescribe a synthetic thyroid called Synthroid or Levoxyl (levothyroxine). Levothyroxine is T4 hormone exclusively. The T4 is then converted in the body to T3, the active thyroid hormone. Unfortunately, some patients don't convert T4 to T3 very well so they can have persistent symptoms of low thyroid.

We have found that patients often have better results with a natural thyroid replacement (Armour or compounded thyroid). These contain both T4 and T3 thyroid hormones. By replacing both T4 and T3, we can optimize blood levels of the active thyroid hormone. Patients usually feel better with this approach.

Interestingly enough, the *New England Journal* had a comparison study years ago that showed most low thyroid patients felt better on natural thyroid (T4 and T3) than they did on synthetic thyroid (T4 only).

DHEA and HGH replacement

Bioidentical hormone therapy is unique in using DHEA (dehydroepiandosterone) and HGH (human growth hormone. These hormones are a major boon toward reaching your antiaging goals.

DHEA is an adrenal gland hormone (adrenal glands sit on top of the kidneys), but it is also produced in the brain and skin. DHEA is the most abundant steroid hormone in the body. As we age, our DHEA levels drop so that by age forty-five, we produce half the level we produced at age twenty.

This hormone is important for normal immune function. It also improves metabolism and insulin sensitivity, has a positive effect on mood, and enhances antioxidant protection.

DHEA is released from the adrenal gland. This is the same gland where the stress hormone cortisol is produced. When we are excessively stressed out, we produce more cortisol and less DHEA, creating imbalance. Combining DHEA supplementation with stress reduction helps slow the aging process in a multitude of ways.

Blood levels of DHEA are best measured with a blood test called DHEA-sulfate. DHEA-sulfate gives us a better assessment of your DHEA level than simply measuring a DHEA level.

HGH is released from the anterior pituitary gland in the brain. It plays a major role in repair and rejuvenation. It keeps us "anabolic" by maintaining bone density, muscle tone, and strength while decreasing body fat. It also supports brain function and a healthy immune system.

Currently, the best way to assess your HGH production is with a blood test called IGF-1, insulin-like growth factor 1. HGH is released from the pituitary gland intermittently, and it is only briefly in the bloodstream. Because of the transient and intermittent release of HGH, it is difficult to precisely measure with a blood test. HGH stimulates the liver to produce growth factors. IGF-1 is a major growth factor that stays in the bloodstream at a consistent level. When we measure IGF-1, it is an indirect but accurate measure of your HGH level. If your IGF-1 level is deficient you may be a candidate for HGH therapy.

HGH is synergistic with testosterone and estrogen in improving health and supporting healthy body composition. HGH therapy requires subcutaneous injections (small painless needle under the skin). Be aware of the marketing of HGH tablets, sprays, and so forth, as they are ineffective. The real deal requires injections.

If your blood tests indicate deficiencies of either HGH or DHEA, then supplementation with these antiaging hormones should be considered. DHEA is easy and relatively inexpensive to supplement. HGH is expensive but is gradually becoming more affordable. (HGH helps with weight loss because if you are on HGH, you can no longer afford food!)

If expense prohibits you from tapping into the diverse benefits of HGH, rest assured that you will still do extremely well with our antiaging program. In addition, we can improve our own HGH levels by following a few basic rules:

- Exercise focusing on high-intensity and short-duration weight lifting. This type of exercise elicits anabolic hormone release.

- Reduce insulin levels with a healthy diet. High insulin levels offset HGH actions.

- Reduce cortisol levels with stress reduction. High cortisol levels decrease HGH effects.

- Adequate protein diet. Protein is required for HGH production.

- Avoid excessive alcohol consumption. Excessive alcohol dampens the release of HGH.

- Quality sleep. Deep sleep is when HGH is released.

Many people are paying good money for HGH but are not aware of simple lifestyle changes that could dramatically improve their results while simultaneously decreasing the required dose and expense.

A final option for optimizing HGH production in the body is with secretagogues. Secretagogues are combinations of amino acids that encourage the pituitary gland to produce more HGH. Younger people usually have a better response to the secretagogues than older people do. There are many products to choose from on the market. I suggest selecting a secretagogue from one of the compounding pharmacies. If you choose to try a secretagogue, get a baseline IGF-1 level prior to starting the secretagogue. After you have used the secretagogue for three to six months, repeat the IGF-1 blood test to assess response.

It is surprising to realize that all of our bioidentical hormones are also natural anti-inflammatory and antioxidants. These attributes decrease the risk of every degenerative disease.

Because of the crucial role bioidentical hormones play throughout the body, it is essential to understand that there is no physiologic benefit to maintaining deficient or low hormone levels. For optimal health, we should measure our hormone levels and correct deficiencies as they develop.

We identify hormone deficiencies by a combination of reviewing symptoms as well as hormone blood levels. We correct hormone deficiencies by working with compounding pharmacies. Compounding pharmacies allow us tremendous flexibility in dosing as well as routes of hormone administration. The pharmacists at compounding pharmacies are able to prepare hormones, supplements, and medications to fill individualized prescriptions. This allows us access to multiple dose and route options.

Depending on the hormones that are deficient, we can offer hormone replacement as topical creams, oral capsules, troches (lozenges that dissolve under the tongue), pellets placed under the skin, or injections.

The different route options allow us to raise hormone levels in the body as naturally as possible. Route options such as creams, troches, and pellets release the hormone directly into the bloodstream, mimicking the release of hormones from the body's organs. The body perceives the elevated blood hormone level as if it were produced naturally in the body. This unique feature of bioidentical hormone therapy is in direct contrast to synthetic hormones usually given by capsule or pill form.

Flexible dosing options allow us to use unlimited dosing options to meet individual patient requirements. The multiple dosing and route options make bioidentical replacement a unique, customized program for each patient. This allows improved patient compliance and results.

We monitor each patient with serial reviews of hormone deficiency symptoms as well as serial measurements of blood hormone levels to ensure patient safety and success. Contrast this approach with the "one-size-fits-all" mentality of traditional synthetic hormone therapy.

Hormone conversion

Another important consideration with hormone supplementation programs is a process called hormone conversion. Hormone conversion means that hormones natural to the body can be converted to other natural hormones in the body.

Prominent examples of hormone conversion include DHEA and testosterone. Some of the DHEA produced by the body is converted into testosterone in women. In addition, some of the testosterone produced in men and women is converted to estrogen.

Patients are usually quite shocked to learn that testosterone can be converted directly into estrogen by the body. Most amazing about this conversion process is realizing that the hormone chemical structure of estrogen is surprisingly similar to the hormone chemical structure of testosterone. So similar, in fact, that the body can easily convert testosterone into estrogen.

Think about that: the body easily changes the "male hormone" into the "female hormone!" Simple changes in structure result in dramatic changes in hormone effect.

For many reasons, it is crucial that you are aware of this conversion process. First, it should reinforce the importance of using only bioidentical hormones. If there is a subtle structural difference that differentiates estrogen from testosterone, then you certainly would not want to use synthetic hormones that are chemically altered. When you change the chemical structure, you change the hormone. So only use the "real deal"— bioidentical hormones.

Second, the conversion process is another reason to strive for hormone balance. In other words, supplementing with one hormone can influence the levels of other hormones. If we focus just on estrogen replacement in women, as has been the tradition in hormone replacement therapy, or if we focus just on testosterone replacement in men, we will miss the cascade effect on other hormones in the body.

When we replace only estrogen in women or only testosterone in men, we take one hormone imbalance and create another hormone imbalance. Because of the persistent hormone imbalances, we can never reach optimal health.

Finally, the hormone conversion process reinforces the importance of following blood levels of all your hormones so we can adjust doses if necessary to maintain healthy hormone balance.

Testosterone to estrogen conversion

Let's look at the testosterone to estrogen conversion in men in more depth. Some testosterone in men is converted to estradiol (estrogen). The enzyme that facilitates this conversion is primarily in fat cells. The more body fat men have, the more estrogen is produced.

As men produce less testosterone, they tend to gain more fat. As they gain more fat, they produce more estrogen. The result is low testosterone levels and high estrogen levels. We even see men with higher estrogen levels than their wives!

Clearly, this low testosterone and high estrogen in men represents an unhealthy hormone balance for the patient. Low testosterone and high estrogen in men increases the risk of prostate problems, heart problems, and worsens body composition. The increase in body fat results in increased estrogen production and sets the stage for low muscle mass, low bone density, and progressively increasing body fat.

When we supplement with testosterone in men, we need to keep this estrogen conversion in mind. Because of this conversion, we measure estradiol levels in men before and during testosterone supplementation. We have the option of utilizing specific nutrient supplementation, as well as prescription medication if necessary, to maintain healthy estrogen levels. These specific nutrients or prescription medications are proven to effectively reduce this testosterone to estrogen conversion.

Testosterone to DHT conversion

An additional consideration with testosterone is that some testosterone is converted to DHT, dihydrotestosterone. DHT is a beneficial testosterone metabolite with many important functions. DHT contributes to male sexual drive and function, body composition, and brain health. However, some evidence links elevated DHT levels with male pattern hair loss and enlargement of the prostate.

Although there is still debate regarding potential negative effects of elevated DHT levels, it makes sense to take nutrients to avoid excessive conversion of testosterone to DHT. Examples of nutrients that help keep both DHT and estrogen balanced in men include fish oil, zinc, indole-3-carbinol, nettle extract, pygeum, chrysin, and selenium. Many of these nutrients can be found together in prostate formulas.

Hormone dosing and routes

Now I will illustrate some of the dosing and route options of bioidentical hormones. The dosing options are endless when we work with compounding pharmacies. We can adjust the dose as much as needed to resolve symptoms and improve blood levels to optimize results.

As we discussed earlier, we can use topical creams, troches that dissolve under the tongue, oral tablets, pellets placed just under the skin, and even injections. Remember, we can combine various hormones together in creams, capsules, or troches to make the dosing of multiple different hormones easier for the patients.

Let's review some route options for each of the major hormones used in bioidentical hormone replacement programs.

Progesterone

All routes of progesterone administration are extremely safe and effective. We decide on capsules, topical creams, or troches primarily based on patient preferences. Whatever is easier for the patient is the route chosen. One thing to note: if a women is sleeping poorly, then we often start with a capsule form of progesterone because it greatly improves sleep. Women with progesterone deficiencies often report improved sleep within a few days of starting progesterone. I have frequently had patients who have gone years with only a few hours of sleep each night suddenly sleeping eight full hours within a few days of starting progesterone. If nothing else, at least they feel younger!

Prior to perimenopause and menopause, progesterone is released primarily during the latter half of the monthly menstrual cycle. Progesterone balances estrogen throughout the body, but specifically at breast and uterine tissue.

When on hormone therapy, many women want to re-create the usual monthly menstrual cycle. To do so requires taking progesterone approximately twelve days monthly. These women may have a menstrual period while off the progesterone.

Other women would prefer not to cycle off progesterone, instead taking progesterone continually throughout the month, either because they would rather not have periods or because they sleep well while on progesterone and don't want to stop taking it.

Estrogen

Bioidentical estrogen includes estradiol, estrone, and estriol. We can utilize just estradiol, or we can use bi-est (estradiol plus estriol) or tri-est (estradiol, estrone, and estriol). We can adjust the dose of each of the three main estrogens depending on specific patient requirements.

Our primary goal with estrogen therapy is to optimize the estradiol levels in the blood. Estradiol is the dominant estrogen prior to menopause, and restoring the healthy ratio of estradiol to the other estrogens is the most physiologic and beneficial for overall health. Pellets placed under the skin (subcutaneous) are a unique way to avoid the "first pass liver effect" (more on this in a moment) as well as to ensure physiologic levels of estradiol. The pellets are placed every four to six months and are extremely convenient for patients.

With bi-est and tri-est, we also utilize troches, topical creams and capsules. However, with estrogen supplementation, we must acknowledge that an oral capsule affects the metabolism of the estrogens.

When we take a capsule of an estrogen, the hormone is absorbed from the intestinal tract and goes directly to the liver. This is called the "first-pass effect," meaning the first pass of the hormone goes to the liver prior to going to the rest of the body.

With bioidentical estrogen, the consequences of the first-pass effect are quite minimal when compared to the consequences of taking a synthetic hormone. Regardless, it is important to acknowledge the possible impact of the liver metabolism of an oral form of estrogen.

The potential consequences of the first-pass effect include the release of clotting factors from the liver, the potential of increased risk of elevated blood pressure, and a slight increase risk of gallbladder problems. Again, this is rarely problematic with bioidentical hormones when compared to synthetic hormones. Regardless, the first-pass effect needs to be discussed so the patient can consider this when selecting the route of hormone administration.

With troches, pellets, and topical routes, we avoid this first-pass effect completely. Despite the potential consequences of an oral estrogen replacement, I rarely see any problems in my clinic with patients who choose an oral bi-est or tri-est. Indeed, I have many patients who request using the capsule form of the estrogens because they find them easier to take, thereby improving their personal compliance with the hormone therapy program.

My preference, however, is to utilize pellets, troches, or creams. For sure, an oral bioidentical estrogen is safe and certainly better than not supplementing at all. But we can dispel any concern regarding the liver effects of oral estrogens by choosing options other than capsules.

Testosterone in women

For testosterone supplementation in women, we favor topical creams, troches, or subcutaneous pellets. Creams are simple to use, and the dose can be adjusted by the patient with ease. We obtain great blood levels with both the cream and the troches. Pellet therapy with testosterone is also very effective and extremely easy for the patients. I don't prescribe oral forms of testosterone because of the liver issue and because the other route options are so effective and better replicate our natural physiology.

Testosterone in men

Many options are available for male testosterone supplementation. Most commonly utilized is a daily topical cream or gel. We also obtain excellent blood levels and results with a weekly injection of testosterone. We teach the patient to administer the injection himself or to have a significant other give the injection. Many men seem to be more compliant with a weekly dose compared to a daily application, but the decision is based on the patient's personal preference.

We greatly improve patient compliance when we utilize subcutaneous pellet therapy. Since the pellets usually last six months between insertions, many men prefer this route. With pellet therapy, we obtain optimal blood levels in a painless, hassle-free fashion.

Pellet therapy is the ideal form to mimic the natural physiology of the body, as the hormone is released directly into the bloodstream.

Chorionic gonadotropin

A third option for testosterone supplementation for men is called human chorionic gonadotropin (HCG). HCG is identical to a hormone produced by the pituitary gland that stimulates the testicles to produce more testosterone. With HCG, the patient's body produces the resulting increase in testosterone completely and naturally.

HCG is administered twice a week in subcutaneous injections (just beneath the skin with a small-gauge needle). The injections are virtually painless. HCG is a great option for many men with suboptimal testosterone levels.

HCG is more effective in younger men with lower testosterone levels; however, it can be tried in older men as well. When we use HCG, I have men recheck their blood level of testosterone after four to six weeks of HCG therapy to assess the response. If we obtain optimal testosterone levels, then we can continue the therapy. If testosterone levels are not optimal, then we discontinue the HCG and utilize testosterone therapy.

DHEA

DHEA is easily supplemented with capsules, troches, or topical creams. Blood levels improve consistently regardless of route chosen. Patient preference dictates the route chosen.

HGH (human growth hormone)

Despite many advertisements that suggest otherwise, the most effective way to supplement HGH is with subcutaneous injections. The daily injections are incredible safe and effective. The cost is the only limiting factor with HGH.

There is a multidose pen that makes HGH supplementation extremely easy. The pen is the size of a ballpoint pen with a fine needle tip. You simply dial in your dose and depress the end button; your HGH is administered automatically.

HGH Secretagogues

Secretagogues can be taken in an oral capsule form, in a topical cream, or in a sublingual (under the tongue) spray. The best secretagogues are obtained from either a physician's office or compounding pharmacies.

Keys to bioidentical hormone therapy:

1) Obtain lab work for specific hormone levels both at onset of therapy and with serial follow-up. Hormone panel for men includes total and free testosterone, DHEA-sulfate, IGF-1(measure of growth hormone), and estradiol (main estrogen). TSH, free T4, and free T3 are thyroid blood tests. Hormone panel for women includes

testosterone, estradiol, FSH, progesterone, IGF-1, and DHEA-sulfate. To completely evaluate thyroid function, we measure a TSH, free T4, and free T3.

2) Work with a physician trained in bioidentical hormone replacement therapy. (A real good doc can be reached at 520-547-2820.)

3) Supplement deficient hormones with bioidentical hormones—no synthetic substitutes. Remember balance.

4) Optimize results by combining symptom reduction with hormone blood levels to gauge dose adjustments.

5) Utilize custom dosing and routes with compounding pharmacies to optimize hormone therapy. Choose hormone delivery routes that mimic the body's physiology.

6) Eat a healthy diet. A whole food diet rich in healthy protein (lean meats, fish, eggs), healthy fat (olive oil, avocados, raw nuts, seeds, fish oil), and healthy carbohydrates (fruits and vegetables). *

7) Avoid or minimize processed foods, chemical food additives, and artificial sweeteners.*

8) Participate in a moderate, consistent exercise program.*

*Healthy nutrition and exercise programs maximize results with hormone supplementation programs.

Hormones used in female hormone therapy programs:

Estradiol

Estriol

Estrone

(Bi-est/tri-est)

Progesterone

Testosterone

DHEA (dehydroepiandosterone)

HGH (human growth hormone)

Thyroid

Hormones used in male hormone therapy programs:

Testosterone
HCG (human chorionic gonadotropin)
DHEA (dehydroepiandosterone)
HGH (growth hormone)
Thyroid

Bioidentical hormone therapy offers a modality that slows the aging process, improves health, and decreases the risk of many degenerative diseases. It will add quality years to your life.

It is important to reinforce the point that there are no physiologic advantages to maintaining low estrogen, progesterone, testosterone, DHEA, or HGH levels.

Problems associated with low estrogen, testosterone, and low progesterone levels in women:

Symptoms of hot flashes and
   night sweats
Mood swings
Depression
Anxiety
Dry skin
Vaginal dryness
Central weight gain
Acne
Bone loss
Lean muscle loss

Increase in body fat
Increased risk of dementia
Poor memory
Fatigue
Increased cholesterol
Increased blood pressure
Increased cardiovascular risk
Incontinence
Arthritis
Insomnia

Problems with low testosterone in men:

Muscle loss
Bone loss
Weight gain
Fatigue
Depression
Decreased libido

Decreased sexual performance
Increased blood pressure
Increased blood glucose levels
Elevated cholesterol levels
Increased risk of dementia
Increased cardiovascular risk

Problems with low growth hormone levels:

Accelerated skin aging

Bone loss

Muscle loss

Increase in body fat

Decreased aerobic capacity

Decreased metabolism

Decreased immune function

Decreased libido and sexual
performance

Increased cardiovascular risk

Decreased skin thickness

Problems with low thyroid levels:

Increase in body fat

Fatigue

Depression

Increase in cholesterol

Lower body temperature

Cold intolerance

Constipation

Dry skin

Benefits of DHEA supplementation:

Improved immune function

Improved metabolism

Improved mood and memory

Improved bone density

Decreased body fat

Advantages of maintaining *deficient* hormone levels:

None

Side effects of bioidentical hormones

I am frequently asked questions about potential side effects of bioidentical hormone replacement. Fortunately, side effects are few and usually transient.

The key with bioidentical hormones is the fact that they are identical to hormones naturally produced in the body. They follow the same metabolic pathways as hormones produced by the body. There is no difference. As a result, any side effects you experience with bioidentical hormone replacement are identical to side effects you could experience from hormone produced naturally by your body! Most of the time side effects of hormones are related to fluctuations in the blood levels.

Most side effects in women include breast tenderness, bloating, vaginal bleeding, irritability, or acne. Again, all of these potential side effects are transient and usually resolve with dose adjustments.

Sometimes as patients start hormones, they will experience mild, transient side effects that simply represent the body's attempt to acclimate to the higher hormone levels. Typically, even if we continue the same dose of hormones in these patients, their side effects will resolve. However, if the side effects are bothersome, we can simply hold the hormones or reduce the doses until symptoms completely resolve. When necessary, we can use nutrient supplementation and even prescription medications to resolve side effects that are more bothersome.

Side effects in men are even less common. Occasionally we see acne with DHEA and/or testosterone supplementation. Acne is transient and resolves with dose adjustments and/or a brief course of medications.

Side effects of excessive estrogen levels: breast tenderness, bloating, vaginal bleeding, and irritability.

Side effects of excessive progesterone levels are rare but typically include breast tenderness, bloating, or fatigue.

Side effects of excessive testosterone levels are limited to oily skin or acne, or rarely, irritability.

Side effects of excessive DHEA are limited to acne.

Side effects of excessive HGH are joint pain or fluid retention (rare and transient) and bankruptcy (common and permanent!).

Side effects of excessive thyroid are palpitations, anxiety, weight loss, sweating.

> Please understand that all of these side effects are transient and easily corrected with dose adjustments.

Bioidentical Hormone Therapy Nuts and Bolts:

1) Utilize bioidentical hormones only, not synthetics.

2) Balance all hormones.

3) Measure blood levels at baseline and after starting hormone therapy or adjusting doses.

4) Use compounded hormones and individualized doses.

5) Understand the perceived risks and the tremendous benefits of hormone therapy.

6) Combine with an appropriate diet, supplement program, and exercise for optimal results.

7) See me!

Remember, hormone deficiencies adversely affect our antiaging goals. When our hormones are out of balance, the benefits of our diet, exercise, and supplement programs are diminished.

CHAPTER 5
QUESTIONS

Student:

I've read that testosterone causes prostate cancer, and estrogen causes breast cancer. What do you think?

Professor:

Both of those topics have been studied extensively. There is no evidence to support those statements.

There is a lot of misinformation regarding hormone therapy. I believe it is a tremendous disservice to patients to deny them the health benefits of bioidentical hormones. No disease process in medicine is impacted by only one variable. We should consider and evaluate all variables that influence our health as well as disease.

We previously covered the misconception regarding bioidentical hormones and cancer. When we perpetuate this myth, patients are denied the multiple health benefits of hormone therapy while simultaneously ignoring proven risk factors for cancer. We must reinforce the fact that deficient levels of your natural hormones adversely affect health. By balancing your hormones to optimal levels, we improve your immune system and decrease your risk of many diseases.

Unfortunately, patients are usually advised to not check their hormone blood levels, to not replace with bioidentical hormones, and to "treat" hormone deficiency symptoms with prescription medications. All this is done with the mistaken belief that you are decreasing your risk of cancer, while simultaneously ignoring other cancer risk factors.

For example, we know sugar and processed carbohydrate consumption elevates our blood glucose level. Elevated blood glucose and insulin levels fuel cancer cells. Despite this knowledge, cancer patients are rarely, if ever, advised to get on a low-glycemic (low-sugar) diet.

It makes no physiologic sense to keep your natural hormone levels in the basement while keeping your sugar levels on the roof; this is a perfect architectural plan for a custom-built home for cancer.

This combination of high sugar and low hormones actually increases glycation, increases inflammation, increases oxidation, increases obesity, suppresses immune function, accelerates aging, and increases cancer risk.

Student:
Will hormone replacement make me gain fat?

Professor:
Not as much as eating that bagel! Actually, many patients are concerned about this issue. Interestingly, most patients increase body fat as their natural hormone levels decline. This is because of the adverse effect that hormone deficiencies have on our metabolisms. In other words, if we don't replenish hormone deficiencies, most patients gain fat.

During menopause and perimenopause, most women have an increase in body fat without hormone therapy. Most patients increase lean body mass and decrease body fat with appropriate bioidentical hormone therapy.

A small percentage of patients have an increase in body fat with HRT. This is minimized by changing the route of administration, i.e., switching from capsules to topical creams or switching to pellets. In addition, staying on an unprocessed, real food "caveman" type diet works synergistically with hormones to improve metabolism, minimizing weight gain.

Student:
I am only thirty-nine years old, and I have a normal menstrual cycle. Over the last two years, I have noticed weight gain and fatigue. In addition, I have poor focus and concentration. My doctor checked my thyroid and said it was in optimal range. Am I too young for hormone problems?

Professor:
I suspect that you have low testosterone levels. I frequently evaluate women in my office with similar complaints. They tell me that despite eating

well and exercising consistently, they have weight gain, fatigue, and low energy. Many also report lower libido and poor focus and concentration.

Testosterone levels in women often drop in their mid-thirties. Testosterone has immense importance on your overall health and well-being.

Come to the office and we will check your testosterone level. If it is low, you will notice dramatic improvement with testosterone supplementation.

Student:

I understand that our natural hormones don't cause cancer, but if we already have breast cancer or prostate cancer, can we still supplement with hormones?

Professor:

Since hormones stimulate breast cells and prostate cells, it is often felt that we should withhold hormone therapy for cancer patients. The literature is conflicting on whether hormones stimulate preexisting cancer growth, but there is no trend in the literature showing consistently that hormones are a risk.

In addition, a number of smaller studies using hormone therapy for patients with preexisting cancers actually show a decreased risk of recurrence and metastasis (spread of the cancer) in those patients on bioidentical hormones!

I believe the best option is to present the information to the patients and allow them to discuss it with their oncologists and make their own decisions. Each case must be looked at on an individual basis. We do have patients with histories of prostate cancer and patients with histories of breast cancer who choose bioidentical hormone therapy for its myriad health benefits.

Student:

My mother has been on Premarin and Provera since she hit menopause. Given the Women's Health Initiative findings, should she stop taking them?

Professor:

I mentioned the flaws in the study during the lecture, but I also want to note that the study actually had benefits for some patients, and as mentioned, the overall risks were quite low. For example, the women on synthetic hormones in the study had fewer cases of osteoporosis and colon cancer than women not on the synthetic hormones.

Additional reviews of the data have revealed some interesting findings. Women who were on just Premarin and not Provera (Provera was not given to women who had a previous hysterectomy) had fewer cases of breast cancer than women on both hormones and fewer cases of breast cancer than women not on hormones. This data suggests that Provera may contribute more to the potential problems of synthetic hormones than Premarin.

When women were started on the hormones early in menopause, instead of waiting a number of years with untreated hormone deficiencies, they were found to have fewer cases of dementia and heart disease than the other patients.

This new data has made many previous opponents of HRT reconsider their previous recommendations. Certainly, it has convinced many people to select bioidentical hormones instead of synthetic hormones to greatly optimize benefits while significantly reducing risk.

So to answer your question, I would give your mother this new information and let her decide. Seeking the counsel of an expert in hormones and menopause is a reasonable approach. A true expert informs you of both the pros and cons of using hormone therapy.

Of course, my advice would be to switch her to bioidentical hormones.

Student:

Do you place all your antiaging patients on hormones?

Professor:

If patients have low hormone levels, then we discuss bioidentical hormone supplementation options. After reviewing the lab tests with the patient, I give my recommendations regarding an individualized hormone program. The decision about starting on a hormone program is completely up to the patient. My goal with each patient is to give information, answer questions, and help with his or her decision.

As with any medical decision, a risk-versus-benefit analysis should take place. It is crucial that we look at the risks and benefits of starting on a hormone program—as well as the risks and benefits of *not* starting on a hormone program. For example, there is no doubt in the medical and science literature that a deficiency of these hormones will increase the risk for dementia, osteoporosis, and heart disease, adversely affecting quality of life. It doesn't mean you will develop these problems; it means your risk is increased.

On the other hand, there is considerable doubt and debate in the medical and scientific literature regarding whether hormone supplementation programs will increase your risk of cancer. If a patient feels this possibility of increased cancer risk outweighs the proven benefits of a hormone therapy program, then that person should not start hormones.

All patients must be well informed so that they are comfortable with their decisions. My job is to make sure they are empowered with the necessary information to make educated decisions. If they choose not to begin hormones, I will continue to work with them to optimize diet, exercise, and supplements for overall health.

Student:

I have many symptoms suggestive of low testosterone; however, when my testosterone level was checked, I was told it was a normal level for a man my age. Can I still go on testosterone supplementation?

Professor:

Your question raises many crucial points of testosterone supplementation.

The first point is that symptoms of low testosterone overlap with symptoms of other medical problems, so we must be sure to check for other medical problems and not simply assume a patient needs testosterone.

The second point is that a "normal" hormone blood test may simply mean that the test is within normal reference range. Normal reference ranges for hormones simply represent the range of blood test results for a large group of people. Normal reference ranges do not define *optimal* hormone ranges. So it is not appropriate to withhold hormone supplementation simply because the test result is within a broad reference range; we want the level within a narrow optimal range.

A third point relates specifically with testosterone blood tests. To accurately measure testosterone levels, we must measure both *total* and *free* testosterone. The total testosterone value represents the amount of testosterone that is circulating in the bloodstream and bound to a protein carrier molecule. The protein carrier molecule is much like a transport ship carrying cargo on the ocean. A free testosterone value represents the portion of testosterone that is not bound to a protein carrier. The free testosterone represents the most biologically active testosterone.

It is crucial to measure both the total and the free testosterone because studies have shown that you could have a "normal" total testosterone at the same time that you have a low or suboptimal free testosterone. Patients with a low free testosterone would benefit greatly with testosterone supplementation therapy.

Bring me a copy of your lab results, and I will give you my recommendation.

Student:

As a male, if I have a low testosterone blood level, is there anything I can do to increase the level without taking hormones?

Professor:

Yes, indeed. Many lifestyle choices can lower your testosterone level and should be addressed, while many other lifestyle choices can improve hormone levels.

Frequently, a poor diet is the culprit. A high-glycemic diet that results in high insulin levels will lower your testosterone production. Also, a deprivation or calorie-restrictive diet with subsequent elevation of cortisol levels will decrease testosterone production. In addition, a low-protein or low-fat diet will result in low testosterone production.

I must point out that when the body produces testosterone, estrogen, progesterone, and DHEA, it starts with cholesterol. That is not a misprint! The first substance in the chemical pathway for the production of these life essential hormones is cholesterol! Remember, cholesterol is essential for life.

Because hormone production requires cholesterol, we must be careful with cholesterol-lowering medications. Studies have shown that if we lower the cholesterol too much, then testosterone production can decline.

High stress levels resulting in high cortisol will lower testosterone production. Think about it. If the body is under stress, it goes into survival mode. When in survival mode, energy is not going to be wasted on testosterone production. Energy is going to be spent on keeping you alive through the stressful event. This is why we see not only low testosterone but also experience low libido when we are stressed out.

Exercise is the final lifestyle influence on testosterone production. Prolonged aerobic exercise will lower testosterone production. High-intensity, short-duration exercise such as interval training or resistance training will augment testosterone (and HGH) production.

Following the *Antiaging 101* program will support hormone production and balance in the body. If testosterone levels are still not optimal despite a healthy lifestyle, then supplementation would be recommended.

Student:

I dislike having my blood drawn. Can I use saliva testing for hormones instead of blood tests?

Professor:

Although there is debate on the blood versus saliva tests, current literature favors blood tests over saliva tests. Yes, saliva tests are painless, but we get a better picture of overall hormone balance with the blood tests.

If a patient has saliva tests done, I will certainly review them and utilize them, but clinically my preference at this time is to use blood levels.

Student:

I was reading a magazine recently and noticed an advertisement for a synthetic hormone replacement that indicated it was derived from natural sources. Is that the same as bioidentical hormones?

Professor:

No, it is not the same. It is an example of clever marketing. For a hormone to be classified as bioidentical, it has to be identical to hormones produced in the body. The bioidentical hormones are natural to the body.

Here is where it can get confusing. Bioidentical hormones are derived from a chemical found in soy or wild yams. (Apparently, "tame" yams are not a good source!) The chemical is synthesized into the same molecular structure of human hormones. The result of this synthesis is hormones that are produced naturally by the human body.

The key point is that we are concerned with the end product. If we start with natural substances but end up with a hormone that is even *slightly* different from human hormones, then they are not bioidentical. Remember, structure matters. Different structures mean different hormones and different effects in the body.

While the advertisement may be accurate in stating that the hormones are derived from natural sources, we only focus on the end product.

Since pharmaceutical companies can't patent a natural substance, they must alter the hormone to make a patentable drug. Of course, when the hormone is altered, it is no longer bioidentical.

The best way to differentiate synthetic from bioidentical is to simply read the label. For an estrogen to be bioidentical, the label must read estradiol, estriol, or estrone (bi-est or tri-est). For progesterone to be bioidentical, the label must read progesterone (not medroxyprogesterone, not progestin, not Provera). For a testosterone to be bioidentical, the label must read testosterone.

Student:

I am allergic to soy; can I still use bioidentical hormones if they are derived from soy?

Professor:

Bioidentical hormones are produced from a chemical found in soy, but the end result is a bioidentical hormone that has no soy in it whatsoever. Therefore, you can still use them without any problem.

Student:

Are there studies supporting the use of bioidentical hormones?

Professor:

Yes, there are clinical studies, scientific studies, animal studies—you name it, they exist. Please check the reference list in your course manual.

In addition, across the world, we have experience from clinics and private physician practices with decades of clinical data.

Student:

My doctor told me a hormone is a hormone. She said all hormones are the same. She said it doesn't matter if the hormone is natural or not. She says all hormones cause cancer. What is your response?

Professor:

Your physician's intentions are probably good, but I believe she has a different perspective on hormone replacement because of problems found with synthetic hormones. I have had many patients quote their doctors with similar statements.

Let's think about this in a logical fashion. Premarin is a horse-derived estrogen. Humans have three types of estrogen in their bodies. Premarin has over twenty-five different types of estrogen. The main type of estrogen in Premarin is called equilin. Equilin is not found in the human body. It is not a human hormone. Estradiol is the main human estrogen. Estradiol is not found in Premarin.

The shape of the hormone determines its action in the body. If the shape is different, then the action is different. Synthetic hormones are shaped differently than bioidentical hormones. Thus, their actions are different in the body.

For all of our adult lives, we have natural, bioidentical hormones in our bodies. Does is make biologic sense that our natural hormones are carcinogens at balanced levels?

Hormones keep us on a normal, balanced path to maintain our wellness and health. When hormones are deficient or out of balance, then we get off the path to good health.

In women, we see more breast cancer the longer they go into menopause without hormone replacement. In other words, more years with low hormone levels supports cancer growth and weakens our immune system.

We see more prostate cancer in older men with low testosterone levels. We find much *less* prostate cancer in younger men with higher testosterone levels.

Most women with breast cancer have *never* been on any hormone replacement.

Most men with prostate cancer have *never* been on any hormone replacement.

Synthetic hormones have been found to increase the risk of cancer. Birth control pills (synthetic hormones) have been found to increase the risk of breast cancer. Bioidentical hormones have been found not to increase the risk of cancer. Some studies show that bioidentical hormones *decrease* the risk of cancer.

Hormones given in a pill form require higher dosages because they are metabolized by the liver prior to getting into the bloodstream. This liver metabolism causes increased risk of blood clotting and increased inflammation. Bioidentical hormones given via creams, troches, or pellets do not increase blood clotting or inflammation.

Finally, which would you choose? Hormones identical to what your body produces or hormones from a pharmaceutical company intentionally created to be different from non-patentable natural hormones?

Conclusion: All hormones are not the same.

Student:

I understand what you are saying about the differences between bioidentical hormones and synthetic hormones. Unfortunately, I am not comfortable starting hormone therapy because of the associations with breast cancer. Is this rational?

Professor:

I appreciate your concerns. My intent is to give you information and let you make the ultimate decision regarding hormone therapy. This is a rational approach. I do think it is necessary to hear the rest of the story regarding hormones and breast cancer.

The risk of breast cancer is present in all women—regardless of whether they go on hormone therapy. In fact, we see more cases of breast cancer the longer a woman is in menopause with hormone deficiencies. As we have stated prior, most women with breast cancer have *never* been on hormone replacement therapy.

When we review the scientific literature, we see that birth control pills, a form of synthetic hormone, slightly increase breast cancer risk. The scientific literature proves that synthetic hormones also slightly increase the risk of breast cancer.

The scientific literature proves that bioidentical hormones do not increase the risk of breast cancer. Some compelling literature reveals that bioidentical hormone therapy may *decrease* the risk of breast cancer.

The scientific literature documents the multiple problems associated with hormone deficiencies, such as osteoporosis, dementia, obesity, and cardiovascular disease.

The scientific literature is overwhelming in documenting the benefits of hormone therapy on osteoporosis, dementia, obesity, and cardiovascular disease.

The scientific literature, as well as clinical evidence, reveals without a doubt that quality of life is enhanced with bioidentical hormone replacement therapy.

Bottom line: if you are a woman, there is a risk of breast cancer, period. I cannot promise you that you won't get breast cancer ... with or without hormones.

However, if we utilize bioidentical hormones, we can give you tremendous health benefits without increasing the risk of cancer.

Student:

I am fifty-two years old, and I have not had a menstrual period for two years. After our last lecture, I had lab tests that showed an FSH of 90, an estradiol of 5, and a testosterone level of 12. My doctor said that my blood tests are normal. What do you think?

Professor:

Your blood tests are "normal" for menopause, but they are not optimal. To support your physiology and overall health, we would start bioidentical hormones. There is no physiologic benefit to you to keep your hormones out of balance. Even if you have minimal hot flashes or night sweats, keeping your hormones low is detrimental to your health.

We aim to improve your estradiol level to over the 70 to 90 range. Improving your estradiol level will lower your FSH. Our goal with the FSH level is to bring it under a level of 20. Your testosterone level should be elevated to over the 50 range. Our goal with your blood test results is to find and correct the hormone deficiencies.

Student:

Would you give some patient examples of hormone supplementation programs?

Professor:

Sure. Please meet our volunteer patients (names have been changed to protect patient privacy):

Emily Estrogen
Paula Progesterone
Tom Testosterone
H. G. Hormone

Emily Estrogen

Emily is a fifty-one-year-old who has not had a menstrual period for the past eight months. She complains of frequent hot flashes during the day and debilitating night sweats that prevent her from getting a good night's sleep. Her moods are unstable; she frequently gets angry one minute and then is crying the next minute. She feels her energy level is low, and her libido level is even lower. She has noticed her waist size is gradually increasing, despite a healthy diet and exercise program. She complains that her skin is dry and itchy. She also reports that her memory is failing, and she feels that she has lost her focus and concentration. Her physician informed her that her blood pressure and cholesterol levels are elevated.

Lab tests reveal:

Low estradiol, high FSH, low progesterone, and low testosterone (menopause)

Plan:

Bioidentical estrogen, progesterone, and testosterone supplementation

Results:

Within weeks: Resolution of hot flashes and night sweats. Sleeping great. Within months: Stable moods, better energy, and "great" libido. Skin dryness has resolved.
After one year: Memory is back. Body weight normal. Blood pressure and cholesterol levels have normalized.
Emily's report: "I feel like I did twenty years ago!"

Paula Progesterone

Paula is a thirty-eight-year-old who reports progressive symptoms over the past two years. She reports that her periods are heavy and erratic. Some months she has heavy menstrual bleeding for several days, usually with uncomfortable cramping. She has started having migraine headaches during the week preceding her period. To add insult to injury, she is having difficulty sleeping at night, especially the week before her menstrual period. Her family has noticed that she has developed a quick temper. Her physician has suggested a hysterectomy because of her heavy menstrual bleeding.

Lab tests reveal:

Low progesterone, normal estradiol and FSH levels

Plan:

Bioidentical progesterone (and no hysterectomy)

Results:

Within weeks: Sleeping well and no migraines
Within months: Restoration of normal menstrual periods, and her "quick temper" has resolved
After one year: "My life is back!"

Thomas Testosterone

Tom is a fifty-five-year-old executive who reports that his overall performance has dwindled over the past four years. His professional drive has gone south, and his energy level is minimal. He used to love going to the gym but now finds it difficult to get motivated. When he does exercise, he seems to have less endurance and strength. He is frustrated because he has developed a gut and is having difficulty losing the extra weight. His wife reports that he takes numerous naps and is less interested in his many hobbies. He also has "zero libido."

Lab tests reveal:

Low testosterone (andropause, a.k.a. male menopause)

Plan:

Bioidentical testosterone with pellet therapy

Results:

Within weeks: Better energy and endurance
Within months: Back in the gym three times a week with great results. No more naps. Libido is high.
After one year: "My gut is gone!" and "I've never felt better!"

H. G. Hormone

H. G. is a fifty-nine-year-old retired pilot who has been on a hormone supplementation program for the past ten years. He is doing well on his age-management program. He is religious about his diet, supplement, and hormone program. During his follow-up appointment, he asked if there was anything else he could do to ensure healthy aging.

Lab tests reveal:

Excellent levels of total and free testosterone as well as levels of DHEA-sulfate. Low-level IGF-1, a measure of HGH.

Plan:

HGH supplementation

Results:

Within weeks: More energy. Shorter exercise recovery and feels stronger in the gym.
Within months: Drop in body fat, better skin tone
After one year: Improved skin tone, "My hair is thicker," and improvement in body composition (on DEXA scan). "I feel like my immune system is optimized; I haven't even caught a cold in the past year."

What does the medical and scientific literature reveal about bioidentical hormones?

❖ A 2001 study of IGF-1 levels (measure of HGH) in older women reported association of low IGF-1 levels with poor muscle strength and mobility in women aged seventy to seventy-nine.

❖ A 2003 study found that growth hormone deficiency results in reduced longevity.

❖ A 1999 study of HGH therapy in elderly women with osteoporosis reported an increase in bone density, increase in lean body mass, and a decrease in body fat.

❖ A 2002 *Endocrinology* study found that HGH therapy decreases abdominal fat by up to 50 percent.

❖ *New England Journal* review article on HGH therapy found *no* increased risk of cancer with HGH therapy.

❖ HGH therapy was found to facilitate glucose metabolism, lower insulin levels, and improve insulin sensitivity.

❖ Study reported that the risk of heart disease increased by 38 percent for every 40 ng/dl decrease of IGF-1 (HGH deficiency increases cardiovascular risk).

❖ *Annals of Internal Medicine* study reported significant increases in bone density with HGH therapy in adult patients with osteoporosis/ osteopenia.

❖ DHEA therapy reduces abdominal fat and improves insulin sensitivity. A study in the *Journal of the American Medical Association* found that DHEA therapy led to significant reductions in abdominal fat as well as significant increases in insulin sensitivity.

❖ Study completed in 1989 demonstrated that "women who used menopause hormones had up to 50 percent fewer heart attacks than non-users of hormones."

❖ A total of 1,064 women received a CAT scan assessment of coronary plaque. Women on estrogen therapy had 30 to 40 percent less coronary calcification than women not on estrogen. Those women on estrogen for at least five years had 60 percent lower levels of coronary calcification.

❖ Postmenopausal women placed on estrogen therapy were shown to quickly demonstrate improvements on cognitive testing and resumption of premenopausal cortical (brain) function patterns on PET scans.

❖ *Neurology* study found that hormone therapy was associated with a significantly reduced risk of Alzheimer's disease, as well as an association between low estrogen levels and Alzheimer's.

❖ Premarin (synthetic estrogen) increases inflammation as measured by CRP, while topical bioidentical estrogen decreases inflammation (remember first-pass liver metabolism).

❖ In a 2005 study of breast cancer risk in relation to different types of hormone replacement therapy, it was found that the risk of breast cancer was significantly greater with HRT containing synthetic progestins (such as Provera) than with HRT containing bioidentical progesterone, the relative risk (RR) being 1.4 and 0.9, respectively. (RR of 1.0 is neutral—that is, the risk of breast cancer in women with no HRT is 1.0.)

❖ A 2006 review of menopausal hormone therapy in patients with breast cancer reported that hormone therapy was not associated with increased cancer recurrence, cancer-related mortality, or total mortality. Seven studies with control groups revealed that patients using hormone therapy had a decreased chance of recurrence and cancer-related mortality compared to the control groups.

❖ Study found that elderly women are at a greater risk of death after a hip fracture than after breast cancer. (Remember, estrogen saves bone tissue.) Osteoporosis causes 1.5 million fractures annually in the United States, including 300,000 hip fractures and 700,000 vertebral fractures.

❖ Testosterone replacement study in 163 men treated for three and a half years found improvement in mood, libido, and sexual performance, and increased lean body mass, muscle strength, and bone density.

❖ Testosterone deprivation therapy (often utilized in prostate cancer patients) results in decreased quality of life, increased body fat, decreased muscle mass, decreased bone density, increased depression, increased risk heart disease, and decreased libido.

❖ Men with low testosterone were 33 percent more likely to die from all causes within eighteen years compared to men with higher testosterone levels.

❖ Researchers assessed hormone levels (IGF-1, DHEA, and testosterone) in 410 men over sixty-five years of age. Men increased their six-year risk of death by 47 percent, 85 percent, and 120 percent if they had lower-than-threshold values of one, two, and three hormones, respectively, compared with men in the higher quartiles.

❖ Researchers treating 4,000 women with a combination of estrogen and testosterone found that only one patient in every 1,000 was diagnosed with cancer by the end of the study (less than half the national average).

❖ Johns Hopkins University study found that women on both estrogen and testosterone had decreased body fat, increased muscle mass, increased muscle strength, and improved libido.

❖ A twelve-year study of 290,827 postmenopausal women found that "all-cause death rates were lower among estrogen users than never users." Breast cancer mortality did not increase with estrogen use.

❖ A 2006 study found that women younger than forty-five years who had prophylactic oophorectomy (removal of both ovaries in attempt to prevent ovarian cancer) and did not receive adequate estrogen replacement therapy had a 70 percent higher mortality risk. (The women who had oophorectomies and did not receive adequate estrogen therapy had an increased risk of mortality from breast and uterine cancers, as well as cardiovascular and neurologic disease.) The study had a thirty-year follow-up period.

❖ A reevaluation of the Women's Health Initiative study found that hormone therapy started early in menopause (before age sixty-five) reduced the risk of all-cause dementia and Alzheimer's disease. Hormone therapy was associated with a 46 percent overall reduction in dementia risk and a 64 percent reduction in Alzheimer's disease.

❖ Study found that men with coronary heart disease had 20 percent lower testosterone levels than those with normal coronary arteries (on angiogram).

❖ In a study of forty-five men, testosterone therapy improved libido in 80 percent.

❖ A Northwestern University study evaluated seventy-three studies on the use of testosterone for erectile dysfunction. Meta-analysis revealed a success rate of 59 percent using testosterone alone.

❖ An extensive review of the medical literature published from 1966 through 1999 found that men with depression had the lowest testosterone levels.

❖ A study of 310 men found that higher levels of testosterone are associated with better cognitive function in older men.

❖ A study of 547 men found that higher testosterone levels and lower estradiol levels predicted better performance on cognitive tests.

❖ Seventy men, age sixty-five years or older, with low testosterone levels received testosterone therapy over a three-year period. Results found that testosterone therapy improved physical performance and strength.

❖ A study of testosterone therapy in men with type 2 diabetes found decreased insulin resistance, improved blood glucose control, improved cholesterol panel, and decreased central body fat.

❖ Japanese women were found to have higher levels of estradiol in their blood yet much lower rates of breast cancer than American women. When Japanese women adapt a Western lifestyle, risk of breast cancer increases.

❖ Research study found a 50 percent reduction in the recurrence of breast cancer in women who used hormone replacement therapy.

❖ A 2006 study of male veterans found men with low testosterone levels had a 68 percent increased risk of death compared to men with normal levels.

❖ UCLA study in 2006 found that older men on a placebo had more prostate cancers than those treated with testosterone therapy.

❖ Study found that in men with congestive heart failure, those with the lowest levels of testosterone and DHEA had the lowest survival rate of 27 percent. Men with congestive heart failure with no hormone deficiencies had the best three-year survival rate of 83 percent.

❖ Johns Hopkins researchers found that men with low to normal testosterone levels are more likely to have diabetes than men with higher levels. Men in the lowest third of testosterone levels were four times more likely to have diabetes than men in the highest third.

❖ Research has shown that men with low testosterone levels double their risk of developing metabolic syndrome.

❖ Studies have shown that men with low levels of testosterone are at increased risk of developing Alzheimer's disease.

❖ A 1993 review of published scientific studies stated that HRT after menopause resulted in a 50 percent decreased risk of heart disease, 28 percent decreased risk of death from heart disease, a 59 percent decreased risk of hip fractures from osteoporosis, and *no* significant increased risk of breast cancer.

❖ A 2001 literature review reported that HRT in menopause produced a 34 percent decrease risk in colon cancer and between a 20 to 60 percent reduction in Alzheimer's disease.

❖ A 1998 report in the *Journal of the American Medical Association* concluded that 99 percent of postmenopausal women would benefit from taking HRT, experiencing a decreased death rate and improved longevity.

❖ A 1996 study found that the death rate from all causes was reduced by 44 percent in women on estrogen therapy.

❖ Study reported in *American Journal of Obstetrics and Gynecology* found that estrogen and testosterone replacement in women provides improvement in psychological and sexual symptoms of menopause.

❖ Research has demonstrated that estrogen positively affects neuronal (brain cell) structure and function and has receptors in areas of the brain especially involved in memory.

❖ Study demonstrated that higher estrogen levels in women improve verbal production, fine motor tasks, visual memory, and articulatory speed and accuracy.

❖ Study found that in menopausal women, lower scores on four measures of cognitive function correlated with significantly lower blood levels of estrogen and testosterone.

❖ A study reported in the *Journal of the American Medical Association* found that women who started hormone replacement therapy around the time of menopause had between a 40 and 80 percent reduction in the incidence of Alzheimer's disease, compared to women not using hormone therapy (remember your risk-versus-benefit analysis).

❖ No studies have reported an increase in situ cases of breast cancer in hormone users (if hormones were causing new breast tumors, we would expect to see an increase in in situ cancers.)

❖ Study found that after ten years of hormone replacement therapy in women, there is a 50 percent reduction in fractures.

❖ A study in the *Journal of the National Cancer Institute* found that women who had taken estrogen for eleven or more years reduced their risk of dying of colon cancer by 46 percent.

And much more …

CHAPTER 6

STRESS REDUCTION

The hormone cortisol is released when we are under stress. Cortisol allows us to survive a stressful situation, and stressful situations confront us on a daily basis. For example, you are driving to work for an important 8:00 AM meeting with your boss. Unfortunately, you are running late. You had a fitful night sleep (stressor #1), and you were too nervous to eat so you skipped breakfast (stressor #2). You are driving to work in heavy traffic (stressor #3), gulping caffeinated coffee (stressor #4). While driving, your cell phone rings, and you hope it's not your boss asking why you are late (stressor #5). You look down briefly to pick up your cell phone. When you look back to the road, you realize that a few feet ahead is a school bus, stopped in the road, boarding young children (stressor #6). Your heart races faster as you slam on the brakes, barely missing the back of the school bus (stressor #7). As your car stops abruptly, your coffee spills all over your lap (stressor #8). Now there is no doubt you are going to miss the meeting (stressor #9). Thoughts of losing your job permeate your brain (stressor #10). Unbelievably, your day has just begun, and your body and health are under siege. The stress response is activated and in full gear. *Red alert!*

Let's discuss what occurs during the stress response. Initially, the sympathetic nervous system is activated (more on this soon). The sympathetic nervous system stimulates the adrenal glands to release adrenaline. The adrenaline aids the acute phase of the stress response. Adrenaline focuses your attention, increases your heart rate and blood pressure, and rapidly mobilizes energy for fuel. Adrenaline protects in the short run of the stress response.

While adrenaline protects us in the first phase of the stress response, cortisol works more slowly. Cortisol works to restore the energy supply, activating the immune system to help us handle the threat of the stressor. Think of it this way: adrenaline helps us in the first half of the "game of stress," while cortisol helps us in the second half of the game.

While the cortisol release helps us acutely, it comes with a price. Cortisol's function is to assist us in dealing with each stressor. Remember, cortisol helps us mobilize energy and support our physiology as we deal with the acute stressor. It is important to understand that we would succumb to any threat or illness if we were unable to produce cortisol.

Problems arise not because we release cortisol but because we release excessive cortisol for prolonged periods. Excessive levels of cortisol are released in response to ongoing chronic stress. The common culprits of chronic stress are psychological stressors such as work difficulties, financial worries, and family problems. Physical stressors such as poor diets, sedentary lifestyle, sleep deprivation, or bad habits such as smoking, drugs, or excessive alcohol consumption also contribute to chronic stress.

Stress reduction equals cortisol control.

Excessive cortisol is an age accelerator, and any efforts we make to minimize the damage of elevated cortisol levels will assist us in slowing the aging process. Excessive cortisol is catabolic. With excessive cortisol levels, we lose muscle and bone and gain body fat.

Paradoxically, high cortisol levels impair our immune systems and make us more vulnerable to illness. High cortisol has been found to dampen our memories and contribute to dementia.

Because of the detrimental impact of excessive or chronically elevated cortisol, we must take active steps to minimize the problem. While it is not possible, or advisable, to avoid stress entirely, we can eliminate or at least minimize the lifestyle habits that stress our health.

Our antiaging program will fortify us and greatly diminish the erosive damage of chronic stress. All the components of our antiaging program will assist and augment how our bodies respond to the multiple stressors we must face on a daily basis.

Stress reduction means controlling cortisol hormone. As stated earlier, high cortisol makes us heavy, slow, sick, and weak. High cortisol will sabotage any attempt at reaching our antiaging goals.

Healthy diet equals cortisol control.

The first step in cortisol control is making sure we are compliant with all components discussed in *Antiaging 101*. First and foremost is diet. Poor diets increase cortisol, so we need to focus on a balanced whole-food diet as covered previously.

Don't restrict or deprive, as doing so will simply activate the stress response and raise your cortisol level. Deprivation diets are a common cause of elevated cortisol so please avoid that trap.

Since our bodies run on protein 24/7, we must remember to try to eat protein at every meal. If we skip meals and don't consume any protein, problems develop, for our bodies still need protein to run, but not enough protein is coming in via the diet. Because the body still has to get a supply of amino acids from somewhere, it will leech protein out of our muscles to help fuel our metabolism. This results in muscle loss, which we want to avoid at all costs.

Another problem with skipping meals is that our blood glucose levels become unstable. The brain desires a stable blood glucose level. A blood glucose drop is a stress to the brain, so the body sends out cortisol and adrenaline hormones to help raise the blood glucose level.

Unfortunately, this stress hormone release increases catabolic breakdown of muscle tissue to help balance out the blood glucose level. This stress hormone surge is beneficial in the short term but detrimental in the long term.

When we eat a healthy, balanced diet, we "reassure" the body and the brain by supplying the necessary nutrients to support our metabolism, growth and repair, and to support balanced blood sugar levels. When we deprive, the body/brain acts as if we are in a famine situation and activates a "red alert" by releasing stress hormones.

By eating as we have outlined in this course, you reassure the body/brain that you are not in a famine, and you stay in "triple **R** mode": relaxation, repair, and rejuvenation. Following our antiaging diet is the foundation for your success with cortisol control.

Nutraceutical supplementation equals cortisol control.

Nutritional deficiencies are also stressors, so in conjunction with your healthy diet, remember to supplement with appropriate vitamins, minerals, fish oil, and targeted nutrients. Establish a routine so you maintain consistency with your supplement program. This is a personal routine, but it could be as simple as storing your supplements near your toothpaste so that you take them twice daily when you brush your teeth.

Whatever it takes to keep you supplementing every day, do it! Make it a lifelong habit. Supply your cells with nutrients as they are working every minute of every day.

Antiaging goals equal stress management.

The combined influences of healthy diet and supplement programs mean reductions in common stressors like elevated glucose, elevated insulin levels, elevated oxidation, and elevated inflammation. Reduction in glycation, inflammation, and oxidation has numerous healthy ramifications throughout the body—all without prescription medications.

Unhealthy diet-induced stressors:

Elevated glucose
Elevated insulin
Elevated oxidation
Elevated inflammation

Intelligent exercise equals cortisol control

This class has reviewed the multiple benefits of a consistent, moderate exercise program. A great stress reducer, exercise will lower your cortisol. However, don't fall into the "calorie trap" and assume that the more calories you burn with exercise, the better.

Excessive, prolonged exercise is a stressor, and it will raise your cortisol level, offsetting benefits. Stick with our recommended resistance training and interval training programs for optimal results. Think "short and sweet" exercise sessions.

As discussed previously, focus on intensity and not on duration. Be consistent. Even a short twenty-minute weight training session is beneficial. When we exercise in this manner, we literally control stress.

With intelligent exercise, we stress our muscles the right amount to stimulate the anabolic repair and rebuild response for healthy body composition. The controlled stress response of exercise allows the body to respond to the stressor of exercise in a beneficial, effective manner.

With prolonged exercise, such as running a marathon, the stress response becomes excessive, high amounts of cortisol are released, and catabolic forces are stimulated to break us down.

We know that just as a balanced diet reassures the body and brain that all is well, short-duration, high-intensity exercise reassures the body that we are not stressed out, running for our lives. Rather, this form of exercise reassures the body that we are young, vibrant, and active. The body will respond to this message with rejuvenation forces and enhanced health and body composition. It will keep you in "triple R mode."

Hormone therapy equals cortisol control.

Hormone therapy is a tremendous addition to stress reduction. When we restore hormone balance with bioidentical hormone therapy, we supply our cells with appropriate instructions for cell function. Cells work efficiently and effectively, with improvement in metabolism, immune function, and brain function.

Clearly, improving our physiologic systems allows our bodies to function efficiently. With physiologic systems in peak condition, we are then able to deal with stressors effectively—ultimately with less cortisol release.

This restoration of hormone balance has some practical day-to-day benefits. For example, with the resulting improvement in brain chemistry and function, our sugar cravings disappear. As difficult as it may be to believe, these sugar cravings are simply the brains attempt at a "Band-Aid" solution to brain chemical imbalances.

Restored hormone balance means restored brain chemical balance and resolution of mood swings, cravings, and depression. The result of this hormone balance is stress reduction. The more we restore our physiology, the less our bodies are "stressed." Bioidentical hormone therapy allows us to restore our physiological balance efficiently.

Bioidentical hormone therapy also cushions the stress response of the body to exercise. Even with our intelligent exercise program, our bodies will release cortisol because of the "stress" of exercise. Indeed, we require activating the stress response to begin the repair and rebuild process.

The anabolic repair response is initiated with the release of cortisol and other stress hormones. When we have bioidentical hormones like testosterone available, the repair process is enhanced and the cortisol response is balanced, so we don't set off those destructive catabolic forces.

By reaching our healthy aging goals with the programs delineated in *Antiaging 101*, great strides toward stress reduction are attained. In fact, many times by reaching our antiaging goals, no additional formal stress-reduction techniques are even required. However, most stress reduction techniques are simple and require minimal amounts of your valuable time.

Sleep equals cortisol control.

Sleep is a much-ignored stress reducer. When we sleep well, cortisol levels are lowered. If we don't get quality sleep, cortisol levels rise. In addition, when we sleep poorly, we rely on stimulants like caffeine to give us temporary energy; of course, these stimulants result in higher cortisol.

Poor sleep will impede progress toward our antiaging goals by creating hormonal imbalances. Not only does poor sleep elevate cortisol, but poor sleep leads to deficient production of growth hormone (HGH). Lower HGH and higher cortisol induce multiple problems by contributing to higher glucose and insulin levels, and ultimately, increased catabolic metabolism. If you consistently sleep poorly, you will be on a road toward accelerated aging.

There are a few simple common sense techniques to improve your sleep pattern. First, avoid caffeinated beverages after midday. Second, follow our healthy diet, exercise, and hormone programs; they will dramatically improve your sleep quality. Finally, devote your bed to sleep (and fun with your significant other).

Make the bedroom a perfect sleep environment. Get the television out of your bedroom; no food in your bedroom; no stereo in your bedroom. Make your bedroom a quiet, dark, and comfortable place to sleep, and eventually your body will jump into sleep mode quickly when you lie down at night.

In addition, listen to what Mom said and get to bed at a decent time. The more hours you sleep before midnight, the better. I don't mean you have to go to bed after the 6:00 PM news, but try to get to bed by 10:00 PM when you can. You will feel better and more restored in the morning if you do.

We should reinforce that during sleep, your body heals, repairs, and restores. By following *Antiaging 101* programs, you will burn fat and build muscle while you sleep! You wake up healthier than when you went to bed. You will feel energetic and happy. Not a bad way to start each day!

Before discussing simple stress-reduction techniques, it is important to acknowledge an important point regarding psychological stress. It isn't the stressor that is the problem—it's your body's response to the stressor.

We all have life stressors that we can't avoid. How we deal with them is the key to stress reduction. For illustration, if a co-worker is a stress in your life, simply by not letting him get to you, you minimize the stress response. I know it sounds too easy, but we are talking about your health here. If you allow his irritating behavior to bother you, then you are letting him win. You are literally allowing him not only to decrease the quality of your life but allowing him to shorten your life as well.

When you realize the destructive power of your co-worker, or other stressors, you are empowered to resist it, to de-stress. Of course, your resistance and tolerance toward his behavior are stronger because of your participation in our healthy aging program.

The nervous system

To understand the body's stress response, we must look at the nervous system in a little more depth. Our nervous systems have two main components. One component is the "voluntary nervous system." The voluntary component of the nervous system, as you can gather from the name, is under one's voluntary control. When you want your body to do something, your thoughts stimulates the brain to send out appropriate signals to the body to execute what you want done. For example, when you want to lift something, wave to a friend, or choke your co-worker, you activate the voluntary nervous system. This is rather straightforward.

The second main component of our nervous system is labeled the "autonomic nervous system." This part of the nervous system is usually quite automatic and less under the control of our thoughts. Breathing is a great example. Our autonomic nervous systems allows us to breathe without being consciously aware that we are breathing. Life is certainly easier if we don't have to think about taking every breath!

However, we can override the autonomic system to some degree. When we practice deep breathing, we are overriding the autonomic system and voluntarily controlling the rate and depth of our breathing.

The autonomic nervous system is responsible for the stress response. The autonomic nervous system sends its nerve fibers to the heart muscle, the endocrine glands (hormone glands), and smooth muscle. Smooth muscle is found in many diverse parts of the body, including the lining of blood vessels, bladder, gastrointestinal tract, and the respiratory tract. You can think of the autonomic nervous system as an on/off switch for organs and muscles throughout the body. The on/off functions of the nervous system work to regulate heart muscle, control smooth muscle contraction, and to stimulate or inhibit endocrine gland hormone release.

One division of the autonomic nervous system is called the sympathetic nervous system; the other division is called the parasympathetic nervous system. In general, the sympathetic nervous system stimulates, while the parasympathetic system relaxes. Part of the autonomic nervous system is turned on to elicit the stress response, and a second part of the autonomic nervous system is turned off during the stress response. The part turned on during stress is the sympathetic nervous system. The part turned off during stress is the parasympathetic nervous system.

When the sympathetic nervous system is turned on, the body prepares immediately for the stressor at hand by activating the fight-or-flight response. Your racing heart, sweaty palms, rapid breathing, and sudden focus occur because of the sympathetic nervous system.

Without activation of the sym**pathetic** nervous system, your stress response would be **pathetic!** When the sympathetic nervous system is activated, the body releases two hormones, epinephrine and norepinephrine, to run the stress response. These hormones are responsible for the proverbial "adrenaline rush" we feel when we are stressed or excited.

This adrenaline rush is crucial for survival. Stress-related problems don't develop because of the adrenaline rush; they develop when we are constantly activating the sympathetic nervous system because of perpetual psychological or physical stress.

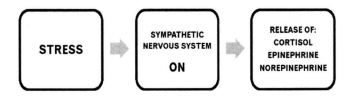

The parasympathetic nervous system has opposite effects than those of the sympathetic nervous system. The parasympathetic system is on when we are calm; it is off when we are stressed. The relaxation response requires activation of the parasympathetic nervous system.

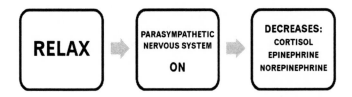

If we are under constant stress, our bodies can't turn on the parasympathetic system, and we can't relax. When the parasympathetic nervous system is activated, our breathing slows, our heart rate slows, and the sweating stops. When the parasympathetic nervous system is activated, we can tap into anabolic metabolism and growth. When we are in sympathetic mode, we are catabolic and experiencing breakdown.

Incessant stress forces the body into a perpetual stress response. Prolonged stress response leads to activation of the sympathetic nervous system. Activation of the sympathetic nervous system produces high cortisol and high epinephrine levels. Elevated cortisol and epinephrine levels promotes catabolic metabolism. Catabolic metabolism results in muscle loss, bone loss, fat gain, and an impaired immune system.

This altered body composition and suppressed immune system contributes to illness and accelerated aging. Of course, illness and accelerated aging leads to more stress and continued activation of the stress response ... Are you getting dizzy?

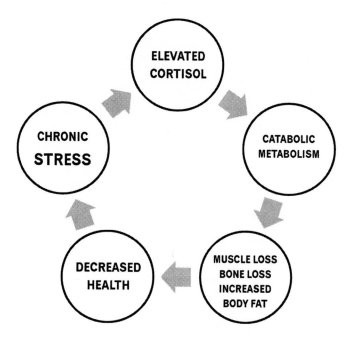

Chronic stress halts progress toward our antiaging goals.

How important is controlling our stress response in our antiaging lifestyle?

Unfortunately, an excessive stress response will sabotage all of our eight antiaging goals. When we activate the hormones involved in the stress response, we do the following:

1. Elevate glucose levels
2. Elevate insulin levels
3. Elevate cortisol levels
4. Impair cell function
5. Increase free radical damage
6. Suppress hormone levels
7. Disrupt anabolic metabolism (and increase catabolic metabolism)
8. Increase inflammation

If we don't control our stress response and frequently elicit the relaxation response, we cannot slow the aging process. Without a stress-reduction program, all of our antiaging modalities will be useless. It is that important.

Fortify your stress response with our antiaging program.

Part of your body's response to stress is determined by the level of anabolic hormones such as HGH, testosterone, and DHEA. These anabolic hormones balance elevated cortisol levels and offset its destructive influence. When we use balanced hormone therapy, we greatly improve our "stress response."

HGH, DHEA, and testosterone balance cortisol.

I mentioned that when we exercise, our cortisol levels rise. With sustained, prolonged aerobic exercise, this cortisol rise occurs without a corresponding rise in our anabolic hormones. In this setting, cortisol proceeds down its destructive path unabated.

In contrast, with resistance training programs such as weight lifting, even though our cortisol is elevated, anabolic hormones offset it. Cortisol is prevented from any negative influence by the concomitant rise in our anabolic hormone levels. This is a main reason why prolonged aerobics is detrimental to health, while short/intense weight training or interval training programs are so beneficial.

Elicit the relaxation response.

I'm a huge basketball fan. Here in Tucson, for over twenty years, we had the privilege of watching the great Hall of Fame coach Lute Olson at work. How does this relate to stress reduction? The answer is simply knowing when to call a "time-out."

In life, we are under constant stress; many people and responsibilities pull us in different directions. Dealing with stressors will, of course, raise our cortisol levels. Since we can't live in a cocoon, we deal with individual stressors as well as we can. Thankfully, our bodies know how to de-stress and repair the damage of chronically elevated cortisol levels.

To tap into the body's de-stress talent, one needs to occasionally take a much-deserved time-out. When we do, we briefly get away from the stressors, and our bodies lower the cortisol levels quickly. This elicits a relaxation response, as we discussed earlier.

Time-Out!

During University of Arizona basketball games, if the players were playing erratically, or if they were not sticking to the game plan, Coach Olson would call a time-out. During this time-out, Coach would simply let the players take a quick break, drink some water, and clear their minds. Or he may have "gently" reminded them of what they were supposed to be doing!

This gives the players a new perspective and reinforces their abilities to play well. Toward the end of close games, the decisions of when to call a time-out greatly affected player performance and helped win ball games.

In life, it is no different. Think of each day as another basketball game against a tough, competitive component. You have prepared well with diet, supplements, exercise, and hormones. When things get tough, take a time-out and relax.

These time outs may simply be taking a short walk; listening to music; meditating; taking some slow, deep breaths; or sharing a few jokes with a friend. The idea is to get away from life stressors, even for a brief period. By doing so, your body will lower cortisol and offset the erosive damages of chronically high cortisol.

It really is a miracle that the body can do this so quickly and efficiently. Unfortunately, many of us forget to take a time-out and never allow the body to reset our stress response. It is crucial to take a time-out every day.

We need to step off the treadmill of life periodically. This can be done in the morning, evening, or at your lunch break. It doesn't matter when; just schedule it into your day, every day. Stress reduction extends your life.

> Cortisol control lengthens your life and improves your health.

Meditation

Many people equate stress reduction with meditation. Indeed, meditation has been shown to have multiple health benefits. *Why?* Because of cortisol reduction.

To many of us, meditation is intimidating. Oftentimes we don't quite understand it, or we view it as some esoteric activity. Thankfully, you can meditate without having to move to Tibet or sit in some bizarre position on the floor.

There are many great how-to resources on meditation. The basics are straightforward. Simply find a comfortable chair in a quiet room where you won't be disturbed. Relax. Close your eyes and clear your mind of everything. (For some of us, this is easier than it is for others.)

Focus on your breathing—slow inhalations and slow exhalations. Sequentially relax all your muscles, starting from your face and moving down to your feet. Briefly tense a muscle group and then feel the muscles relax. Do this from head to toe until you are completely relaxed.

If you start thinking of something, erase it and clear your mind immediately. Sometimes repeating a thought, or prayer, or even a word or "mantra" repeatedly will help keep your mind clear. Some people find listening to relaxing music helpful. Meditate for fifteen minutes and you're done.

You will find this to be reenergizing and an effective stress reducer. Be consistent, and you will slow the aging process and greatly improve your health.

Breathing

As crazy as it may sound, our breathing patterns become dysfunctional when we are tense or under stress. We tend to take shallow, ineffective breaths that lead to poor oxygen to our cells and an increased stress response.

This is easy to rectify. A few times during the day, take a few minutes to focus on your breathing. Take slow deep breaths through your nose and exhale slowly through your mouth. You can remember this by the expression "Smell the roses and blow out the candles." In through the nose, out through the mouth. *Slowly.*

Focus on expanding your chest and lowering your diaphragm as you inhale, then exhale slowly as you feel your chest contract. This is extremely effective at eliciting a quick relaxation response.

So remember to breathe well throughout the day and prior to or during stressful situations. You will immediately notice feeling relaxed and less stressed.

Attitude

Tell all your friends that your professor says it is okay to have attitude! I'm sure you are wondering what I mean by attitude, and how it relates to stress reduction and cortisol control. As it turns out, research has repeatedly shown the importance of the mind-body connection. Your thoughts greatly influence your body and health.[7]

In medicine, we know that patients who believe in their therapy heal better and faster than patients who don't believe in their therapy. In antiaging medicine, we know that people who believe they can become healthier and biologically younger become healthier and younger. The best part about your thoughts and attitude is that they are completely free!

So let's look at attitude. You want to maintain an attitude that supports your health and lowers your cortisol response. An antiaging attitude means you are optimistic, not pessimistic. You see the good in people instead of focusing on the bad.

Since how we perceive stress impacts our health as much as the stressor itself, we can reduce the negative impacts of excessive stress by simply adjusting our attitudes.

Medical studies find a decreased incidence of virtually all degenerative diseases in optimistic patients. You will be less likely to develop most degenerative diseases simply by maintaining a healthy attitude, especially combined with our antiaging lifestyle. Recent studies find less dementia in optimistic people with positive attitudes, and more dementia in pessimistic patients with negative attitudes.[1]

How we can nurture a healthy attitude?

Like anything else, it takes practice. Try to make someone laugh every day. Do something nice for someone without expecting anything in return. Help a stranger, help a friend, volunteer … whatever it takes, just do it, and do it every day.

You will find that when you change your attitude, it becomes extremely fulfilling, and in time you will develop an even better attitude and maintain it for longer periods of time. Within days to months, you will have a healthy attitude virtually all the time.

As you begin your antiaging program, it is absolutely essential that you apply your new attitude to ensure the success of your entire program. For example, when you start your new diet, focus on what you can eat, not on what you can't eat. People who fail new diets tend to focus on what they are missing instead of following the new diet. They only think negatively, constantly reinforcing their own deprivation and sacrifice. This will doom them to failure.

Instead, learn to love the new foods you are eating. Always remember that you are eating for health and longevity. Focus on how good the healthy food tastes, how much better your energy level is, and how much better you feel. The diet will then become second nature, and you won't miss any part of your old way of eating. *Your old way of eating makes you old.*

Another negative attitude trap that we fall into with new diet and exercise programs is an excessive focus on "weight loss." If weight loss is slower than expected, people get disappointed and discouraged and end up quitting the program. It is of paramount importance to avoid this trap. Remember that it took you a long time to get unhealthy and to gain excess body fat. You can't expect instantaneous results. It is going to take time for your metabolism to be corrected and restored so you can burn fat efficiently.

Don't set unrealistic goals about your weight loss. Instead, focus your sights on the eight antiaging goals and know that as you reach these goals you will become healthier and leaner.

Think about your improved energy and vitality. Think about your improved strength and muscle tone. Think positive.

Winning Attitude

Successful athletes share two common characteristics. One, they prepare well and train for their sport. Two, they know they can and will win. It's called a winning attitude.

Many teams are coached well and prepare well, but they still don't have winning programs. Winning teams know and believe that they will win, and they usually do. They have willpower.

If they don't win, they maintain a successful attitude. Instead of getting dejected with a loss, they use the loss as a learning experience for the next contest. They learn from and get better with time.

With your antiaging program, you will prepare well by taking this course. To be successful with your program, you must know you will get healthier and younger. You eat well most of the time, you exercise well most of the time, you take your supplements and hormones most of the time, and you utilize stress-reduction techniques most of the time.

If you occasionally eat an unhealthy meal or snack, miss a workout, skip your supplements, or become stressed, get over it and move on. As my Italian uncle would say, "Forget about it." It's not a big deal. Learn from your mistake and get back on your program.

Maintain an antiaging attitude. You will get younger with time.

Brain Health

Stress reduction and cortisol control are crucial for optimizing brain health. As noted in our earlier discussions, excessive cortisol directly harms areas of the brain required to formulate memory. Simple stress-reduction techniques will offset the damage to your brain and memory.

Maintaining and enhancing our brain health is a priority for everyone following an antiaging program. In traditional health care, we tend to look for a prescription medication that can somehow enhance our brain health. We want a prescription medication that diminishes our chances of developing dementia or becoming senile.

While research into potential pharmaceutical agents is worthwhile, it does not make sense to ignore the many brain benefits of our antiaging program while waiting for a pharmaceutical agent to become available. Benefits that you can capitalize on now, prior to any damage occurring to your brain cells, will be much more effective. Fortunately, all of our antiaging goals will definitely improve and optimize our brain health.

It is reassuring to know that when you balance your hormones, control your glucose and insulin, support healthy cell function, and support metabolism, you enhance your brain structure and function.

As we discuss our brain health, it is a good time to repeat and reinforce the impact of each of our antiaging goals on our brains. Glycation, oxidation, inflammation, nutrient deficiencies, hormone imbalances, and impaired metabolism all diminish our brain cell function and brain health.

Individually, each of our antiaging goals will enhance brain health. Together, all of our antiaging goals have a dramatic synergistic impact on our brain health. We can significantly delay, and very likely avoid, the onset of dementia with our seven antiaging goals. Just this knowledge alone should be ample motivation to lead a healthy lifestyle.

Recent medical literature has shown us that our brain cells (neurons) have the ability to increase in number and improve in efficiency.[1-6] (This is called neuroplasticity.) In medicine, it was believed forever that neurons were unable to form new neural connections. In other words, once there was injury to neurons, there was no way to improve the affected area of the injured brain.

It is exciting to utilize this recently gained knowledge of the brain to keep our brains vibrant and healthy. Again, reaching our antiaging goals will allow us to hang on to all of our neurons and keep them working in top-notch condition.

The brain is much like our muscles. When we exercise our muscles, they become stronger and more efficient. When we exercise our brains, we become more intelligent, have better memories, and stay young.

Exercise has been shown to stimulate the release of neuronal growth factors. These growth factors literally help build your brain. This knowledge should be ample motivation to get out there and exercise!

Just as our muscles respond best to short-duration, high-intensity exercise, our brains respond best to exercises that require concentration (i.e., high intensity) and are of shorter duration.

When we exercise, we don't want to do the same thing over and over again—for example, long-duration aerobic exercise. This type of prolonged exercise does not produce the stimuli our muscles need to get stronger and more efficient.

The stimuli that build our muscle also build our brains. When we do the same things repeatedly, our brain cells are not appropriately stimulated. We need to do something new, something that requires concentration and focus, to encourage the formation of new neurons and to increase the connections of neurons to each other.

Try to learn new things. Learning something new requires focus, concentration, and intense thought, all perfect stimuli to the brain. Examples of the ideal forms of "brain exercises" are learning to speak a new language, learning to play a musical instrument, visiting a new part of the country, or traveling out of the country.

These types of activities force us to concentrate and focus, providing the stimulation for stronger brains. If we just watch television every night, the brain gets minimal exercise. When we read about a new hobby or activity, we learn, and the brain formulates more "circuits" to assist us in learning and remembering the new activity.

The brain is appropriately stimulated with these types of activities to stay young and efficient, just as our muscles are appropriately stimulated with resistance training to stay young and efficient.

This is antiaging at its finest—optimizing our health, improving our performance, and delaying and avoiding the onset of degenerative diseases.

> Live young, get young, and stay young with our antiaging lifestyle.

Stress Reduction Nuts and Bolts:

1) Stress accelerates aging.

2) Stress makes you slow, heavy, weak, and sick.

3) Tap into the body's ability to "de-stress" every day by eliciting the relaxation response.

4) Stress reduction controls cortisol levels. Cortisol control improves health and slows aging.

5) Comply with all components of *Antiaging 101* for optimal health to fortify your stress response.

The most significant benefit of stress reductions is toward goal #3: cortisol control. By controlling cortisol, we improve blood glucose and insulin control, help control free radicals, and contribute toward optimal metabolism.

Poor stress and cortisol control will sabotage your healthy aging goals.
You must control the **rage**, or you will **rapidly age!**
If you are not at **ease**, you will get dis**ease**.

CHAPTER 6

QUESTIONS

Student:

I have a prescription for an antianxiety medication. Wouldn't that be an effective stress reducer?

Professor:

We all have stress. Our responses to stress are the key. Taking a prescription to blunt the stress response does not fortify our wellness. Eliciting the relaxation response with stress-reduction techniques allows your body to de-stress without sedating medications. Our goal would be to gradually wean you off the antianxiety medication.

Student:

Do I have to meditate? I think it's boring.

Professor:

Meditation is proven to decrease your risk of many health problems, primarily because of its ability to lower cortisol levels. However, it is not the only effective stress reducer.

What is most important is to do something just for you every day. Take at least twenty to thirty minutes to relax, read, walk, garden, do a crossword puzzle, have sex, have sex while doing a crossword puzzle ... whatever you enjoy. Just do it every day to elicit the relaxation response.

Student:

I have had a lifelong struggle with my weight. I must admit I am constantly stressed and never take time to smell the roses. Do you think my constant stress level is contributing to my weight gain?

Professor:

Yes, I do. I am impressed that you have made the connection, because most of us don't. Without a doubt, stress increases and maintains body fat. High cortisol from chronic stress adversely affects metabolism, lowers lean body mass, and increases body fat. If you eat well and follow a stress-reduction program, you will lose excess body fat. No doubt, stress reduction will result in fat loss.

Student:

Why does stress-induced illness often involve our digestive system?

Professor:

Stress-induced illness can and does affect every system in the body. We do see many digestive symptoms because of stress. Abdominal pain, bloating, ulcers, bleeding, nausea, diarrhea, and constipation are frequently stress-related complaints.

Remember the influences of the sympathetic and parasympathetic components of the nervous system. The parasympathetic system supports normal digestion. The sympathetic system, because it only activates body systems needed for immediate survival, actually shuts off the digestive system. When we constantly activate the sympathetic system with stress, we impair normal digestion of food, and we impair the normal function of the stomach, colon, and digestive enzymes.

When we elicit the relaxation response, we activate the parasympathetic nervous system with subsequent improvement of normal digestive functions.

Stress can increase the risk of any disease, including cancer, dementia, and heart disease. Because stress impairs our immune system function, we are susceptible to all types of illness.

Student:

Since exercise is stressful to the body, why do you consider it an effective stress reducer?

Professor:

The right type and duration of exercise is an amazing stress reducer. Yes, exercise is a stress to the body, but with an intelligent exercise program, as we discussed, the body responds to this exercise-induced stimulus to become stronger, leaner, and healthier.

Exercise is a great way to burn off nervous energy. Think again about the body's sympathetic stress response. The goal of the sympathetic response is to ready us for a fight-or-flight. When we do neither, our bodies try to keep us tense and ready to battle the stressor.

Exercise is the body's natural way of utilizing this sympathetic response in an effective manner. We use this pent-up nervous energy during our exercise session and defuse the stress response in a productive manner. When we remain sedentary, this nervous energy builds up and gradually breaks us down. A sedentary lifestyle accelerates the aging process.

Student:

I understand the benefits of stress-reduction techniques but find it difficult to fit them into my schedule. Any tips?

Professor:

Stress-reduction techniques truly do not require much time. One suggestion is to add some breathing exercises a few times during the day. Do the following three or four times daily: Clear your mind. Focus only on your breathing. Take three slow, deep breaths. Breathe in through your nose and out through your mouth. Breathe in slowly and exhale slowly. Think only about your breathing. If you start thinking about something else before completing three slow breaths, then start over again. You will find this very relaxing.

I do this when I wake up in the morning before getting out of bed. I do it again while driving to and from work, when stopped at red lights. Then I try to do it a few times at work during the day, especially during stressful periods. It is simple, brief, effective and takes minimal time.

At first, you will find that you start thinking about something else before you complete three breaths. If so, start again. Eventually, you will be able to clear your mind, take the slow, deep breaths, and feel restored.

Student:

I read that married people live longer than single people. Is that because married life is less stressful?

Professor:

Yes ... or it could be that life just *seems* longer when you are married!

What does the medical and scientific literature reveal about stress?

❖ Death rates from heart disease and cancer are four to seven times higher among people who harbor hostile attitudes.

❖ People who reported a history of workplace stress over the previous ten-year period developed colon and rectal cancer at a rate 5.5 times greater than that of unstressed people.

❖ A study on meditation showed that twice-daily meditation reduces the thickness of the blood vessel–obstructing plaques (atherosclerosis) that form in carotid arteries.

❖ Meditation can lower the blood pressure in hypertensive people down to blood pressure levels comparable to those achieved with prescription drugs.

❖ Studies show that people who meditate on a daily basis reduce their health-care utilization by 50 to 55 percent compared with people who do not meditate.

❖ Multiple studies confirm improved cortisol control with meditation.

❖ Analysts estimate that $200 billion a year is lost to industry from stress-related ailments.

❖ Sleep deprived people have increased blood pressure, increased blood glucose levels, and increased markers of inflammation (i.e., increased C-reactive protein.)

❖ People who consistently get six hours or less sleep per day have shorter life spans than people who sleep seven to eight hours a day.

❖ Sleep deprivation increases rate of obesity.

❖ People who are sleep deprived have physiologic abnormalities that increase appetite and caloric intake.

- A University of California study found that chronic stress adversely affects three biological factors involved with cellular aging.

- Depression increases inflammation and impairs immune function.

- Depressed people had a fourfold greater risk of heart attack compared to nondepressed people.

- Higher levels of inflammatory markers were measured in patients with major depression.

- High levels of stress hormones cortisol and norepinephrine contribute to the development of metabolic syndrome.

- Both depression and heart disease are associated with low concentrations of omega-3 fatty acids in red blood cells.

- Depressed people have higher blood levels of homocysteine (a cardiac risk factor.)

- A Duke University study found that heart patients who exercise and learn anger management are less likely to suffer angina episodes.

- A 1996 study measured cortisol levels in women with both early-stage and metastatic breast cancer. Both groups had higher levels of cortisol compared to women without breast cancer. In addition, those with metastatic breast cancer had higher cortisol levels than women with early-stage breast cancer.

- The journal *Lancet Oncology* reported that evidence from both animal and human studies suggests that stress and depression impair the immune system and might promote the initiation and progression of some types of cancer.

- Mayo Clinic researchers reported a study revealing that heart disease patients with the highest stress levels had markedly increased rates of rehospitalization and reoccurrence of further heart disease–related problems, including heart attacks and cardiac arrest.

❖ The *European Heart Journal* reported a twenty-one-year study of approximately 14,000 patients that found chronic stress is an independent risk factor for heart disease and stroke.

❖ Research found that high cortisol levels can promote degeneration and death of neurons (brain cells) as well as decreased memory in healthy elderly people.

❖ The journal *Neurology* reported that chronic stress is associated with the risk of developing Alzheimer's disease. The study found that people who were prone to experiencing high levels of stress had twice the risk of developing Alzheimer's disease compared to those who were not prone to stress.

❖ Study found that exercise training can reduce the cortisol response to stress as well as the higher levels of cortisol found with aging.

❖ Vitamin C has been shown to decrease stress-induced cortisol levels. One study found that marathon runners who supplemented with vitamin C had significantly lower post-race cortisol levels compared to those runners taking a placebo.

❖ A study discovered that people who were given vitamin C supplementation before being subjected to psychological stress had lower blood pressure and lower cortisol levels compared to those who were given placebos.

❖ Research found that fish oil supplementation reduced cortisol levels of people subjected to a battery of mental stress tests.

❖ Multiple studies report a link between central obesity (abdominal fat) and elevated cortisol levels.

❖ Published studies have demonstrated that high levels of stress are significantly linked to the frequency of respiratory infections, rates of exacerbations of multiple sclerosis, and irritable bowel syndrome.

And much more …

CONCLUSION

I hope you have enjoyed the class. You have learned how to change your health and your life. You now understand what you need to do to allow you to reclaim and maintain your health.

The results are indeed amazing—better energy, better moods, better bodies. You will be stronger, leaner, and more resistant to illness. You will dramatically decrease the risk of obesity, diabetes, heart disease, osteoporosis, and cancer. In fact, you will rarely even catch a cold or the flu.

You will look and feel significantly younger because you will be biologically younger. You will lead an active life. You will not only be there for your children and grandchildren, but you will also be an active participant in their lives. A grandfather playing basketball with his grandson … a grandmother playing tennis with her granddaughter … we want you spending your life being active and feeling your best instead of sitting in a waiting room feeling unwell.

Apply what you have learned in this course. Don't allow the media or "government recommendations" confuse you about what is healthy. And certainly don't let the pharmaceutical companies convince you that multiple prescription medications are required for good health.

Here is a guarantee for you: none of the top ten prescription medications will improve your health. Getting on prescription medications becomes a snowball effect. You take one pill, develop side effects, and need a second pill to decrease the side effects. The second pill gives you other problems, and you then need a third pill … on and on it goes—until you are financially drained and no healthier than when you started.

Certainly, some of us require prescription medications for the rest of our lives. Yes, I prescribe medications when they are necessary for pain control, to fight infection, to control erratic hearts, to open wheezing lungs, to stop seizures. But a short course of a medication to treat an acute medical condition is vastly different from taking daily medications for the rest of your life. Our goal is to minimize or eliminate these chronic medications traditionally used for health and well-being.

With our antiaging lifestyle, we can often eliminate prescription medications. Frequently after patients participate in our diet, supplement, hormone, and exercise programs, we find significant improvements in blood pressure, cholesterol levels, blood glucose levels, and body weight. Because of these objective improvements, patients are able to wean off blood pressure and cholesterol medications, or at the minimum, we can reduce dosages of these medications. Even in diabetic patients on oral diabetic medications, we can quite often reduce dosages or eliminate these medications completely.

With our bioidentical hormone replacement programs, we find that patients increase their bone density each year. Because of this increased bone density, we usually eliminate expensive medications that only decrease the rate of bone loss. With hormone replacement, especially with the bioidentical hormone pellet program, we have had patients previously diagnosed with osteopenia or osteoporosis restore normal bone density.

There are numerous sources of health and wellness information available. Some sources are outstanding; others are, frankly, worthless. Don't let the variability in quality deter you from learning about wellness. With your new knowledge, you will be able to discriminate quality information from poor-quality information.

No doubt you will be exposed to health and aging advice from books, magazines, Internet, friends, families, various health professionals, and health authorities like your neighbors. By all means, read, listen, and learn. See if the information is consistent with your healthy aging goals. If it is, go for it. If not, ignore it.

By learning the eight healthy aging goals, you have empowered yourself to make healthy decisions for the rest of your life.

Just think—this program encourages you to do the following so you can be healthy:

Eat more.
Exercise less.
Relax more.
Spend more money. (Oops!)

Don't forget your goals:

1) Control insulin levels.
2) Control glucose levels.
3) Control cortisol levels.
4) Optimize cell function.
5) Control free radicals.
6) Control hormone levels.
7) Optimize metabolism.
8) Control inflammation.

> Stay on target and age well.

FINAL QUESTIONS

Student:

My father has a vintage mustang that he treats like a baby. He keeps it tuned and clean and always takes care of it. It looks new. Your *Antiaging 101* program seems to take care of our bodies just as my father takes care of his car. Any thoughts?

Professor:

I think it raises a great analogy, and it also raises some interesting points. Most of us treat our cars better than we treat ourselves. We only use the best fuel for our cars, yet we don't hesitate to put "junk" in our bodies. We get frequent tune-ups and oil changes but never bother to check our own blood tests. We know when our car filters were changed, when we last changed the oil, and when we last rotated the tires, but we don't know our own glucose levels, insulin levels, or hormone levels.

We would never drive with low fuel or oil, but we go hours with low nutrient levels. We would never take our sports cars off-road, but we constantly veer off the road to health.

We know that if we follow the maintenance program for our vehicles, we will maximize the car's performance. Yet we hesitate to get on a healthy antiaging program to enhance our own performance.

Certainly, our bodies are a much more complex machine than even the most expensive automobile. If we stay on our healthy aging program, we will get more miles and show less signs of wear and tear. We may not "look new," but we will look, feel, and be younger.

Student:

You have been an emergency physician for over twenty years, and you still practice emergency medicine—so how did you get involved with antiaging medicine? Also, don't the two philosophies conflict with each other?

Professor:

I love acute care medicine and enjoy working with and learning from physicians from other specialties. These physicians have devoted many years of their lives in training to give the best medical care possible.

I have always been interested in wellness. Specifically with what can be done to stay healthy and to slow the aging process.

Over the twenty-plus years that I have been an emergency physician, the biggest impact on my healthy-aging philosophy has been watching patients change over the years. More and more patients are obese. More and more patients are morbidly obese. More young people have diabetes, high blood pressure, and heart disease. Most of the patients are on multiple prescription medications.

I am amazed at how people in their twenties and thirties look ten to twenty years older than they actually are. It seems the health of most people in this country is going in the wrong direction, yet we have better medical technology, better treatment options, and better medications.

There is a disconnect between the advances in health care and the deteriorating health care of patients. By witnessing this change in patients' health over the years, it became apparent to me that many of the patients' health issues could have avoided. Many of the health problems that brought them into the ER could have been eliminated, or at least improved, with some basic lifestyle adjustments.

For many patients, simply changing to a healthy diet while simultaneously avoiding chemicals in processed foods could have a dramatic impact on their overall health. For other patients, simply participating in an exercise program could change their health.

It is true that time restrictions in medicine really don't allow physicians a chance to take the time necessary to explain a healthy diet or healthy exercise program. By setting up a separate antiaging practice, I have the luxury of spending time with patients to "tune up" their lifestyles in order to improve health.

In the ER, I will deal with acute medical problems in a timely fashion. In the office, I will take extra time to explain how our day-to-day lifestyle decisions can dramatically improve our health and decrease the chance of ending up in the ER.

Student:

Our medical system is highly subspecialized. Do you think antiaging medicine will become subspecialized?

Professor:

There are certainly numerous benefits, given the vast expansion of medical breakthroughs, to subspecialization. These subspecialists can do amazing procedures to help heart attack or stroke victims, or to repair a traumatized limb or injured brain.

The advances in critical care medicine and transplant surgery alone are truly astounding. The advances throughout all medical specialties are overwhelming.

However, while medicine is broken down into specific specialists, our bodies are not. The trillions of cells in the body communicate with each other. What is good for heart cells is good for brain cells is good for skin cells ... and so on. This leads us to a unifying approach of "cellular medicine," which is more beneficial for preventative care.

So while specialists are essential when things are "broken," a unifying approach to aging and wellness is more effective for keeping us healthy in the first place.

As we learn more about what makes us tick, we will find more common ground for wellness and optimal health. The eight goals of healthy aging are perfect examples of how unifying themes affect all areas of health and aging.

Student:

Many of the suggestions regarding diet, exercise, supplements, and hormones in *Antiaging 101* are quite a bit different from "mainstream" opinions and, in fact, are often polar opposite opinions of those I have heard or read before. Do you think there are a lot of myths regarding wellness ... or just disagreements about the best plans?

Professor:

Your question is insightful. I believe there are numerous "myths" regarding diet, exercise, supplements, and hormone therapy. These myths are difficult to dispute, as they have become entrenched within the wellness world. Here is a list of some of the most common wellness myths:

Eating fat makes you fat.
Dietary fat raises your cholesterol level.
Dietary fat causes heart disease.
Cholesterol causes heart disease.
The calorie theory of weight loss is an effective tool for losing weight.
Vegetarian diets are the healthiest diets.
Red meat is unhealthy.
Aerobics is the best cardiovascular exercise.
Aerobics is the best exercise for weight loss.
You get all the nutrients you need from your diet.
Grains are good for your health.
The food pyramid has been proven to improve health.
Your cancer risk is primarily determined by genetics.
Your risk of heart disease is primarily determined by genetics.
Bioidentical hormones cause cancer.
High-protein diets cause kidney failure.

Student:

Given that long list of myths, how do we know what to believe?

Professor:

If you want to pass this course, you'd better believe me! Seriously, though, it is a difficult question to answer briefly. Many of the myths are simply assumptions that have been passed on over time. For example, it would seem logical that eating fat makes you fat. There is just one problem with that logic: it is erroneous. It does not make biochemical sense.

When we look at the science, none of these common myths survive. However, when people have a vested interest in any of these myths, it is difficult to change minds, regardless of science. Remember, the earth is flat and the sun revolves around the earth. Many former "truths" in science and medicine have taken decades, even centuries, until they were finally disproved. Frankly, with antiaging, I don't want to wait until society catches up.

Probably the best approach with any of these myths is to look at them from a perspective of how the body works. Does a statement or theory seem logical if we look at the physiology of the body and, specifically, how cells function?

If every cell in the body is enveloped in a fat-filled membrane, does it make sense to limit healthy fat intake?

If the brain is sixty percent fat, does it make sense to be on a low-fat diet? If the body produces 90 percent of its cholesterol, regardless of the amount of cholesterol in the diet, does it make sense to limit cholesterol intake?

If over 50 percent of heart attack patients have normal cholesterol, does it seem logical that cholesterol is a major cause of heart disease?

If every cell in the body requires hormones for optimal function, would it be beneficial to have deficient hormone levels?

Since we have an exponential rise in the number of obese and diabetic patients, most of whom have high glucose and insulin levels, does it make sense to keep them on a low-fat, high-carbohydrate diet—a diet proven to raise glucose and insulin levels?

I could continue, but I think you get the picture.

Another option is to simply evaluate how you feel ... and your response to any of the above myths. If it is good for your body, you will feel well over time, and you will notice a positive impact on your health and well-being. Specifically, you will have improvement in the antiaging goals outlined in this course.

Finally, prior to starting a diet, exercise program, or hormone program, obtain some objective lab tests. Get a body scan to measure body fat and muscle mass. Draw blood for a fasting glucose, insulin, and lipid panel. Try the new program for six months and then repeat the tests. Find out if your results improve. The body scans and blood tests don't lie.

Student:

What about the gold standard double-blinded, placebo-controlled studies?

Professor:

What are you, a spy for the drug companies?

A double-blinded, placebo-controlled study requires control of all variables except one. In other words, if we are testing a medication or supplement, everything and everyone should be the same except that some take the tested product and some take a placebo (sugar pill).

It is impossible to control for all variables. With a study of a diet or supplement, imagine finding a group of people where each has the same metabolism, same stress levels, same genetics, same body weight, same exercise level, same alcohol use, same prescription drug use … It is not going to happen.

Yes, we can and should look at those studies, but they can't be the only source of research information.

We must also remember that just because a double-blinded, placebo-controlled study has not been done does not mean that a diet, supplement, hormone isn't beneficial.

We must look at all the scientific evidence as well as all the clinical evidence to assess a lifestyle decision fully.

Student:

How about waiting for FDA endorsement before starting on something?

Professor:

Because you will die waiting.

The FDA's job is to evaluate the safety of a drug or supplement, not to find the best treatment or option available. For example, they will determine if a medication is safe enough to give to the public, but they will not determine if there are better or healthier options. Remember, your natural hormones are not drugs; the D in FDA is for *drug* evaluation.

Student:

Why do you feel that counting calories doesn't matter?

Professor:

Calorie counting is a waste of your time. Following the calorie theory of weight loss is ineffective. More important than counting the number of calories in your diet, or counting the number of calories you burn with exercise, is eating nutrient-dense real food and avoiding nutrient-poor processed foods.

Certainly, eating too few calories is unhealthy and eating excessive amounts of high-calorie processed foods is unhealthy, but assuming that all calories are created equal leads to unhealthy diets.

Let's look into calories and metabolism to give you a better idea of what I'm talking about. Calories are simply a unit of measure of the amount of energy released when the body breaks down food. Carbohydrates and protein have four calories per gram, and fat has nine calories per gram.

The number of calories per gram does not tell you anything about how the body utilizes specific macronutrients (fat, protein, carbohydrates), nor does it give you any information on the impact the macronutrients have on metabolism.

The number of calories in a meal or snack gives us no useful information on how those calories impact your metabolism, your blood glucose level, your insulin level, or your cortisol level.

To avoid fat because it has more calories per gram than carbohydrates will be detrimental to your health, yet this is encouraged by many nutritionists, physicians, and other health professionals.

We need to focus on supplying the body with appropriate nutrients instead of counting calories. Of course, I don't want you eating excessive calories, but if you eat real food as we discussed in this course, your calorie intake will actually decrease and become self-regulating.

The most common misconception is that creating a calorie deficit, i.e., fewer calories in, with more calories burned, will lead to burning fat. Most of the calories burned during a twenty-four-hour day are burned from "basal metabolism." This is the amount of calories required to run the body and keep you breathing, thinking, moving, and even sleeping.

The basal metabolism represents the majority of calories burned every day. Physical activity burns a small percentage of calories. The high-calorie requirement of your basal metabolism, and the minimal percentage of calories burned with physical exercise, is important to understand for two reasons.

First, if you eat fewer calories than needed for your basal metabolism, your body will go into starvation mode and you will become catabolic. This will lead to bone loss, muscle loss, suppressed immune function, and poor health.

Second, if you chase the calorie theory by exercising obsessively, you will become frustrated and catabolic. By combining calorie restriction with excessive exercise, you will become an elite member of the "pale and frail" club.

Your body is hardwired to keep you eating to supply the body with needed nutrients. Restricting calories stresses your body. No matter how much willpower you think you have, your body will send numerous signals for you to eat—because if you don't eat, your body knows you will die. This will lead to tremendous food cravings and, ultimately, poor food choices.

Support your body and your health: Eat real food and avoid junk food. Don't worry about calories in versus calories out. Become a proactive eater of healthy proteins, healthy carbohydrates, and healthy fats.

Student:

If I follow the *Antiaging 101* program, can I stop my prescription medications?

Professor:

Don't stop any medications without medical guidance. After all, if I am sued, I won't be able to teach this class or write the course manual for the 202-level courses!

However, in most situations, you will dramatically reduce the need for prescription medications—and frequently eliminate them completely.

Prescription medications are great when needed. You certainly should not stop needed medications without input from your physician. Some of us will require prescription medications for the rest of our lives.

I am not against prescription medications, and I prescribe them on a daily basis. I am against using prescription medications when lifestyle modalities are a more effective option.

If a patient is not willing to change his diet or start an exercise program, or consistently take supplements or necessary hormones, then a prescription may be the only option. Medications may be needed if lifestyle changes aren't successful enough in improving your health.

Student:

I always thought antiaging was about living as long as possible, but this course seems to emphasize living healthy as opposed to living longer. Do you agree?

Professor:

I would definitely agree. Many antiaging practitioners dislike the term "antiaging," as it implies a negative connotation regarding aging. Many people assume that the antiaging focus is about extending lifespan.

You will notice other terminology such as "age management" or "quality of life medicine" or even "rejuvenation medicine." This other nomenclature is an attempt to remove the negative connotation implicit in the term "antiaging."

Although you will maximize your life span with this type of program, the real goal is to improve your "health span." In other words, we strive to keep you healthy for as long as possible. *What is the point of life extension without quality of life and optimal health?*

In addition, it is important to realize that none of the *Antiaging 101* modalities would lengthen your life at the expense of jeopardizing the quality of your life or your health. We don't recommend any supplements, hormones, or lifestyle changes that would increase your risk of health problems.

Everything suggested is safe and works to improve health and decrease the risk of all degenerative diseases. The main goal is to slow the accelerated aging process that is so prevalent. The second goal is to promote healthy aging.

Student:

I have noticed that many supplements are marketed as having "antiaging" benefits. How do we know if they are legitimate?

Professor:

Indeed, many antiaging supplements exist. Many are beneficial; many are worthless.

We did review some great supplements in this course. Although you won't wake up ten years younger with these supplements, they can slow the aging process. In fact, a recent study found that people who simply supplement daily with a multivitamin have longer telomeres. Longer telomeres translate into longer life.

If the supplements positively influence any of our eight antiaging goals, then they will help slow the deterioration of the aging process. For example, if the supplement lowers glycation, inflammation, or oxidation, then it will contribute to healthy aging.

Student:

Isn't an antiaging program expensive?

Professor:

Yes, but you're worth it!

Student:

Would you give us a sample week on an antiaging program, including meal examples as well as frequency of exercise and stress-reduction sessions? I'm not sure I can do all this every day.

Professor:

Sure. It is important to understand that this new lifestyle is not time consuming nor difficult to maintain. Remember, it is not about perfection.

Some things you should attempt to do daily, but many antiaging modalities are effective even if you are not compliant every day. Just do your best to make the program a habit.

Try to take your supplements and any prescribed hormones every day. Try to eat well, exercise, and practice stress-reduction techniques on most days.

A week in the life of an antiaging program

MONDAY

8:00 AM
Breakfast: vegetable, three-egg omelet, grapefruit, coffee, water
Dose of supplements
Dose of bioidentical hormones (if directed)

Noon
Lunch: chicken Caesar salad, bowl of berries, iced tea

3:00 PM
Snack: apple slices dipped in natural peanut butter, water

5:00 PM
Exercise: thirty-minute weight training session

6:00 PM
Dinner: grilled salmon, salad with oil and vinegar, green beans, bowl of blueberries, glass of red wine, water
Dose of supplements

8:00 PM
Snack: cup of raw almonds

9:00 PM
Stress reducer: reading for pleasure for one hour

10:00 PM
Dose of hormones
Lights out

TUESDAY

7:00 AM
Exercise: twenty-minute interval-training session

8:00 AM
Breakfast: three fried eggs, plain organic yogurt with berries, coffee, water
Dose of supplements
Dose of hormones (if directed)

10:00 AM
Snack: protein shake, handful of raw walnuts

Noon
Lunch: tuna salad with almonds, vegetables, pine nuts, whole orange, water

12:30 PM
Stress reducer: fifteen-minute walk

4:00 PM
Snack: organic cottage cheese with sliced peaches

7:00 PM
Dinner: grilled chicken breasts, broccoli, salad with oil and vinegar, bowel of berries, water
Dose of supplements

10:00 PM
Dose of hormones
Lights out

WEDNESDAY

7:00 AM

Breakfast: three-egg omelet with Canadian bacon, grapefruit, coffee, water
Dose of supplements
Dose of hormones (if directed)

8:00 AM

Exercise: thirty-minute weight training session

10:00 AM

Snack: protein shake, apple

Noon

Lunch: open-faced turkey sandwich on organic rye bread; side salad with sunflower seeds, tomatoes, olive oil; green tea; water

3:00 PM

Snack: whole apple, handful of raw cashews, water

6:00 PM

Dinner: grilled steak fillet, salad with oil and vinegar, asparagus, bowel of berries, red wine, water
Dose of supplements

7:00 PM

Stress reducer: enjoy a comedy on DVD

11:00 PM

Dose of hormones
Lights out

THURSDAY

8:00 AM

Breakfast: protein smoothie (whey protein, berries, plain yogurt, coconut)
Dose supplements
Dose hormones

11:00 AM

Snack: grapes and almonds

Noon

Lunch: chicken lettuce wrap, broccoli, cherries, iced tea

2:00 PM

Exercise: twenty-minute interval training (power walk)

4:00 PM

Snack: apple slices with natural almond butter

6:00 PM

Dinner: grilled halibut; salsa; dinner salad with tomatoes, cucumbers, and garbanzo beans; fruit plate, water
Dose supplements

7:00 PM

Stress reducer: watch sunset while enjoying glass of wine with cheese

10:30 PM

Dose hormones
Lights out

FRIDAY

8:00 AM

Breakfast: three scrambled eggs, plain organic yogurt with berries, turkey bacon
Dose supplements
Dose hormones

11:00 AM

Stress reducer: fifteen-minute meditation session

Noon

Lunch: large Cobb salad, iced tea, fruit slices

4:00 PM

Snack: protein bar

5:30 PM

Exercise: thirty-minute weight training session

7:00 PM

Dinner: two grilled hamburgers (no bun) with lettuce, mustard, onions; dinner salad with oil and vinegar; white beans; bowl of blueberries, water
Dose supplements

9:00 PM

Snack: glass of wine, raw pistachios

11:00 PM

Dose hormones
Lights out

SATURDAY

9:00 AM
Breakfast: three-cheese omelet, pineapple slices, hot tea
Dose supplements
Dose hormones (if directed)

11:00 AM
Exercise and stress reducer: bike ride for thirty minutes

12:30 PM
Lunch: roasted turkey slices, spinach salad with pecans and beans, orange slices, water

4:00 PM
Snack: celery sticks, cheese slices, raw cashews

6:00 PM
Dinner: grilled steak fillet; salad with cucumbers, tomatoes, onions, vinaigrette; steamed cauliflower, pineapple slices
Dose supplements

11:00 PM
Dose hormones
Lights out

SUNDAY

8:00 AM
Breakfast: three-egg omelet with turkey bacon and cheese, melon slices, coffee or tea
Dose supplements
Dose hormones (if directed)

Noon
Lunch: tuna salad, organic cottage cheese, apple, iced tea

3:00 PM
Snack: protein smoothie with favorite fruit

4:00 PM
Exercise and stress reducer: hike Sabino Canyon for thirty minutes

5:00 PM
Snack: organic trail mix with raw nuts, sunflower seeds, flaxseed, water

7:00 PM
Dinner: favorite meal and favorite desert, glass of favorite wine
Dose supplements

10:00 PM
Dose hormones
Lights out

METABOLISM

In *Antiaging 101*, we have discussed the importance of maintaining an efficient metabolism. Every modality in this course impacts and improves our metabolism.

Many people complain of low energy and excess body fat. Most of these people will tell you that they have tried different diets, exercise programs, and supplements, to no avail. Becoming frustrated with these many futile attempts to get healthy, they surrender their efforts.

A natural response to this frustration is to believe that they are genetically inclined to have high body fat and low energy, and as a result, they erroneously decide that it is their destiny.

It is critical that we understand that if someone has excess body fat and/or low energy levels, it is because of an impaired metabolism. When we "fix" the impaired metabolism, excess body fat is burned and energy levels are restored.

It is no one's destiny to be heavy, weak, and exhausted! Remember the bottom line: if you have excess body fat and/or low energy, it is because your metabolism is impaired.

To restore metabolism to prime condition, we must first acknowledge that many different factors impair metabolism. All or some of these many different factors may be to blame for an individual's impaired metabolism.

To repair metabolism effectively requires that we look at all potential metabolic disruptors. It may be one factor for you yet multiple factors for someone else. When we are aware of all the possibilities, then we can correct the problems.

Let's look at the main metabolic disruptors. Most metabolic disruptors are linked to diet errors, hormone imbalances, stress, chemicals, or exercise patterns. All these disruptors are eliminated with our antiaging programs.

Most of us with excess body fat and/or low energy assume it is because we eat too much and exercise too little. Before we make that assumption, we must look deeply into the categories of metabolic disruptors.

Metabolic disruptors

Diet factors:

Protein deficiencies
Fat deficiencies
Excess processed carbohydrates
Vitamin and mineral deficiencies
Chemicals in processed foods (MSG, aspartame, trans fats, preservatives)
Deprivation diets
Excess grains
Alcohol (excessive)
High-fructose corn syrup

Chemical factors:

Artificial sweeteners
MSG
Preservatives
Smoking
Alcohol (excessive)
Sugar
Medications (prescription and nonprescription)
High-fructose corn syrup

Hormonal factors:

Thyroid deficiency
Testosterone deficiencies in men and women
Estrogen deficiency in women
Estrogen excess in men
DHEA deficiency
HGH deficiency
Cortisol excess
Insulin excess

Stress factors:

Prolonged stress response
Insufficient relaxation response
Deprivation diets
Excessive/prolonged exercise

Exercise factors:

Prolonged aerobics
Sedentary lifestyle
Insufficient resistance training

As we have discussed in class, all of these metabolic disruptors fuel catabolic metabolism and accelerate aging. Some of us are very sensitive to these metabolic disruptors, while some of us are more resistant to their influences. Regardless of our sensitivities to the metabolic disruptors, we all would be healthier if we eliminated them from our lifestyles.

When we evaluate the multiple factors involved in an impaired metabolism, we better understand why a diet program may dramatically help one person but have minimal impact on another person.

If someone has impaired metabolism from high insulin, then a low-glycemic diet with improved insulin control would be life changing.

If someone has impaired metabolism because of excess chemicals in processed foods, then elimination of those foods would have dramatic effects.

When we look at all possible factors with impaired metabolism, we can more effectively streamline our efforts. For example, I commonly see patients with impaired metabolism from hormone imbalances trying to lose excess body fat with deprivation diets. Not only is a deprivation diet unhealthy, it would have zero impact on the root cause of their excess body fat. They would become more and more frustrated with their weight loss efforts.

I frequently see patients with impaired metabolism and excess body fat go to extremes with an exercise program. Oftentimes they will spend inordinate amounts of time running or following some other prolonged aerobic program without any significant results. When we decrease their aerobic sessions and switch them to weight lifting and/or interval training, they begin to lose excess body fat and immediately restore energy levels. They get better results with less time expenditure.

When we identify the specific factors contributing to our impaired metabolism, we can create effective solutions and eliminate the frustrations of other ineffective options. When you start seeing results with your new program, it becomes self-fulfilling and self-motivating. When it works, you stay with it. When you stay with it, the program becomes a way of life instead of a temporary measure. It becomes a lifestyle.

The following is a list of anabolic metabolic enhancers and catabolic metabolic disruptors:

Anabolic	Catabolic
Interval training	Prolonged aerobics
Resistance training	Running marathons
Real, natural foods	Processed foods
Supplement program	Nutrient deficiencies
Healthy proteins	Processed foods
Healthy fats	Trans fats
Stress reduction	Stress response
Bioidentical hormones	Synthetic hormones
Organic foods	Chemical additives
Insulin control	High insulin levels
Cortisol control	High cortisol levels
Antioxidants	High fructose corn syrup

Anabolic	Catabolic
Vegetables	Aspartame
Whole fruits	Sucralose
Healthy carbohydrates	Processed grains
Organic foods	Diet foods
Whole fruits	Sugar
Olive oil	Processed oils
Water	Corn oil
Fish oil	Soda
Hormone balance	Hormone imbalances
Antioxidants	Excessive free radicals
Healthy carbohydrates	High-glycemic foods

What about telomeres?

Telomeres, the genetic material at the end of chromosomes, become progressively shorter with aging. Telomere length has been proposed as a marker of biological aging. With telomeres, length matters!

The following things shorten telomeres:

Weight gain
Insulin resistance
Excessive oxidation
Inflammation
Sedentary lifestyle (catabolic metabolism)
Excessive cortisol

The following things lengthen telomeres:

Resveratrol
Vitamin D
Reaching our antiaging goals:
Lowering inflammation
Lowering oxidative stress
Lowering glycation
Lowering cortisol
Nutraceutical supplementation

ANTIAGING TESTS

The following should be checked every six to twelve months:

1) Fasting insulin level (goal of 5 or less)

2) Fasting glucose level (goal of 70–90)

3) Hemoglobin A1C (goal of less than 5)

4) AM cortisol level (goal of 9–14)

5) Fatty acid profile (goal: omega-6 to omega-3 ratio of two to one)

6) Female hormone levels:
    Estradiol (goal minimum 70–110)
    Progesterone (goal minimum 10–15)
    Testosterone (goal minimum 50–70)
    FSH (goal less than 20)
    DHEA (goal minimum 150–350)
    IGF-1 (goal 250–290)
    TSH (goal 0.5-2.0)
    Free T3 (goal 3.0–4.0)

7) Male hormone levels:
    Total testosterone (goal 700–900)
    Free testosterone level (goal 25–35)
    DHEA-sulfate (goal 250–450)
    Estradiol (goal less than 40)
    TSH (goal 0.5–2.0)
    Free T3 (goal 3.0–4.0)
    IGF-1 (goal 250–290)

8) DEXA SCAN:
    Female body fat 20 to 25 percent
    Male body fat 15 to 20 percent
    Bone density (goal T score over -1.0)

READING LIST FOR ANTIAGING 101

Adams, Mike. *Grocery Warning.* Truth Publishing, 2005.

Agatston, Arthur. *The South Beach Diet: The Delicious, Doctor-Designed, Foolproof Plan for Fast and Healthy Weight Loss.* New York: Random House, 2003.

Arem, Ridha. *The Thyroid Solution: A Mind-Body Program for Beating Depression and Regaining Your Emotional and Physical Health.* Westminster: Ballantine Books, 1999.

Atkins, Robert C. *Dr. Atkins' Age-Defying Diet Revolution: A Powerful New Dietary Defense against Aging.* New York: Saint Martin's Press LLC, 2000.

Barnes, Broda. *Hypothyroidism: the Unsuspected Illness.* HarperCollins, 1976.

Cordain, Loren. *The Paleo Diet: Lose Weight and Get Healthy by Eating the Food You Were Designed to Eat.* Wiley, John & Sons, Incorporated, 2002.

Crayhon, Robert. *Robert Crayhon's Nutrition Made Simple: A Comprehensive Guide to the Latest Findings in Optimal Nutrition.* New York: M. Evans, 1994.

Eades, Michael R., and Mary Dan Eades. *Protein Power.* New York: Bantam Books, 1996.

Eades, Michael R., and Mary Dan Eades. *Protein Power Life Plan: A New Comprehensive Blueprint for Optimal Health.* Grand Central Publishing, 2000.

Enig, Mary G. *Know Your Fats: The Complete Primer for Understanding the Nutrition of Fats, Oils and Cholesterol*. Silver Spring: Bethesda Press, 2000.

Erasmus, Udo. *Fats That Heal, Fats That Kill: The Complete Guide to Fats, Oils, Cholesterol and Human Health*. Summertown: Alive Books, 1993.

Gittleman, Ann Louise. *The Fat Flush Plan*. McGraw-Hill Companies, 2001.

Hyman, Mark. *UltraMetabolism: The Simple Plan for Automatic Weight Loss*. New York: Simon & Schuster, 2006.

Mercola, Joseph, and Alison Rose Levy. *The No-Grain Diet: Conquer Carbohydrate Addiction and Stay Slim for Life*. New York: Penguin Group, 2004.

Ravnskov, Uffe. *The Cholesterol Myths: Exposing the Fallacy That Saturated Fat and Cholesterol Cause Heart Disease*. Washington: New Trends Publishing, 2000.

Rouzier, Neal. *How to Achieve Healthy Aging*. WorldLink Medical Publishing, 2001.

Rosedale, Ron, and Carol Colman. *The Rosedale Diet*. New York: HarperCollins, 2004.

Rubin, Jordan, and Charles F. Stanley. *The Maker's Diet*. New York: Penguin Group, 2005.

Schwarzbein, Diana, and Nancy Deville. *The Schwarzbein Principle*. Deerfield Beach: HCI, 1999.

Sears, Barry. *The Zone: A Dietary Road Map to Lose Weight Permanently: Reset Your Genetic Code: Prevent Disease: Achieve Maximum Physical Performance*. New York: HarperCollins, 1995.

Sears, Barry. *Mastering the Zone: The Next Step in Achieving SuperHealth and Permanent Fat Loss*. New York: HarperCollins, 1997.

Sears, Barry. *The Antiaging Zone*. New York: HarperCollins, 1999.

Sears, Barry. *The Omega Rx Zone: The Miracle of New High-Dose Fish Oil*. New York: HarperCollins, 2002.

Sears, Barry. *The Anti-Inflammation Zone: Reversing the Silent Epidemic That's Destroying Our Health*. New York: HarperCollins, 2005.

Taubes, Gary. *Good Calories, Bad Calories: Fats, Carbs, and the Controversial Science of Diet and Health*. New York: Anchor Books, 2007.

Ullis, Karlis, and Joshua Shackman. *The Hormone Revolution Weight-Loss Plan*. Avery, 2003.

Vliet, Elizabeth Lee. *Screaming to Be Heard: Hormonal Connections Women Suspect & Doctors Ignore.* New York: M. Evans and Company, 1995.

Wright, Jonathan, and Lane Lenard. *Maximize Your Vitality & Potency: For Men Over 40.* Smart Publications, 1999.

Supplements

Allport, Susan. *The Queen of Fats: Why Omega-3s Were Removed from the Western Diet and What We Can Do to Replace Them.* University of California Press, 2006.

Bernstein, Richard, *Dr. Bernstein's Diabetes Solution: A Complete Guide to Achieving Normal Blood Sugars.* Boston: Little Brown and Company, 1997.

Challem, Jack. *The Inflammation Syndrome: The Complete Nutritional Program to Prevent and Reverse Heart Disease, Arthritis, Diabetes, Allergies, and Asthma.* Somerset: John Wiley & Sons, 2003.

Challem, Jack, Burt Berkson, and Melissa Diane Smith. *Syndrome X: The Complete Nutritional Program to Prevent and Reverse Insulin Resistance.* Somerset: John Wiley & Sons, 2000.

Firshein, Richard. *The Nutraceutical Revolution.* Riverhead Books, 1999.

Mondoa, Emil I., and Mindy Kitei. *Sugars That Heal: The New Healing Science of Glyconutrients.* New York: Ballantine Books, 2001.

Hormones

Corio, Laura E. *The Change Before the Change: Everything You Need to Know to Stay Healthy in the Decade Before Menopause.* Westminster: Bantam Books, 2000.

Hertoghe, Thierry. *The Hormone Handbook.* International Medical Books, 2006.

Reiss, Uzzi, and Martin Zucker. *Natural Hormone Balance for Women: Look Younger, Feel Stronger, and Live Life with Exuberance.* Atria, 2001.

Shippen, Eugene, and William Fryer. *Testosterone Syndrome: The Critical Factor for Energy, Health, & Sexuality—Reversing the Male Menopause.* M. Evans and Company, 1998.

Ullis, Karlis, and Joshua Shackman. *The Hormone Revolution Weight-Loss Plan.* Avery, 2003.

Exercise

Connelly, Scott, and Carol Colman. *Body RX: Dr. Scott Connelly's 6-Pack Prescription.* Penguin Group, 2001.

Darden, Ellington. *The New High-Intensity Training: The Best Muscle-Building System You've Never Tried.* Emmaus: Rodale Press, 2004.

King, Ian, Lou Schuler, and Frederick Deluvier. *Men's Health Book of Muscle: The World's Most Complete Guide to Building Your Body.* Saint Martin's Press LLC, 2003.

Schuler, Lou, Adam Campbell, and Jeff Volek. *The Testosterone Advantage Plan: Lose Weight, Gain Muscle, Boost Energy.* Rodale Press, 2002.

Zim, Steve, and Mark Laska. *Hot Point Fitness: The Revolutionary New Program for Fast and Total Body Transformation.* Da Capo Press, 2001.

Antiaging

Cherniske, Stephen. *The Metabolic Plan: Stay Younger Longer.* New York: Random House, 2003.

Evans, William, Jacqueline Thompson, and Irwin H. Rosenberg *Biomarkers: the 10 determinants of aging you can control.* Simon & Schuster, 1991.

Klatz, Ronald, Bob Goldman, and Cherly Hirsch. *Stopping the Clock: Longevity for the New Millennium.* North Bergen: Basic Health Publications, 1996.

Kurzweil, Ray, and Terry Grossman. *Fantastic Voyage: Live Long Enough to Live Forever.* Rodale Press, 2004.

Miller, Philip Lee, Monica Reinagle, *The Life Extension Revolution: The New Science of Growing Older without Aging.* Random House, 2005.

Stress Reduction

Khalsa, Dharma Singh, and Cameron Stauth. *Meditation as Medicine: Activate the Power of Your Natural Healing Force.* Simon & Schuster, 2001.

Sapolsky, Robert. *Why Zebras Don't Get Ulcers: An Updated Guide to Stress, Stress-Related Diseases, and Coping.* W. H. Freeman Company, 1994.

HEALTHY AGING/WELLNESS WEB SITES

www.Alsearsmd.com (Al Sears, MD) Great information on benefits of caveman diet, interval training, and antiaging.

www.DrSinatra.com (Steven Sinatra, MD)

www.DrWhitaker.com (Julian Whitaker, MD)

(Dr. Sears, Dr. Whitaker, and Dr. Sinatra have excellent newsletters)

www.Bioidenticalhormonesociety.com (great source of medical references)

www.Agemed.org (Age Management Medial Group)

www.Lef.org (Life Extension)

www.Fuctionalmedicine.org (Institute for Functional Medicine)

NOTES

INTRODUCTION

1) Ebersberger, I. "Genomewide comparison of DNA sequences between human and chimpanzees." *Am J Hum Genet* 2002 Jun;70(6):1490-7.

2) Britton, RJ. "Divergence between samples of chimpanzee and human DNA sequences is 5 percent, counting indels." *Proc Natl Acad Sci* 2002 Oct 15;99(21):13633-5.

3) Sibley, CG. "The phylogeny of the hominoid primates, as indicated by DNA-DNA hybridization." *J Mol Evol* 1984;20(1):2-15.

4) Chen, FC. "Genomic divergences between humans and other hominoids and the effective population size of the common ancestor of humans and chimpanzees." *Am J Hum Genet* 2001 Feb;68(2):444-56.

5) Futterman, AD. "Immunological and physiological changes associated with induced positive and negative mood." *Psychosom Med* 1984 Nov-Dec;56(6):499-511.

6) Pray, LA. "Epigenetics: Genome, meet your environment." *The Scientist* Jul 2004;18(13):14-20 .

7) Robert, L. "Genetic, epigenetic, and posttranslational mechanisms of aging." *Biogerontology* 2010 Feb 16 (Epub ahead of print)

8) Surani, MA. "Reprogramming of genome function through epigenetic inheritance." *Nature* 2001 Nov 1;14(6859):122-8.

9) Waterland, RA. "Transposable elements: Targets for early nutritional effects on epigenetic gene regulation." *Mol Cell Biol* 2003 Aug 23(15):5293-300.

10) Willet, WC. "Balancing lifestyle and genomics research for disease prevention." *Science* 2002 Apr;296(5568):695-8.

11) Helmuth, L. "Neuroscience. Boosting brain activity from the outside in." *Science* 2001 May 18;292(5520):1284-6.

12) Javierre, BM. "Changes in the pattern of DNA methylation associate with twin discordance in systemic lupus erythematosus." *Genome Res.* 2010 Feb;20(2):170-9.

13) Pert, C. *Molecules of Emotion: The Science Behind Mind-Body Medicine.* New York: Scribner, 1993.

CHAPTER 1: GOALS OF ANTIAGING

1) Botion, LM. "Long-term regulation of lipolysis and hormone-sensitive lipase by insulin and glucose." *Diabetes* 1999 Sep;48(9):1691-7.

2) Yalow, RS. "Plasma insulin and growth hormone levels in obesity and diabetes." *Ann N Y Acad Sci* 1965 Oct 8;131(1):357-73.

3) Reaven, GM. "Role of insulin in endogenous hypertriglyceridemia." *J Clin Invest* Nov;46(11):1756-7.

4) Fontbonne, A. "Why can high insulin levels indicate a risk for coronary heart disease?" *Diabetologia* 1994 Sep;37(9):953-5.

5) Foster, D. "Insulin resistance—a secret killer?" *N Engl J Med* 1989 Mar 16;320(11):733-4.

6) Gertler, MM. "Ischemic heart disease, insulin, carbohydrate and lipid inter-relationship." *Circulation* 1972 Jul;46(1):103-11.

7) Stern, MP. "Body fat distribution and hyperinsulinemia as risk factors for diabetes and cardiovascular disease." *Arteriosclerosis* 1986 Mar-Apr;6(2):123-30.

8) Reaven, GM. "The insulin resistance syndrome: definition and dietary approaches to treatment." *Annu Rev Nutr* 2005;25:391-406.

9) Bao, W. "Persistent elevation of plasma insulin levels is associated with increased cardiovascular risk in children and young adults." *Circulation* 1996 Jan 1;93(1):54-9.

10) Mobbs, CV. "Genetic influences on glucose neurotoxicity, aging and diabetes: a possible role for glucose hysteresis." *Genetica* 1993;91(1-3):239–253.

11) Duimetiere, P. "Relationship of plasma insulin to the incidence of myocardial infarction and coronary heart disease mortality in a middle-aged population." *Diabetologia* 1980 Sep;19(3):205-10.

12) Depres, JP. "Hyperinsulinemia as an independent risk factor for ischemic heart disease." *N Engl J Med* 1996 Apr11;334(15):952-7.

13) Fontbonne, A. "Hyperisulinemia as a predictor of coronary heart disease mortality in a healthy population: the Paris Prospective Study, 15-year follow-up." *Diabetolgia* 1991 May;34(5):41-6.

14) Kaplan, NM. "The deadly quartet and the insulin resistance syndrome: an historical perspective." *Hypertens Res* 1996 Jun;19(Suppl 1):S9-11.

15) Laws, A. "Evidence for an independent relationship between insulin resistance and fasting HDL-cholesterol, triglyceride and insulin concentrations." *J Intern Med* 1992 Jan;231(1):25-30.

16) Tiley, SL. "Mixed messages: modulation of inflammation and immune responses by prostaglandins and thromboxanes." *J Clin Invest* 2001 Jul;108(1):15-23.

17) Metz S. "Lipoxygenase pathway in islet endocrine cells. Oxidative metabolism of arachidonic acid promotes insulin release." *J Clin Invest* 1983 May;71(5):1191-205.

18) Metz S. "Modulation of insulin secretion by cyclic AMP and prostaglandin E: the effects of theophylline, sodium salicylate and tolbutamide." *Metabolism* 1982 Oct;31(10):1014-103.

19) Oates, JA., "Clinical implications of prostaglandin and thrombaxane A2 formation (1)." *N Engl J Med* 1988 Sep 15;319(11):689-98.

20) Horrobin, DF. "Loss of delta-6-desaturase activity as a key factor in aging." *Med Hypothesis* 1981 Sep;7(9):1211-20.

21) Serhan, CN. "Lipoxin biosynthesis and its impact in inflammatory and vascular events." *Biochem Biophys Acta* 1994 Apr 14;1212(1):1-25.

22) Stone, KJ. "The metabolism of dihomo-gamma-linolenic acid in men." *Lipids* 1979 Feb;14(2):174-80.

23) Raheja, BS. "Significance of the N-6/N-3 ratio for insulin action in diabetes." *Ann N Y Acad Sci* 1993 Jun14;683:258-71.

24) Reaven, GM. "Banting Lecture 1988. Role of insulin resistance in human disease. 1988" *Nutrition* 1997 Jan;13(1):65.

25) Reaven, GM. "The insulin resistance syndrome: definition and dietary approaches to treatment." *Ann Rev Nutr* 2005;25: 391-406.

26) Eaton, SB. "Stone agers in the fast lane: chronic degenerative diseases in evolutionary perspective." *Am J Med* 1988 Apr;84(4):739-49.

27) Baynes, JW. "The Maillard hypothesis on aging: time to focus on DNA." *Ann N Y Acad Sci* 2002 Apr;959:360-7.

28) Cerami, A., "Glucose and aging." *Sci Am* 1987 May;256(5):90–6.

29) Chlouverakis, C. "Glucose tolerance, age, and circulating insulin." *Lancet* Apr 15;1(7494):8069.

30) Parr, T."Insulin exposure controls the rate of mammalian aging." *Mech Ageing Dev* 1996 Jul 5;88(1-2):75-82.

31) Haffner, SM. "Relationship of proinsulin and insulin to cardiovascular risk factors in nondiabetic subjects." *Diabetes* 1993 Sep;42(9):1297-302.

32) Reaven, GM. "Role of insulin resistance in human disease (syndrome X): an expanded definition." *Annu Rev Med* 1993;44:121-31.

33) Yam, D. "Insulin-cancer relationships: possible dietary implication." *Med Hypothesis* 1992 Jun;35(2):111-7.

34) LeRoith, D. "Insulin-like growth factors and cancer." *Ann Intern Med* 1995 Jan 1;122(1):54–9.

35) Pollak, MN. " Insulin and insulin-like growth factor signaling in neoplasia." *Nat Rev Cancer* 2008 Dec;8(12):915-28.

36) Baserga R. "The IGF-1 receptor in cancer biology." *Int J Cancer* 2003 Dec 20;107(6):873-7.

37) Osborne, CK. "Hormone responsive breast cancer in long-term tissue culture: effect of insulin." *Proc Natl Acad Sci* 1976 Dec;73(12):4536-40.

38) Craft, S. "Memory improvement following induced hyperinsulinemia in Alzheimer's disease." *Neurobiol Aging* 1996 Jan-Feb;17(1):123-30.

39) Arvanitakis, Z. "Diabetes mellitus and risk of Alzheimer disease and decline in cognitive function." *Arch Neurol* 2004 May;61(5):661-6.

40) Xu, W. "Mid- and late-life diabetes in relation to risk of dementia: a population-based twin study." *Diabetes* 2009 Jan;58(1):71-7.

41) Bunn, HF. "The glycosylation of hemoglobin: relevance to diabetes mellitus." *Science.* 1978 April 7;200(4337):21-7.

42) Bunn, HF. "Reaction of monosaccharides with proteins: possible evolutionary significance." *Science* 1981 Jul 10;213(4504):222-4.

43) Cerami, A. "Glucose and aging." *Sci Am* 1987 May;256(5):90-6.

44) Jenkins, DJ. Glycemic index of foods: a physiological basis for carbohydrate exchange." *Am J Clin Nutr* 1981 Mar;34(3):362-6.

45) Warburg, O. "On the origin of cancer cells." *Science* 1956 Feb 24;123(3191): 309-14.

46) Fantin,VR. "Attenuation of LDH-A expression uncovers a link between glycolysis, mitochondrial physiology, and tumor maintenance." *Cancer Cell* 2006 Jun;9(6):425-34.

47) Vaughn, AE. "Glucose metabolism inhibits apoptosis in neurons and cancer cells by redox inactivation of cytochrome c." *Nat Cell Biol* 2008 Dec;10(12):1477-83.

48) Selye, H."Studies in adaptation." *Endocrinology* 1937;21(2):169-88.

49) Orth, DN. "Cushing's syndrome." *N Engl J Med* 1995 Mar 23;332(12):791-803.

50) Simmons, PS. "Increased proteolysis. An affect of increases in plasma cortisol within the physiologic range." *J Clin Invest* 1984 Feb;73(2):412-20.

51) Epel, ES. "Stress and body shape: stress-induced cortisol secretion is consistently greater among women with central fat." *Psychosom Med* 2000 Sep-Oct;62(5):623-32.

52) Bjorntorp, P. "Do stress reactions cause abdominal obesity and comorbidities?" *Obes Rev* 2001 May;2(2):73–86.

53) Cupps, TR. "Corticosteroid-mediated immunoregulation in man." *Immunol Rev* 1982;65:133-55.

54) Sapolsky, RM. "Prolonged glucocorticoid exposure reduces hippocampal neuron number: Implications for aging." *J Neurosci* 1985 May;5(5):1222-7.

55) Sapolsky, RM. "Hippocampal damage associated with prolonged glucocorticoid exposure in primates." *J Neurosci* 1990 Sep;10(9):2897-902.

56) Lupien, SJ. "Cortisol levels during human aging predict hippocampal atrophy and memory deficits." *Nat Neurosci* 1998 May;1(1):69-73.

57) Sapolsky, RM. "The neuroendocrinology of stress and aging: the glucocorticoid cascade hypothesis." *Endocr Rev* 1986 Aug;7(3):284-301.

58) Ehrenfeucht, A. "Computation in living cells: gene assembly in ciliats." 2004.

59) Knowles, JR. "Enzyme-catalyzed phosphoryl transfer reactions." *Annu Rev Biochem.* 1980;49:877-919.

60) Singer, SJ. "The fluid mosaic model of the structure of cell membranes." *Science* 1972 Feb 18;175(23):720-31.

61) Alberts, B. *Molecular Biology of the Cell.* New York: Garland Science 2002.

62) Kovacic, P. "Mechanisms of carcinogenesis: focus on oxidative stress and electron transfer." *Curr Med Chem* 2001 Jun;8(7):773-96.

63) Harman, D. "Aging: a theory based on free radical and radiation biology." *J Gerontol* 1956;11(3):298-300.

64) McCord, JM. "Superoxide dismutase. An enzymic function for erythrocuprein." *J Biol Chem* 1969 Nov 25;244(27):6049-55.

65) Orr, WC. "Extension of life span by overexpression of superoxide dismutase and catalase in drosophila melanogaster. *Science* 1994 Feb 25;263(5150):1128-30.

66) Kristal, BS. "An emerging hypothesis: synergistic induction of aging by free radicals and Maillard reactions." *J Gerontol* 1992 Jul;47(4):B107-14.

67) Bunn, HF. "Reaction of monosaccharides with proteins: possible evolutionary significance." *Science*. 1981 Jul10;213(4504):222-4.

68) Cerami, A. "Glucose and aging." *Sci Am* 1987 May;256(5):90-6.

69) Bruning, PF. "Insulin resistance and breast-cancer risk." *Int J Cancer* 1992 Oct 21;52(4):511-6.

70) Lamberts, SW. "The endocrinology of aging." *Science* 1997 Oct 17;278(5337): 419-24.

71) Paddon-Jones, D. "Role of dietary protein in the sarcopenia of aging." *Am J Clin Nutr* 2008 May;87(5):1562S-66S.

72) Young, VR. "Protein intake and requirements with reference to diet and health." *Am J Clin Nutr*. 1987 May;45(5 Suppl):1323-43.

73) Young VR. "A theoretical basis for increasing current estimates of the amino acid requirements in adult man, with experimental support." *Am J Clin Nutr* 1989 Jul;50(1):80-92.

74) Bales, CW. "Sarcopenia, weight loss, and nutritional frailty in the elderly." *Annu Rev Nutr*. 2002;22:309-23.

75) Janssen, I. "Linking age-related changes in skeletal muscle mass and composition with metabolism and disease." *J Nutr Health Aging* 2008 Nov-Dec;9(6):408-19.

76) Becker, AE. "The role of inflammation and infection in coronary heart disease." *Annu Rev Med* 2001;52:289-97.

77) Ridker, PM. "Inflammation, aspirin, and the risk of cardiovascular events in apparently healthy men." *N Engl J Med* 1997 Apr 3;336(14):973-9.

78) Harjai, KJ. "Potential new cardiovascular risk factors: left ventricular hypertrophy,homocysteine,lipoprotein (a), and fibrinogen." *Ann Intern Med* 1999 Sep 7;131(5):376-86.

79) Lagrand, WK. "C-reactive protein as a cardiovascular risk factor: more than an epiphenomenon?" *Circulation* 1999 Jul 6;100:96-102.

80) Rader, DJ. "Inflammatory markers of coronary risk." *N Engl J Med* 2000 Oct 19;343(160:1179-82.

81) Ridker, PM. "C-reactive protein, inflammation, and coronary risk." *Cardiol Clin* 2003 Aug;21(3):315-25.

82) Rifai, N."High-sensitivity C-reactive protein: a novel and promising marker of coronary heart disease." *Clin Chem* 2001 Mar;47(3):403-11.

83) Van Lente, "Markers of inflammation as predictors of cardiovascular disease." *Clin Chim Acta* 22000 Mar;293(1-2):31-52.

84) Yudkin, JS. "Inflammation, obesity, stress, and coronary heart disease: is interleukin-6 the link?" *Atherosclerosis* 2000 Feb;148(2):209-14.

85) Serhan, CN. "Lipoxins biosynthesis and its impact on inflammatory and vascular events." *Biochem Biophys Acta* 1994;1212(1):1-25.

86) Cleland, SJ. "Endothelial dysfunction as a possible link between C-reactive protein and cardiovascular disease." *Clin Sci (Lond)* 2000 May;98(5):531-5.

87) deLongeril, M. "Mediterranean diet, traditional risk factors, and the rate of cardiovascular complications after myocardial infarction: final report of the Lyon Diet Heart Study. *Circulation* 1999 Feb 16;99(6):779-85.

88) Dreon, DM. "A very low-fat diet is not associated with improved lipoprotein profiles in men with a predominance of large, low-density lipoproteins." *Am J Clin Nut* 1999 Mar;69(3):411-18.

89) Gillman, MW "Inverse association of dietary fat with development of ischemic stroke in men." *JAMA* 1997 Dec 24-31;278(24):2145-50.

90) Hudgins, LC. "Human fatty acid synthesis is stimulated by a eucaloric low fat, high carbohydrate diet." *J Clin Invest* 1996 May 1;97(9):2081-91.

91) Jeppesen, J."Effects of low-fat, high-carbohydrate diets on risk factors for ischemic heart disease in postmenopausal women." *Am J Clin Nutr.* 1997 Apr;65(4):1027-33.

92) Katan, MB. "Should a low-fat, high-carbohydrate diet be recommended for everyone. Beyond low-fat diets." *N Engl J Med* 1997 Aug 21;337(8):563-66.

93) Ornish, D. "Serum lipids after a low-fat diet." *JAMA* 1998 May 6;279(17):1345-6.

94) Thompson, PD. "More on low-fat diets." *N Engl J Med* 1998 May 28;338(27):1623-4.

95) Williams, PT. "Low-fat diets, lipoprotein subclasses, and heart disease risk." *Am J Clin Nutr* 1999 Dec;70(6):949-50.

CHAPTER 2: OPTIMAL DIET

1) Eaton, SB. "Paleolithic nutrition revisited: a twelve-year retrospective on its nature and implications." *Eur J Clin Nutr* 1997 Apr;51(4):207-16.

2) Eaton, SB. "An evolutionary perspective enhances understanding of human nutritional requirements." *J Nutr* 1996 Jun;126(6):1732-40.

3) Cerami, A. "Glucose and aging." *Sci Am* 1987 May;256(5):90-6.

4) Rasmussen, OW. "Effects on blood pressure, glucose, and lipid levels of a high-monounsaturated fat diet compared with a high-carbohydrate diet in NIDDM subjects." *Diabetes Care* 1963 Dec;16(12):1565-71.

5) Coulston, AM. "Plasma glucose, insulin and lipid responses to high-carbohydrate, low-fat diets in normal humans." *Metabolism* 1983 Jan;32(1):52-6.

6) Farquhar, JW. "Glucose, insulin, and triglyceride responses to high- and low-carbohydrate diets in man." *J Clin Invest* 1966;45:1648-56.

7) Hudgins, LC. "Human fatty acid synthesis is stimulated by a eucaloric, high-carbohydrate diet." *J Clin Invest* 1996 May 1;97(9):2081-91.

8) Reaven, GM. "Abnormalities of carbohydrate metabolism may play a role in the etiology and clinical course of hypertension. *Trends Pharmacol Sci* 1988 Mar;9(3):78-9.

9) Wellborn, TA "Coronary heart disease incidence and cardiovascular mortality in Busselton with reference to glucose and insulin concentrations." *Diabetes Care* 1979 Mar-Apr;2(2):154-60.

10) Zavaroni, I. "Risk factors for coronary artery disease in healthy persons with hyperinsulinemia and normal glucose tolerance." *N Engl J Med* Mar 16;326(11):702-6.

11) Brownlee, M. "Negative consequences of glycation." *Metabolism* 2000 Feb;49(2 Suppl 1):9-13.

12) Eaton, SB. "*The Paleolithic Prescription.*" New York: Harper and Row, 1988.

13) Eaton, SB. "Stone agers in the fast lane: chronic degenerative diseases and evolutionary implications." *Am J Med* 1988 Apr;84(4):739-49.

14) Kekwick, A. "Metabolic study in human obesity with isocaloric diets high in fat, protein, or carbohydrate. *Metabolism* 1957 Sep;6(5):447-60.

15) Kekwick, A. "Calorie intake in relation to body-weight changes in the obese." *Lancet* 1956 Jul 28;271(6935):155-61

16) Bray, GA. "The myth of diet in the management of obesity." *Am J of Clin Nutr* 1970 Sep;23(9):1141-8.

17) Bray, GA. "Effect of caloric restriction on energy expenditure in obese patients." *Lancet* 1969 Aug 23;2(7617):397-8.

18) Evans, FA. "The treatment of obesity with low-calorie diets." *JAMA* 1931;97(15):1063-9.

19) Hirsch, J. "*Recent Advances in Obesity Research: IV.*" London: John Libbey, 1985.

20) Garrow, JS. *Energy Balance and Obesity in Man.* New York: Elsevier/North-Holland Biomedical Press,1978.

21) Stunkard, A. "The results of treatment for obesity: a review of the literature and a report of a series." *Arch Intern Med* 1959 Jan;103(1):79-85.

22) Feinstein, AR. "Treatment of obesity: an analysis of methods, results, and factors which influence success." *J Chronic Dis.* 1960 Apr;11:349-93.

23) Shetty, PS. "Adaptation to low energy intakes: the responses and limits to low intakes in infants, children and adults." *Eur J Clin Nutr.* 1999 Apr;53(Suppl 1):S14-33.

24) Gordon, ES. "Metabolic aspects of obesity." *Adv Metab Disord.* 1970;4:229-96.

25) Fruhbeck, G. "The adipocyte: a model for integration of endocrine and metabolic signaling in energy metabolism and regulation." *Am J Physiol Endocrinol Metab* 2001 Jun;286(6):E827-47.

26) Pollan, M. *The Omnivore's Dilemma.* New York: Penguin Press, 2006.

27) Pollan, M. "This Steer's Life." *New York Times Magazine.* March 31: 44,2002.

28) Unger, RH. "Glucagon and the insulin glucagon ratio in diabetes and other catabolic illnesses." *Diabetes* 1971 Dec;20(12):834-8.

29) Sadur, CN. "Insulin stimulation of adipose tissue lipoprotein lipase. Use of the euglycemic clamp technique." *J Clin Invest.* 1982 May;69(5):1119-25.

30) Westphal, SA. "Metabolic response to glucose ingested with various amounts of protein." *Am J Clin Nutr* 1990 Aug;52(2):267-72.

31) Cahill, GF. "Effects of insulin on adipose tissue." *Ann NY Acad Sci* 1959 Sept 25;82:4303-11.

32) Rabinowitz, D. "Forearm metabolism in obesity and its response to intra-arterial insulin: characterization of insulin resistance and evidence for adaptive hyperinsulinism." *J Clin Invest* 1962 Dec;41:2173–81.

33) Sims, EA. "Endocrine and metabolic adaptation to obesity and starvation." *Am J Clin Nutr* 1968 Dec;21(12):1455-70.

34) Sims, EA. "Role of insulin in obesity. *Isr J Med Sci* 1974 Oct;10(10):1222-9.

35) Unger, RH. "Glucagon and the insulin glucagon ratio in diabetes and other catabolic illnesses." *Diabetes* 1971 Dec;20(12):834-8.

36) Frayn, KN. *Metabolic Regulation: A Human Perspective.* London: Portland Press, 1996.

37) Brenner, RR. "Nutrition and hormonal factors influencing desaturation of essential fatty acids." *Prog Lipid Res* 1981;20:41-7.

38) Burr, GO. "A new deficiency disease produced by rigid exclusion of fat from the diet." *J Biol Chem* 1929 May 1;82:345-67.

39) Adam, O. "Polyenoic fatty acid metabolism and effects on prostaglandin biosynthesis in adults and aged persons." *Polyunsaturated Fatty Acids Eicosanoids*. American Oil Chemical Society Press: 213-9, 1987.

40) Kirtland, SJ. "Prostaglandin E1: a review." *Prostaglandins Leukot Essent Fatty Acids* 1988;32(3):165-74.

41) Hamberg, M. "Thromboxanes: A new group of biologically active compounds derived from prostaglandins endoperoxides." *Proc Nat Acad Sci* USA 1975 Aug;75(8):2994-8.

42) Meydani, SN. "Modulation of cytokine production by dietary polyunsaturated fatty acids." *Proc Soc Exp Biol Med* 1992 Jan;200(2):189-93.

43) Murota, S. "Involvement of eicosanoids in angiogenesis." *Adv Prostaglandin, Thromboxane Leukot Res* 1991;21:623-6.

44) Oates, JA. "Clinical implications of prostaglandin and thromboxane A2 formation(2)." *N Engl J Med.* 1988 Sep 22;319(12):761-7.

45) Reich, R. "Identification of arachidonic acid pathways required for the invasive and metastatic activity of malignant tumor cells." *Prostaglandins* 1996 Jan;51(1) :1-17.

46) Zipser, RD. "Prostaglandins, thromboxanes and leukotrienes in clinical medicine. *West J Med* 1985 Oct;143(4):485-97.

47) Clarke, SD. "Polyunsaturated fatty acid regulation of gene transcription: a mechanism to improve energy balance and insulin resistance." *Br J Nutr* 2000 Mar;83(Suppl 1):S59-66.

48) Cupps, TR. "Corticosteroid-mediated immunoregulation in man." *Immunol Rev* 1982;65:133-55. 49) Munch, A. "Glucocorticoid-induced lymphocyte death." *Cell Death in Biology and Pathology*. New York: Chapman and Hall, 329–57, 1981.

50) Sapolsky, RM. "The neuroendocrinology of stress and aging: the glucocorticoid cascade hypothesis." *Endocr Rev.* 1986 Aug;7(3):284-301.

51) Orth, DN. "Cushing's syndrome." *N Engl J Med.* 1995 Mar 23;332(12):791-803.

52) Woods, SC. Insulin and the set-point regulation of body weight. In, Novin, Wyrwicka and Bray, eds. 273–80, 1976.

53) Eckel, RH. Obesity: a disease or a physiological adaptation for survival? *Obesity: mechanisms for clinical management*. Eckel, ed. 3-30. (2003)

54) Cahill, GF. "Effects of insulin on adipose tissue." *Ann NY Acad Sci.* 1959 Sep;25:4303-11.

55) Rodin, J. "Insulin levels, hunger, and food intake: an example of feedback loops in body weight regulation." *Health Psychol.* 1985;4(1):1–24.

56) Sims, EA. "Role of insulin in obesity." *Isr J Med Sci.* 1974 Oct;10(10):1222-9.

57) Wertheimer, E. "Influence of hormones on adipose tissue as a center of fat metabolism." *Recent Prog Horm Res* 1960;16:467–95.

58) Renold, AE."Hormonal control of adipose tissue metabolism, with special reference to the effects of insulin." *Diabetologia* 1964 Aug;1(1):1432-8.

59) Zavaroni, I. "Hyperinsulinemia, obesity, and syndrome X." *J Intern Med* 1994 Jan;235(1):51-6.

60) Ascherio, A. "Trans fatty acid intake and risk of myocardial infarction." *Circulation* 1994 Jan;89(1):94-101.

61) Hill, EG. "Perturbation of the metabolism of essential fatty acids by dietary partially hydrogenated vegetable oils." *Proc Nat Acad Sci* USA 1982 Feb;79(4):953-7.

62) Laino, C. "Trans-fatty acids in margarine can increase MI risk." *Circulation* 1994;89:94-101.

63) Mensink, RP. "Effect of dietary trans fatty acids on high-density and low-density lipoproteins levels in healthy subjects." *N Engl J Med* 1980 Aug 16;323(7):439-45.

64) Willet, WC. "Intake of trans fatty acids and risk of coronary heart disease among women." *Lancet* 1993 Mar 6;341(8845):581-5.

65) Kekwick, A. "Metabolic study in human obesity with isocaloric diets high in fat, protein and carbohydrate." *Metabolism* 1957 Sep;6(5):447-60.

66) Ebbeling, CB. "Effects of a low-glycemic load vs. low-fat diet in obese young adults: a randomized trial." *JAMA* 2007 May 16;297(19):2092-102..

67) Johnston, CS. "Postprandial thermogenesis is increased 100% on a high-protein, low-fat diet versus a high-carbohydrate, low-fat diet in healthy young women." *J Am Coll Nutr* 2002 Feb;21(1);56-61.

68) Johnston, CS. "High-protein, low-fat diets are effective for weight loss and favorably alter biomarkers in healthy adults." *J Nutr* 2004 Mar;134(3):586-91.

69) Layman, DK. "Increased dietary protein modifies glucose and insulin homeostasis in adult women during weight loss." *J Nutr* 2003 Feb;133(2):405-10.

70) Layman, DK. "A reduced ratio of dietary carbohydrate to protein improves body composition and blood lipid profiles during weight loss in adult women." *J Nutr* 2003 Feb 133(2):411-7.

71) Skov, AR. "Randomized trial on protein vs. carbohydrate in ad libitum fat – reduced diet for treatment of obesity." *Int J Obes Relat Metab Disord* 1999 May;23(5):528-36.

72) Kemp, R. "The over-all picture of obesity." *Practitioner* Nov;209(253):654-60.

73) Krehl, WA. "Some metabolic changes induced by low-carbohydrate diets." *Am J Clin Nutr* 1967 Feb;20(2):139-48.

74) Hanssen, P. "Treatment of obesity by a diet relatively poor in carbohydrates." *Acta Med Scand.* 1936;88:97-106.

75) Pennington, AW. "Obesity. Overnutrition or disease of metabolism." *Am J Dig Dis.* 1953 Sep;20(9):268-72.

76) Pennington, AW. "Treatment of obesity with calorie unrestricted diets." *Am J Clin Nutr.* 1953 Jul-Aug;1(5):343-8.

77) Silverstone, JT. "The value of a low-carbohydrate diet in obese diabetics. *Metabolism* 1963 Aug;12(8):710-3.

78) Ohlson, MA. *Weight Control Through Nutritionally Adequate Diets.* In Eppright et al., eds., 170–87 (1955).

79) Thorpe, GL. "Treating overweight patients." *JAMA* 1957 Nov 16 16;165(11):1361-5.

80) Pena, L. "A comparative study of two diets in the treatment of primary exogenous obesity in children." *Acta Paediatr Acad Sci Hung.* 1979;20(1):99-03.

81) Wilder, RM. "Diseases of metabolism and nutrition." *Arch Intern Med* 1936;57(2):422-71.

82) Yudkin, J. "The low-carbohydrate diet in the treatment of obesity." *Postgrad Med.* 1972 May;51(5);151-4.

83) Young, CM. "Weight reduction using a moderate-fat diet.1. Clinical responses and energy metabolism." *J Am Diet Assoc* 1952 May;28(5):410-6.

84) Leith, W. "Experiences with the Pennington diet in the management of obesity." *Can Med Assoc* 1961 Jun 24;84:1411-4.

85) Epstein, SS. "Unlabeled milk from cows treated with biosynthetic growth hormones: a case of regulatory abdication." *Int J Health Serv* 1996;26(1):173-85.

86) Epstien, SS. "The chemical jungle: today's beef industry.) *Int J Health Serv* 1990;20(2):277-80.

87) Epstein, SS. "Potential public health hazards of biosynthetic milk hormones." *Int J Health Serv* 1990;20(1):73-84.

88) Hasler, WL. "Celiac sprue as a possible cause of symptoms in presumed irritable bowel syndrome." *Gastroenterology* 2002 Jun;122(7):2086-7.

89) Hoey, J. "Irritable bowel syndrome: could it be celiac disease?" *CMAJ* Feb 19(166)4:479-80.

90) Radlovic, N. "Effect of gluten-free diet on the growth and nutritional status of children with celiac disease." *Srp Arh Celok Lek* 2009 Nov–Dec;137(11–12):622-7.

91) Zwolinska-Wcislo, M. "Celiac disease and other autoimmunological disorders coexistance." *Przegl Lek* 2009;66(7):370-2.

92) Blaylock, R. *"Excitotoxins: The Taste That Kills."* New Mexico: Health Press, 2006.

93) Olney, JW. "Increasing brain tumor rates: is there a link to aspartame?" *J Neuropath Exp Neurol* 1996 Nov;55(11):1115-23.

94) Hall, WL. "Physiological mechanisms mediating aspartame-induced satiety." *Physiol Behav* 2003 Apr;78(4-5):557-62.

CHAPTER 3: NUTRACEUTICAL SUPPLEMENTATION

1) Xu, Q."Multivitamin use and telomere length in women." *Am J Clin Nutr* 2009 Jun;89(6):1857-63.

2) Bouwens, M. "Fish-oil supplementation induces anti-inflammatory gene expression profiles in human mononuclear cells." *Am J Clin Nutr* 2009 Aug;90(2):415-24.

3) Imal, SI. A possibility of nutraceutical as an antiaging intervention. Activation of sirtuins by promoting mammalian NAD biosynthesis. *Pharm Res* (epub ahead of print) (2010 Jan 18).

4) Frojdo, S. "Metabolic effects of resveratrol in mammals—a link between improved insulin action and aging." *Curr Aging Sci.* 2008 Dec;1(3):145–51.

5) Farzaneh-Far, R. "Association of marine omega-3 fatty acid levels with telomeric aging in patients with coronary heart disease." *JAMA* 2010 303(3):250-7.

6) Harman, D. "Aging: a theory based on free radical and radiation chemistry. *J Gerontol 1956* Jul;11(3):298–300.

7) Harman, D. "The biological clock: the mitochondria?" *J Am Geriatr Soc* 1972 Apr;20(4):145-7.

8) Kirkwood, TB. "A network theory of aging: the interactions of defective mitochondria, aberrant proteins, free radicals and scavengers in the aging process." *Mutat Res* 1996 May;316(5-6):209-36.

9) Hagen, TM. "Feeding acetyl-L-carnitine and lipoic acid to old rats significantly improves metabolic function and ambulatory activity." *Proc Natl Acad Sci* 2002 99:1870-5.

10) Fletcher, RH. "Vitamins for chronic disease prevention in adults." *JAMA* 2002 Jun 19;287(23):3127-9.

11) Nestle, M. *Food Politics*. Berkeley: University of California Press, 2002.

12) Panel of Dietary Antioxidants and Related Compounds. *Dietary Reference Intakes for Vitamin C, Vitamin E, Selenium and Carotenoids*. Washington, D.C.:National Academy Press (2000).

13) Alberts, B. *Molecular Biology of the Cell*. New York: Garland Publishing, Inc., 1934.

14) Voet, D. *Fundamentals of Biochemistry*, 2nd ed. John Wiley and sons, Inc., 547, 2008.

15) Harper, A. "Defining the Essentiality of Nutrients." *Modern Nutrition in Health and Disease*, 9th ed., M. E. Shills, ed. Baltimore, MD: Williams and Wilkins, 1999.

16) Decombaz, J. "Effect of L-carnitine on submaximal exercise metabolism after depletion of muscle glycogen." *Med Sci Sports Exerc* 1993 Jan;25(6):733-40.

17) Hagen, TM. "Acetyl-L-carnitine fed to old rats partially restores mitochondrial function and ambulatory activity." *Proc Natl Acad Sci* 1998 Aug;95)16):9562-6.

18) Hagen, TM. "Feeding acetyl-L-carnitine and lipoic acid to old rats significantly improves metabolic function while decreasing oxidative stress." *Proc Natl Acad Sci* 2002 Feb 19;99(4):1870-5.

19) Fosslien, E. "Mitochondrial medicine—molecular pathology of defective oxidative phosphorylation." *Ann Clin Lab Sci* 2001 Jan;7(1):25-67.

20) Packer, L. "Vitamin E is nature's master antioxidant." *Sci Am: Sci Med* 1994 April 1(1):54-63.

21) Pedrielli, P. "Antioxidant synergy and regeneration effect of quercetin, (-)- epicatechin, and (+)-catechin on alpha-tocopherol in homogenous solutions of peroxidating methyl linoleate." *Agric Food Chem* 2002 Nov 20;50(24):7138-44.

22) Tanaka, T. "Chemoprevention of mouse urinary bladder carcinogenesis by the naturally occurring carotenoid astaxanthin." *Carcinogenesis* 1994 Jan;15(1):15-9.

23) Jyonouchi, H. "Immunomodulatory actions of carotenoids: enhancement of in vivo and in vitro antibody production to T-dependent antigens." *Nutr Cancer* 1994;21(1):47-58.

24) Gerster, H. "Antioxidant protection of the ageing macula." *Age Ageing* 1991 Jan;20(1):60-9.

25) Aoi, W. "Astaxanthin limits exercise-induced skeletal and cardiac muscle damage in mice." *Antioxid Reduc Signals* 2003 Feb;5:139-44.

26) Rousseau, EJ. "Protection by beta-carotene and related compounds against oxygen-mediated cytotoxicity and genotoxicity: implications for carcinogenesis and anticarcinogenesis." *Free Radic Biol Med* 1992 Oct;13(4):407-23.

27) Connor, WE. "Importance of n-3 fatty acids in health and disease." *Am J Clin Nutr* 2000 Jan;71(1 Suppl):171S-5S.

28) Eaton, SB. "Dietary intake of long-chain polyunsaturated fatty acids during the paleolithic." *World Rev Nutr Diet* 1998;83:12–23.

29) Willis, AL. *Handbook of Eicosanoids, Prostaglandins, and Related Lipids.* Boca Raton: CRC Press, 1987.

30) Ariza-Ariza, R. "Omega-3 fatty acids in rheumatoid arthritis: an overview." *Sem Arthritis Rheum* 1998;27(6):366-70.

31) Babcok, T. "Eicosapentaenoic acid(EPA): an anti-inflammatory omega-3 fat with potential clinical applications." *Nutrition* 2000 Nov-Dec;16(11-12):1116-8.

32) Belluzzi, A. "Effect of an enteric-coated fish-oil preparation on relapses in Crohn's disease." *N Engl J Med* 1996 Jun 13;334:1557-60.

33) Belluzzi, A. "Polyunsaturated fatty acids and inflammatory bowel disease." *Am J Clin Nutr* Jan;71(1 Suppl):339S-42S.

34) Blok, WL. "Modulation of inflammation and cytokine production by dietary (n-3) fatty acids." *J Nutr* 1996 Jun;126(6):1515-33.

35) Fogh, K. "Eicosanoids in inflammatory skin diseases." *Prostaglandins Other Lipid Mediat* 2000 Nov;63(1-2):43–54.

36) Robinson, DR. "Suppression of autoimmune disease by dietary n-3 fatty acids." *J Lipid Res* 1993 Aug;34(8):1435-44.

37) Bertozzi, RW. "Chemical Glycobiology." *Science* 2001 Mar 23;291(5512):2357-64.

38) Sheng-Ce, T. "Lectin microarrays identify cell-specific and functionally significant cell surface glycan markers." *Glycobiology* Jul 14;18(10):761-9.

39) Makoto, T. "Structures and functional roles of the sugar chains of human erythropoietins." *Glycobiology* 1991 Sep 1(4):337-46.

40) McGeer, EG. "The importance of inflammatory mechanisms in Alzheimer's disease." *Exp Gerontol* 1998 Aug;33(5):371-8.

41) Nunomura, A. "Involvement of oxidative stress in Alzheimer's disease." *J Neuropathol Exp Neurol* 2006 Jul;65(7):631-41.

42) Kovacic, P. "Mechanisms of carcinogenesis: focus on oxidative stress and electron transfer." *Curr Med Chem* 2001 Jun;8(7):773-96.

43) Greenberg, ER. "A clinical trial of antioxidant vitamins to prevent colorectal adenoma. Polyp Prevention Study Group." *N Engl J Med* 1994 Jul 21;331(3):141-7.

44) Rimm, EB. "Vitamin E consumption and the risk of coronary disease in men." *N Engl J Med* 1993 May 20;328:1450-6.

45) Aruoma, O. Nutrition and health aspects of free radicals and antioxidants. *Food Chem Toxicol* 1994 Jul;32(7):671–83.

46) Youn, HS. "Suppression of MyD88- and TRIF-dependent signaling pathways of Toll-like receptor by (-)- epigallocatechin-3-gallate, a polyphenol component of green tea." *Biochem Pharmacol* 2006 Sep 28;72(7):850-9.

47) Lagouge, M. "Resveratrol improves mitochondrial function and protects against metabolic disease by activating SIRT1 and PGC-1alpha. *Cell* 2006 Dec 15;127(6):1109-22.

48) Baur, JA. "Resveratrol improves health and survival of mice on a high-calorie diet. *Nature* 2006 Nov 16;444(7117):337-42.

49) Ng, TP. "Curry consumption and cognitive function in the elderly." *Am J Epidemiol* 2006 Nov 1;164(9):898-906.

50) Kulkarni, R. "Treatment of osteoarthritis with a herbomineral formulation: a double-blind, placebo-controlled, cross-over study." *J Enthnopharmocol* 1991 May-Jun;33(1-2):91-5.

51) Epstein, J. "Curcumin as a therapeutic agent: the evidence from in vitro, animal and human studies." *Br J Nutr* 2010 Jun;103(11):1545-57.

52) Brinkhaus, B. "Herbal medicine with curcumin and fumitory in the treatment of irritable bowel syndrome: a randomized, placebo-controlled, double-blind clinical trial. *Scand J Gastroenterol* 2005 Aug;40(8):936-43.

CHAPTER 4: EXERCISE

1) Kraemer, WJ. "Effects of heavy-resistance training on hormonal response patterns in younger vs. older men." *J Appl Physiol* 1999 Sep;87(3):982-92.

2) Galbo, HJ. "Glucagon and plasma catecholamine response to graded and prolonged exercise in man." *J Appl Physiol* 1975 Jan;38(1):70-6.

3) Galbo, HJ. "The effect of different diets and of insulin on the hormonal response to prolonged exercise." *Acta Physiol Scand* 1979 Sep;107(1):19-32.

4) Weltman, A. "Endurance training amplifies the pulsatile release of growth hormone: effects of training intensity." *J Appl Physiol* 1992 Jun;72(6):2188-96.

5) Vanhelder, WP. "Effect of anaerobic and aerobic exercise of equal duration and work expenditure on plasma growth hormone levels." *Eur J Appl Physiol* 1984;52(3):255-7.

6) Goldfarb, AH. "Beta-endorphin response to exercise. An update." *Sports Med* 1997 Jul;24(1):8-16.

7) Wojtaszewski, JF. "Insulin signaling and insulin sensitivity after exercise in human skeletal muscle." *Diabetes* 2000 Mar;49(3):325-31.

8) Mayer-Davis, EJ. "Intensity and amount of physical activity in relation to insulin sensitivity: the Insulin Resistance Atherosclerosis Study." *JAMA* 1998 Mar 4;279(9):669-74.

9) Viru, A. Hormones in Muscular Activity: Vol. 1. *Hormonal Ensemble in Exercise.* Boca Raton, FL: CRC Press (1983).

10) Viru, A. Hormones in Muscular Activity: Vol. II. *Adaptive Effects of Hormones in Exercise.* Boca Raton, FL: CRC Press,1983.

11) Helmrich, SP. "Physical activity and reduced occurrence of non-insulin dependent diabetes mellitus." *N Engl J Med* 1991 Jul 18;325(3):147-52.

12) Kelley, DE. "Effects of physical activity on insulin action and glucose tolerance in obesity." Med Sci Sports Exer. 1999 Nov;31(11 Suppl):S619-23.

13) Adlercreutz, H. "Effect of training on plasma anabolic and catabolic steroid hormones and the response during physical exercise." *Int J Sports Med* 1986 Jun;7(Suppl 1):27-8.

14) Hooper, SL. "Hormonal responses of elite swimmers to overtraining." *Med Sci Sport Exerc.* 1993 Jun;25(6):741-3.

15) Cumming, DC. "Hormones and athletic performance," in *Endocrinology and Metabolism,* 3rd ed. New York: McGraw-Hill, 1995.

16) Kamei, TY. "Decrease in serum cortisol during yoga exercise is correlated with alpha wave activation." *Percept Mot Skills* 2000 Jun;90(3 Pt 1):1027-32.

17) Myer, TL. "Exercise and endogenous opiates," in *Contemporary Endocrinology: Sports Endocrinology.* 31-42 Totowa, NJ.: Humana Press 31–42, 1999.

18) Lee, IM. "Associations of light, moderate, and vigorous intensity physical activity with longevity." *A J Epidemiol* 2000 151(3):293-9.

19) Smith, LL. "Cytokine hypothesis of overtraining: a physiological adaptation to excessive stress?" *Med Sci Sports Exerc.* 2000 Feb;32(2):317-31.

20) Viru, A. "Hormones in Muscular Activity," Vol. 2, *Adaptive Effects of Hormones in Exercise.* Boca Raton, FL: CRC Press, 1983.

21) Brillon, DJ. "Effect of cortisol on energy expenditure and amino acid metabolism in humans." *Am J Physiol* 1995 Mar;268(3 Pt 1):E501-13.

22) Fielding, RA. "High-velocity resistance training increases skeletal muscle peak power in older women." *J Am Geriatric Soc.* 2002 Apr;50(4):655-62.

23) Pyka, G. "Muscle strength and fiber adaptations to year-long resistance training program in elderly men and women." *J Gerontol* 1979 Jan;49(1):M22-7.

24) Fleg, JL. "Role of muscle loss in the age-associated reduction in VO$_2$ max." *J Appl Physiol* 1988 Sep;65(7):1147-51.

25) Evans, WJ. "Reversing sarcopenia: how weight training can build strength and vitality." *Geriatrics* 1996 May;51(5):46-7.

26) Siegel, A. "Effect of marathon running on Inflammatory and hemostatic markers." *Am J Cardiol.* 2001 Oct 15;88(8):918-20.

27) Lehman, M. "Training-overtraining: performance and hormone levels after a defined increase in training volume vs. intensity in middle- and long-distance runners." *Br J Sports Med* 1992;26:233-42.

28) Church, TS. "Association between cardiorespiratory fitness and C-reactive protein in men." *Arterioscler Thromb Biol* 2002 Nov 1;22(11):1869-76.

29) Simmons, PS. "Increased proteolysis: an effect of increases in plasma cortisol within the physiological range." *J Clin Invest* 1984 Feb;73(2):412-20.

30) Roland Rosmond, MF. "Stress-related cortisol secretion in men: relationships with abdominal obesity and endocrine, metabolic and hemodynamic abnormalities." *J Clin Endocrinol Metab* 1998;83(6):1853-9.

31) Irving, BA. "Effect of exercise training intensity on abdominal-visceral fat and body composition." *Med Sci Sports Exerc* 2008 Nov;40(11):1863-72.

32) Hagerman, FC. "High-intensity resistance training on untrained older men. 1. Strength, cardiovascular, and metabolic responses." *J Gerontol A Biol Sci* 2000 Jul;55(7):8336-46.

33) Tabata, I. "Effects of moderate-intensity endurance and high-intensity intermittent training on anaerobic capacity and VO_2 max." *Med Sci Sports Exerc* 1996 Oct;28(10):1327-30.

CHAPTER 5: HORMONE THERAPY

1) Kuhl, H. "Pharmacokinetics of estrogens and progestogens: influence of different routes of administration." Clinacteric 2005 Aug;8(Suppl 1):3-63.

2) Thom, M. "Hormone profiles in post-menopausal women after therapy with subcutaneous implants." *Br J Obstet Gynecol* 1981(88):426-53.

3) Espie, M. "Breast cancer in postmenopausal women with and without hormone replacement therapy: Preliminary results of the MISSION study." *Gynecol Endocrinol*. 2006 22(8):423-31.

4) www.breastcancer.org/risk

5) www.breastcancer.org/risk. Understanding breast cancer risk.

CHAPTER 6: STRESS REDUCTION

1) Bach-y-Rita, P. "Sensory plasticity: applications to a vision substitution system." *Acta Neurol Scand*. 1967;43:417-26.

2) Kercel, SW. "Some radical implications of Bach-y-Rita's discoveries." *J Integr Neurosci* 2005 Dec;4(4):551-65.

3) Staudt, M. "Brain plasticity following early life brain injury: insights from neuroimaging." Semin Perinatol 2010 Feb;34(1):87-92.

4) Aguilar, MJ. "Recovery of motor function after unilateral infarction of the basis pontis. Report of a case." *Am J Phys Med* 1969 Dec;48(6):279-88.

5) Rosenzweig, MR. "Effects of environmental complexity and training on brain chemistry and anatomy: a replication and extension." *J Comp Physiol Psychol* 1962 Aug;55:429-37.

6) Jacobs, B. "A quantitative dendritic analysis of Wernicke's area in humans. II. Gender, hemispheric, and environmental factors." *J Comp Neurol* 1993 Jan 1;327(1):97-111.

7) Wang, XH. "Personality and lifestyle in relation to dementia incidence." *Neurology* 2009 20;72(3):253-9.

REFERENCES

Testosterone/men

Abate, N. "Sex steroid hormones, upper body obesity, and insulin resistance." *J Clin Endocrinol Metab.* 2002 Oct;87(10):4522-7.

Agarwal, PK. "Testosterone replacement therapy after primary treatment for prostate cancer." *J Urology.* 2005 Feb;173(2):533-6.

Ahmed, SR. "Transdermal testosterone therapy in the treatment of male hypogonadism." *J Clin Endocrinol Metab.* 1988 Mar;66(3):546-51

Ahibom, E. "Testosterone protects cerebellar granule cells from oxidative stress-induced cell death through a receptor mediated mechanism." *Brain Res.* 2001 Feb 23;892(2):255-62. (Testosterone has antioxidant activity.)

Alexandersen, P. "The relationship of natural androgens to coronary heart disease in males: a review." *Atherosclerosis.* 1996 Aug 23;125(1):1-13

Almeida, OP. "One-year follow-up study of association between chemical castration, sex hormones, beta-amyloid, memory and depression in men." *Psychoneuroendocrinology.* 2004 Sep;29(3):1071-81.

Altschule, MD. "The use of testosterone in the treatment of depression." *N Engl J Med.* 1948;239:1036-8.

Amin, S. "Estradiol, testosterone, and the risk for hip fractures in elderly men from the Framingham study." *Ann J Med.* 2006 May;119(5):426-33

Anderson FH. "Androgen supplementation in eugonadal men with osteoporosis:effects of 6 months of treatment on bone mineral density and cardiovascular risk factors." *Bone.* 1996 Feb;18(2):171-7.

Araujo, AB. "Sex steroids and all-cause and cause-specific mortality in men." *Arch Intern Med.* 2007 Jun;167(12):1252-60.

Arnlov, J. "Endogenous sex hormones and cardiovascular disease incidence in men." *Ann Intern Med.* 2006 Aug 1;145(3):176-84.

Arver, S. "Improvement in sexual function in testosterone deficient men treated for one year with a permeation enhanced testosterone transdermal system." *J Urol.* 1996 May;155(5):1604-8.

Arver, S. "Long-term efficacy and safety of a permeation-enhanced testosterone transdermal system in hypogonadal men." *Clin Endo (Oxf).* 1997 Dec;47(6):727-37.

Aversa, A. "Androgens and penile erection: evidence for a direct relationship between free testosterone and cavernous vasodilatation in men with erectile dysfunction." *Clin Endocrinol (Oxf).* 2000 Oct;53(4):517-22.

Bals-Pratsch, M. "Transdermal testosterone substitution therapy in the treatment of male hypogonadism." *Lancet.* 1986 Oct;25(8513):943-6.

Barrett-Connor, E. "Lower endogenous androgen levels and dyslipidemia in men with non-insulin dependent diabetes mellitus." *Ann Intern Med.* 1992 Nov 15;117 (10):807-11

Barrett-Connor, E. "Bioavailable testosterone and depressed mood in older men. The Rancho Bernardo Study."*J Clin Endocrinol Metab.* 1999 Feb;84(2):573-7.

Basaria, S. "Risks versus benefits of testosterone therapy in elderly men." *Drugs Aging.* 1999 Aug;15(2):131-42

Behre, HM. "Prostate volume in testosterone-treated and untreated hypogonadal men in comparison to age-matched controls." *Clin Endo (Oxf).* 1994 Mar;40(3):341-9.

Bhasin, S. "Age-associated sarcopenia-issues in the use of testosterone as an anabolic agent in older men." *J Clin Endo Metab.* 1997 Jun;82(6):1659-60. (Sarcopenia equals muscle loss.)

Bhasin, S. "Testosterone dose-response relationships in healthy young men." *Am J Physiol Endocrinol Metab.* 2001 Dec;281(6):E1172-81.

Bhasin, S. "The dose-dependent effects of testosterone on sexual function and on muscle mass and function." *Mayo Clin Proc.* 2000 Jan;75 Suppl:S70-5

Bhasin, S. "The mechanisms of androgen effects on body composition: mesenchymal pluripotent cell as the target of androgen actions." *J Gerontol A Biol Sci Med Sci.* 2003 Dec;58(12):M1103-10.

Bhasin, S. "Managing the risks of prostate disease during testosterone replacement therapy in older men: recommendations for a standardized monitoring plan." *J Androl*. 2003 May-June;24(3)299-311.

Bhasin, S. "Testosterone replacement increases fat-free mass and muscle size in hypogonadal men." *J Clin Endocrinol Metab*. 1997 Feb;82(2):407-13.

Bhasin, S. "Effects of testosterone administration on fat distribution, insulin sensitivity, and atherosclerosis progression." *Clin Infect Dis*. 2003;37 Suppl 2:S142-9.

Bhasin, S. "The effects of supraphysiologic doses of testosterone on muscle size and strength in normal men." *N Eng J Med*. 1996 July 4;325(1):1-7.

Biundo, B. "Testosterone deficiency in men: new treatments for andropause." *In J Pharm Comp*. 2000;4(6):429-31.

Boyanov, MA. "Testosterone supplementation in men with type 2 diabetes, visceral obesity and partial androgen deficiency." *Aging Male*. 2003 Mar;6(1):1-7.

Bremner, WJ. "Loss of circadian rhythmicity in blood testosterone levels with aging in normal men." *J Clin Endocrinol Metab*. 1983 Jun;56(6):1278-81.

Brodsky, IG. "Effects of testosterone replacement on muscle mass and muscle protein synthesis in hypogonadal men—a clinical research center study." *J Clin Endocrinol Metab*. 1996 Oct;81(10);3469-75.

Cantrill, J. "Which testosterone replacement therapy?" *Clin Endocrinol (Oxf)*. 1984 Aug;21(2):97-107.

Carey, PO. "Transdermal testosterone treatment of hypogonadal men." *J Urol*. 1988 Jun;107(6):722-6.

Carpenter, WR. "Getting over testosterone: Postulating a fresh start for etiologic studies of prostate cancer." *J Na Cancer Inst*. 2008 Feb;100(3):158-9.

Carter, HB. "Longitudinal evaluation of serum androgen levels in men with and without prostate cancer." *Prostate*. 1995 Jul;27(1):15-31.

Chandel, A. "Testosterone concentrations in young patients with diabetes mellitus." *Diabetes Care*. 2008 Oct;31(10):2013-7.

Chearskul, S. "Study of plasma hormones and lipids in healthy elderly Thais compared to patients with chronic diseases: diabetes mellitus, essential hypertension and coronary heart disease." *J Med Assoc Thai*. 2000 Mar;83(3):266-77.

Chen, C. "Endogenous sex hormones and prostate cancer risk: a case-control study nested within the Carotene and retinol efficacy trial." *Cancer Epidemiol Biomarkers Prev.* 2003 Dec;12(12):1410-6. (Low testosterone associated with increased prostate cancer risk.)

Chen, AC. "Complications of androgen-deprivation therapy in men with prostate cancer." *Curr Urol Rep.* 2005 May;6(3):210-6. (complications include sexual side effects, hot flashes, gynecomastia, changes in body composition, osteoporosis, anemia, psychiatric and cognitive problems, fatigue and diminished quality of life.)

Cherrier, MM. "Relationship between testosterone supplementation and insulin-like growth factor-I and cognition in healthy older men." *Psychoneuroendocrinology.* 2004 Jan;29(1):65-82.

Cherrier, MM. "Cognitive effects of short-term manipulation of serum sex steroids in healthy young men." *J Clin Endocrinol Metab.* 2002 Jul;87(7):3090-6.

Cherrier, MM. "Cognitive changes associated with supplementation of testosterone or dihydrotestosterone in mildly hypogonadal men: a preliminary report." *J Androl.* 2003 Jul-Aug;24(4):568-76.

Cherrier, MM. "Testosterone supplementation improves spatial and verbal memory in healthy older men." *Neurology.* 2001 Jul 10;57(1):80-8.

Choong, K. "The physiological and pharmacological basis for the ergogenic effects of androgens in elite sports." *Asian J Androl.* 2008 May;10(3):351-63.

Cooper, MA. "Testosterone replacement therapy for anxiety." *Am J Psychiatry* 2000 Nov;157(11):1884.

Cooper, CS. "Effect of exogenous testosterone on prostate volume, serum and semen PSA levels in healthy young men." *J Urol.*1996 Aug;156(2 Pt 1);438-41. (No effect from testosterone therapy.)

Corrales, JJ. "Partial androgen deficiency in aging type 2 diabetic men and its relationship to glycemic control." *Metabolism.* 2004 May;53(5):666-72.

Crawford, BA. "Randomized placebo-controlled trial of androgen effects on muscle and bone in men requiring long-term systemic glucocorticoid treatment." *J Clin Endo Metab.* 2003 July;88(7):3167-76.

Cutolo, M. "Androgens and estrogens modulate the immune and inflammatory responses in rheumatoid arthritis." *Ann NY Acad Sci.* 2002 June;966:131-42.

Cutolo, M. "Sex hormone status of male patients with rheumatoid arthritis: evidence of low serum concentrations of testosterone at baseline and after HCG stimulation." *Arthritis Rheum.* 1988 Oct;31(10):1314-7.

Cutolo, M. "Androgen replacement therapy in male patients with rheumatoid arthritis." *Arthritis Rheum.* 1991 Jan;34(1):1-5.

Dandona, P. "Low testosterone a problem in young diabetic men." *Diabetes Care.* 2008 Oct (About one-third of young adult men with type 2 diabetes have low testosterone levels.)

Debing, E. "Men with atherosclerotic stenosis of the carotid artery have lower testosterone levels compared with controls." *Int Angiol.* 2008 Apr;27(2):135-41.

Deslypere, JP. "Influence of age on steroid concentrations in skin and striated muscle in women and in cardiac muscle and lung tissue in men." *J Clin Endo Metab.* 1985 Oct;61(4):648-53.

Dobs, AS. "Pharmacokinetics, efficacy, and safety of permeation-enhanced testosterone transdermal system in comparison with bi-weekly injections of testosterone enanthate for the treatment of hypogonadal men." *J Clin Endo Metab.* 1999 Oct;84(10):3469-78.

Dockery, F. "Testosterone suppression in men with prostate cancer is associated with increased arterial stiffness." *Aging Male.* 2002 Dec;5(4):216-22.

Dockery, F. "The relationship between androgens and arterial stiffness in older men." *J Am Geriatr Soc.* 2003 Nov;51(11):1627-32.

Drafta, D. "Age-related changes of plasma steroids in normal adult males." *J Steroid Biochem.* 1982 Dec;17(6):683-7.

Driscoll, I. "Testosterone and cognition in normal aging and Alzheimer's disease: an update." *Curr Alzheimer Res.* 2007 Feb;4(1):33-45.

Dunajska, K. "Evaluation of sex hormone levels and some metabolic factors in men with coronary atherosclerosis." *Aging Male.* 2004 Sep;7(3):197-204. (Men with coronary artery disease had low testosterone and high estradiol.)

Eastell, R. "Management of male osteoporosis: Report of the UK Consensus Group." *QJM.* 1998 Feb;91(2):71-92.

Ebert, T. "The current status of therapy for symptomatic late-onset hypogonadism with transdermal testosterone gel." *Eur Urol.* 2005 Feb 47(2):137-46.

Edwards, I. "Testosterone propionate as a therapeutic agent in patients with organic disease of peripheral vessels." *N Eng J Med.* 1939;220:865-9.

Elwan, O. "Hormonal changes in cerebral infarction in the young and elderly." *J Neurol Sci.* 1990 Sep;98(2-3):235-43.

English, KM. "Low-dose transdermal testosterone therapy improves angina threshold in men with chronic stable angina." *Circulation.* 2000 Oct 17;102(16):1906-11.

English, KM. "Men with coronary artery disease have lower levels of androgens than men with normal coronary angiograms." *Eur Heart J.* 2000 Jun;21(11):890-4.

Findlay, JC. "Treatment of primary hypogonadism in men by the transdermal administration of testosterone." *J Clin Endocrinol Metab.* 1989 Feb;68(2):369-73.

Flamm, J. "An urodynamic study of patients with benign prostatic hypertrophy treated conservatively with phytotherapy or testosterone." *Wien Klin Wochenschr.*1979 Sept 28;91(18):622-7. (Testosterone therapy reduced prostate dysfunction complaints.)

Freedman, DS. "Relation of serum testosterone levels to high density lipoprotein cholesterol and other characteristics in men." *Arterioscler Thromb.* 1991Mar-Apr;11(2):307-15.

Furuya, Y. "Low serum testosterone level predicts worse response to endocrine therapy in Japanese patients with metastatic prostate cancer." *Endocr J.* 2002 Feb;49(1):85-90. (Low T predicts worse response to suppression therapy.)

Gann, PH. "A prospective study of plasma hormone levels, non-hormonal factors, and development of benign prostatic hyperplasia."*Prostate.* 1995 Jan;26(1):40-9.

Gann, PH. "Prospective study of sex hormone levels and risk of prostate cancer." *J Natl Cancer Inst.* 1996 Aug21;88(16):1118-26.

Glueck, CJ. "Endogenous testosterone, fibrinolysis, and coronary heart disease risk in hyperlipidemic men." *J Lab Clin Med.* 1993 Oct;122(4):412-20.

Gouchie, C. "The relationship between testosterone levels and cognitive ability patterns." *Psychoneuroendocrinology.* 199116(4):323-34.

Gooren, L. "Androgen deficiency in the aging male: benefits and risks of androgen supplementation." *J Steroid Biochem Mol Biol.* 2003 Jun;85(2-5):349-55.

Gouras, GK. "Testosterone reduces neuronal secretion of Alzheimer's beta-amyloid peptides." *Proc Natl Acad Sci.* 2000 Feb1;97(3):1202-5.

Greenstein, A. "Does sildenafil combined with testosterone gel improve erectile dysfunction in hypogonadal men in whom testosterone supplement therapy alone failed?" *J Urol.* 2005 Feb;173(2):530-2.

Griggs, RC. "Effect of testosterone on muscle mass and muscle protein synthesis." *J Appl Physiol.* 1989 Jan;66(1):498-503.

Grinspoon, S. "Loss of lean body and muscle mass correlates with androgen levels in hypogonadal men with acquired immunodeficiency syndrome and wasting." *J Clin Endo Metab.*1996 Nov;81(11):4051-8.

Grinspoon, S. "Effects of androgen administration on the growth hormone-insulin-like growth factor 1 axis in men with acquired immunodeficiency syndrome wasting." *J Clin Endocrinol Metab* 1998 Dec;83(12):4251-6.

Grossman, M. "Low Testosterone levels are common and associated with insulin resistance in men with diabetes." *J Clin Endocrinol Metab.* 2008 May;93(5):1834-40.

Gruenewald, DA. "Testosterone supplementation therapy for older men: potential benefits and risks." *J Am Geriatr Soc.* 2003 Jan;51(1):101-15.

Guay, AT. "Testosterone treatment in hypogonadal men: prostate-specific antigen level and risk of prostate cancer." *Endocr Pract.* 2000 Mar-Apr;6(2):132-8.

Gould, DC. "The male menopause: does it exist?:some men need investigation and treatment" *West J Med.* 2000 Aug;173(2):76-8.

Gunawarden, K. "Testosterone is a potential augmentor of antioxidant-induced apoptosis in human prostate cancer cells." *Cancer Detect Prev.*2002;26(2):105-13.

Gutai, J. "Plasma testosterone, high-density lipoprotein cholesterol and other lipoprotein fractions." *Am J Cardiol.* 1981Nov;48(5):897-902.

Haapiainen, R. "Pretreatment plasma levels of testosterone and sex hormone binding globulin binding capacity in relation to clinical staging and survival in prostatic cancer patients." *Prostate.* 1988 12(4):325-32. (Increased risk with low testosterone levels.)

Hajjar, RR. "Outcomes of long-term testosterone replacement in older hypogonadal males: a retrospective analysis." *J Clin Endocrinol Metab.* 1997 Nov;82(11):3793-6.

Hak, AE. "Low levels of endogenous androgens increase the risk of atherosclerosis in elderly men: the Rotterdam study." *J Clin Endo Metab.* 2002 Aug;87(8):3632-9.

Hamalainen, E. "Serum lipoproteins, sex hormones and sex hormone binding globulin in middle-aged men of different physical fitness and risk of coronary heart disease." *Atherosclerosis.* 1987 Oct;67(2-3):155-62.

Hamm, L. "Testosterone propionate in the treatment of angina pectoris." *J Clin Endo.* 1942;2(5):325-28.

Handelsman, D. "Suppression of human spermatogenesis by testosterone implants." *J Clin Endocrinol Metab.*1992 Nov;75(5):1326-32.

Handelsman, D. "Pharmacokinetics and pharmacodynamics of testosterone implants." *J Clin Endocrinol Metab.* 1990 Jul;71(1):216-22.

Harman, SM. "Longitudinal effects of aging on serum total and free testosterone levels in healthy men: Baltimore Longitudinal Study of Aging." *J Clin Endocrinol Metab.* 2001 Feb;86(2):724-31.

Heller, CG. "The male climacteric, its symptomology, diagnosis and treatment." *JAMA.* 1944;126:472-77.

Hoffman, MA. "Is low serum free testosterone a marker for high-grade prostate cancer?" *J Urol.* 2000 Mar;163(3):824-7.

Hogervorst, E. "Serum total testosterone is lower in men with Alzheimer's disease." *Neuro Endocrinol Lett.* 2001 Jun;22(3):163-8.

Hogervorst, E. "Testosterone and gonadotropin levels in men with dementia." *Neuro Endocrinol Lett.* 2003 Jun-Aug;24(3-4):203-8.

Howell, S. J. "Randomized placebo-controlled trial of testosterone replacement in men with mild Leydig cell insufficiency following cytotoxic chemotherapy." *Clin Endo* (Oxf). 2001 Sep;55(3):315-24.

Hsing, AW. "Hormones and prostate cancer: what's next?" Epidemiol Rev. 2001;23(1):42-58.

Hsing, AW. Androgen and prostate cancer: is the hypothesis dead? *Cancer Epidemiol Biomarkers Prev.* 2008 Oct;17(10):2525-30.

Hulka, BS. "Serum hormone levels among patients with prostatic carcinoma or benign prostatic hyperplasia and clinic controls." *Prostate.* 1987 11;(2):171-82.(Association with low testosterone levels)

Hwang, TI. "Combined use of androgen and sildenafil for hypogonadal patients unresponsive to sildenafil alone." *Int J Impot Res.* 2006 Jul-Aug;18(4):400-4.

Imamoto, T. "Pretreatment serum testosterone level as a predictive factor of pathological stage in localized prostate cancer patients treated with radical prostatectomy." *Eur Urol.* 2005 Mar;47(3):308-12. (Metastatic prostate cancer associated with low testosterone.)

Isaia, G. "Effect of testosterone on bone in hypogonadal males." *Maturitas.* 1992 Aug;15(1):47-51.

Isbarn, H. "Testosterone and prostate cancer: revisiting old paradigms." *Eur Urol.* 2009 Jul;56(1):48-56.

Isidori, AM. "Effects of testosterone on body composition, bone metabolism and serum lipid profile in middle-aged men: a meta-analysis." *Clin Endcrinol* (Oxf). 2005 Sep;63(3):280-93.

Iversen, P. "Serum testosterone as a prognostic factor in patients with advanced prostatic carcinoma." *Scan J Urol Nephrol Suppl.*1994;157:41-7.

Jain, P. "Testosterone supplementation for erectile dysfunction: results of a meta-analysis." *J Urol.* 2000 Aug;164(2):371-5.

Jannini, EA. "Lack of sexual activity from erectile dysfunction is associated with a reversible reduction in serum testosterone." *Int J Androl.*1999 Dec;22(6):385-92.

Janowsky, JS. "Testosterone influences spatial cognition in older men." *Behav Neurosci.* 1994 Apr;108(2):325-32.

Jeppesen, LL. "Decreased serum testosterone in men with acute ischemic stroke." *Arterio Thromb Vasc Biol.* 1996 Jun;16(6):749-54.

Joly-Pharaboz, MO. "Androgens inhibit the proliferation of a variant of the human prostate cancer cell line LNCaP." *J Steroid Biochem Mol Biol.* 1995 Oct;55(1):67-76.

Katznelson, L. "Increase in bone density and lean body mass during testosterone administration in men with acquired hypogonadism." *J Clin Endocrinol Metab.* 1996 Dec;81(12):4358-65.

Kaufman, JM. "Androgen replacement after curative radical prostatectomy for prostate cancer in hypogonadal men." *J Urol.* 2004 Sep;172(3):920-2.

Kenny, AM. "Short-term effects of intramuscular and transdermal testosterone on bone turnover, prostate symptoms, cholesterol, and hematocrit in men over age 70 with low testosterone levels." *Endocr Res.* 2000 May;26(2):153-68.

Kenny, AM. "Effects of transdermal testosterone on bone and muscle in older men with low bioavailable testosterone levels." *J Gerontol A Biol Sci Med Sci.* 2001May;56(5):M266-72.

Khaw, KT. "Endogenous sex hormones, HDL cholesterol, and other lipoprotein fractions in men." *Arterioscler Thromb.* 1991May-Jun;11(3):489-94.

Khaw, KT. "Endogenous testosterone and mortality due to all causes, cardiovascular disease, and cancer in men: European prospective investigation into cancer in Norfolk Prospective Population Study." *Circulation.* 2007 Dec;116(23):2694-701. (Increased testosterone associated with decreased mortality and less cancer.)

Kumar, V. L. "Androgen, estrogen, and progesterone receptor contents and serum hormone profiles in patients with benign hypertrophy and carcinoma of the prostate." *J Surg Oncol.* 1990 Jun;44(2):122-8. (Association with low testosterone levels)

Kupelian, V. "Low sex hormone binding globulin, total testosterone, and symptomatic androgen deficiency are associated with development of the metabolic syndrome in non-obese men." *J Clin Endocrinol Metab.* 2006 Mar;91(3):843-50.

Laaksonen, DE. "Sex hormones, inflammation and the metabolic syndrome: a population-based study." *Eur J Endocrinol.* 2003 Dec149(6):601-8.

Lazarou, S. "Hypogonadism in the man with erectile dysfunction: what to look for and when to treat." *Curr Urol Rep.* 2005 Nov;6(6):476-81.

Leder, BZ. "Effects of aromatase inhibition in elderly men with low or borderline-low serum testosterone levels." *J Clin Endocrinol Metab.* 2004 Mar;89(3):1174-80.

Leifke, E. "Low serum levels of testosterone in men with minimal traumatic hip fractures." *Exp Clin Endocrinol Diabetes.* 2005 Apr;113(4):208-13.

Lesser, MA. "Testosterone propionate therapy in one hundred cases of angina pectoris." *J Clin Endcrinol.* 1946;(8):549-55.

Lesser, MA. "Effect of testosterone propionate on the prostate gland of patients over 45 years." *J Clin Endcrinol Metab.* 1955;15(3):297-300.

Levin S. "The therapeutic value of testosterone propionate in angina pectoris." *N Engl J Med.* 1943;228:770-72.

Lu, PH. "Effects of testosterone on cognition and mood in male patients with mild Alzheimer's disease and healthy elderly men." *Arch Neurol.* 2006 Feb;63(2):177-85.

Lund, BC. "Testosterone and andropause: the feasibility of testosterone replacement therapy in elderly men." *Pharmacotherapy.* 1999 Aug;19(8):951-6.

Maggio, M. "The relationship between testosterone and molecular markers of inflammation in older men." *J Endocrinol Invest.* 2005;28(11Suppl Proceedings):116-9.

Malkin, CJ. "The effect of testosterone replacement on endogenous inflammatory cytokines and lipid profiles in hypogonadal men." *J Clin Endocrinol Metab.* 2004 Jul;89(7):3313-8.

Malken, CJ. "Testosterone replacement in hypogonadal men with angina improves ischemic threshold and quality of life." *Heart.* 2004 Aug;90(8):871-6.

Marin, P. "Testosterone and regional fat distribution." *Obes Res.* 1995 Nov;3(Suppl 4):609S-612S) (Improvement with testosterone therapy)

Marin, P. "The effects of testosterone treatment on body composition and metabolism in middle-aged obese men." *Int J Obes Relat Metab Disord.* 1992 Dec;16(12):991-7.

Marin, P. "Androgen treatment of middle-aged, obese men: effects on metabolism, muscle and adipose tissues." *Eur J Med.* 1992 Oct;1(6):329-36.

Marks, LS. "Effect of testosterone replacement therapy on prostate tissue in men with late-onset hypogonadism: a randomized controlled trial." *JAMA.* 2006 Nov15;296(19):2351-61.

Mauras, N. "Testosterone deficiency in young men: marked alterations in whole body protein kinetics, strength, and adiposity." *J Clin Endocrinol Metab.* 1998 Jun;83(6):1886-92.

McNicholas, TA. "A novel testosterone gel formulation normalizes androgen levels in hypogonadal men, with improvements in body composition and sexual function." *BJU Int.* 2003 Jan;91(1):69-74.

Meikle, AW. "Familial prostatic cancer risk and low testosterone." *J Clin Endocrinol Metab.* 1982 Jun;54(6):1104-8.

Miner, MM. "Testosterone and aging: what have we learned since the Institute of Medicine report and what lies ahead?" *Int J Clin Pract.* 2007 Apr;61(4):622-32.

Moffat, SD. "Free testosterone and risk for Alzheimer's disease in older men." *Neurology.* 2004 Jan 27;62(2):188-93.

Moffat, SD. "Longitudinal assessment of serum free testosterone concentration predicts memory performance and cognitive status in elderly men." *J Clin Endocrinol Metab.* 2002 Nov;87(11):5001-7.

Mohamad, MJ. "Serum levels of sex hormones in men with acute myocardial infarction." *Neuro Endocrinol Lett.* 2007 Apr;28(2):182-6. (Lower testosterone levels and higher estradiol levels in men with acute myocardial infarction versus men without coronary disease.)

Monath, JR. "Physiologic variations of serum testosterone with the normal range do not affect serum prostate specific antigen." *Urology.* 1995 Jul;46(1):58-61.

Monda, JM. "The correlation between serum prostate-specific antigen and prostate cancer is not influenced by the serum testosterone concentration." *Urology.* 1995 Jul;46(1):62-4.

Morales, A. "Androgen therapy in advanced carcinoma of the prostate." *Can Med Assoc J.* 1971 Jul 10;105(1):71-2. (Improvement with testosterone therapy.)

Morales, A. "Testosterone supplementation for hypogonadal impotence: assessment of biochemical measures and therapeutic outcomes." *J Urol.* 1997 Mar;157(3):849-54.

Morales, A. "Monitoring androgen replacement therapy: testosterone and prostate safety." *J Endocrinol Invest.* 2005;28(3 Suppl):122-7.

Moretti, C. "Androgens and body composition in the aging male." *J Endocrinol Invest.* 2005;28(3 Suppl):56-64.

Morgentaler, A. "Testosterone replacement therapy and prostate cancer." *Urol Clin North Am.* 2007 Nov;34(4):555-63,vii.

Morgentaler, A. "Occult prostate cancer in men with low testosterone levels." *JAMA.* 1996 Dec 18;276(23):1904-6.

Morgentaler, A. "Male impotence." *Lancet.* 1999 Nov 13;354(9191):1713-8.

Morgentaler, A. "Testosterone replacement therapy and prostate risks: where's the beef?" *Can J Urol.* 2006 Feb;13(Suppl 1):40-3.

Morgentaler, A. "Testosterone therapy for men at risk for or with history of prostate cancer." *Curr Treat Options Oncol.* 2006 Sep;7(5):363-9.

Morgentaler, A. "Guilt by association: a historical perspective on Huggins, testosterone therapy, and prostate cancer." *J Sex Med.* 2008 Aug;5(8):1834-40.

Morgentaler, A. "Prevalence of prostate cancer among hypogonadal men with prostate-specific antigen of 4.0 or less." *Urology.* 2006 Dec;68(6):1263-7.

Morgentaler, A. "Shifting the paradigm of testosterone and prostate cancer: the saturation model and the limits of androgen-dependent growth. *Eur Urol.* Feb;55(2):310-21.

Morgentaler, A. "Cultural biases and scientific squabbles: the challenges to acceptance of testosterone therapy as a mainstream medical treatment." *Aging Male.* 2007 Mar;10(1):1-2.

Morgentaler, A. "Guideline for male testosterone therapy: A clinician's perspective." *J Clin Endocrinol Metab.* 2007 Feb;92(2):416-7.

Morgentaler, A. "Testosterone deficiency and prostate cancer: emerging recognition of an important and troubling relationship." *Eur Urol.* 2007 Sep;52(3):623-5.

Morley, JE. "Longitudinal changes in testosterone, luteinizing hormone, and follicle stimulating hormone in healthy older men. Metabolism." 1997 Apr;46(4):410-13.

Morley, JE. "Testosterone and frailty." *Clin Geriatr Med.* 1997 Nov;13(4):685-95.

Morley, JE. "Potentially predictive and manipulable blood serum correlates of aging in the healthy human male: progressive decreases in bioavailable testosterone, dehydroepiandosterone sulfate, and the ratio of insulin-like growth factor1 to growth hormone." *Proc Natl Acad Sci.* 1997 Jul 8;94(14):7537-42.

Muller, M. "Endogenous sex hormones and progression of carotid atherosclerosis in elderly men." *Circulation.* 2004 May 4;109(17):2074-9.

Nachtigall, LB. "Adult onset idiopathic hypogonadotropic hypogonadism—a treatable form of male infertility." *N Eng J Med.* 1997 Feb 6;336(6):410-5.

Nieschlag, E. "Bioavailability and LH-suppressing effect of different testosterone preparations in normal and hypogonadal men." *Horm Res.* 1976;7(3):138-45.

Nieschlag, E. "Investigation, treatment and monitoring of late-onset hypogonadism in males. ISA, ISSAM, and EAU recommendations." *J Androl.*2006 Mar-Apr;27(2):135-7.

Nomura, A. "Prediagnostic serum hormones and the risk of prostate cancer." *Cancer Res.* 1988 Jun 15;48(12):3515-7.

Novak, A. "Andropause and quality of life: findings from patient focus groups and clinical experts." *Marturitas.* 2002 Dec 10;43(4):231-7.

O'Carroll, R. "Androgens, behavior and nocturnal erection in hypogonadal men: the effects of varying the replacement dose." *Clin Endocrinol.* 1985 Nov;23(5):527-38.

Okun, MS. "Refractory nonmotor symptoms in male patients with Parkinson disease due to testosterone deficiency: a common unrecognized comorbidity." *Arch Neurol.* 2002 May;59(5):807-11.

Oh, JY. "Endogenous sex hormones and the development of type 2 diabetes in older men and women: the Rancho Bernardo Study." *Diabetes Care.* 2002 Jan;25(1):55-60.

Penotti, M. "Effects of androgen supplementation of HRT on the vascular reactivity of cerebral arteries." *Fertil Steril.* 2001 Aug;76(2):235-40.

Poggi, UL. "Plasma testosterone and serum lipids in male survivors of myocardial infarction." *J Steroid Biochem.* 1976 Mar;7(3):229-31.

Pope, HG. "Testosterone gel supplementation for men with refractory depression: a randomized, placebo-controlled trial." *Am J Psychiatry.* 2003 Jan;160(1):105-11.

Phillips, GB. "Sex hormones and hemostatic risk factors for coronary heart disease in men with hypertension." *J Hypertension.* 1993 Jul;11(7):699-702.

Phillips, GB. "Is atherosclerotic cardiovascular disease an endocrinological disorder? The estrogen-androgen paradox." *J Clin Endocrinol Metab.* 2005 May;90(5):2708-11.

Prehn, RT. "On the prevention and therapy of prostate cancer by androgen administration." *Cancer Res.* 1999 Sep1;59(17):4161-4.

Prout, GR. "Response of men with advanced prostatic carcinoma to exogenous administration of testosterone." *Cancer.* 1967 Nov;20(11):1871-8. (Improvement in survival with testosterone therapy.)

Pugh, PJ. "Bio-available testosterone levels fall acutely following myocardial infarction in men: association with fibrinolytic factors." *Endocr Res.* 2002 Aug;28(3):161-73.

Rabkin, JG. "A double-blind, placebo-controlled trial of testosterone therapy for HIV-positive men with hypogonadal symptoms." *Arch Gen Psychiatry.* 2000 Feb;57(2):141-7.

Rakic, Z. "Testosterone treatment in men with erectile disorder and low levels of total testosterone in serum." *Arch Sex Behav.* 1997 Oct;26(5):495-504.

Raynaud, JP. "Prostate cancer risk in testosterone-treated men." *J Steroid Biochem Mol Biol.* 2006 Dec;102(1-5):261-6.

Rebuffe-Scrive, M. "Effect of testosterone on abdominal adipose tissue in men." *Int J Obes.* 1991 Nov;15(11):791-5.

Rhoden, EL. "Androgen replacement in men undergoing treatment for prostate cancer." *J Sex Med*. 2008 Sep;5(9):2202-8.

Rhoden, EL. "Testosterone replacement therapy in hypogonadal men at high risk for prostate cancer: results of 1 year of treatment in men with prostatic intraepithelial neoplasia." *J Urol*. 2003 Dec;170(6 Pt 1):2348-51.

Rhoden, EL. "Influence of demographic factors and biochemical characteristics on the prostatic-specific antigen response to testosterone replacement therapy." *Int J Impot Res*. 2006 Mar-Apr;18(2):201-5.

Ribeiro, M. "Low serum testosterone and a younger age predict for a poor outcome in metastatic prostate cancer." *Am J Clin Oncol*. 1997 Dec;20(6):605-8.

Roddam, AW. "Endogenous hormones and prostate cancer collaborative group. Endogenous sex hormones and prostate cancer: a collaborative analysis of 18 prospective studies" *J Natl Cancer Inst*. 2008 Feb;100(6):170-83. (Evaluated eighteen studies of 3,886 men with prostate cancer and 6,438 controls and found that serum concentrations of sex hormones were not associated with the risk of prostate cancer.)

Rosano, GM. "Acute anti-ischemic effect of testosterone in men with coronary artery disease." *Circulation*. 1999 Apr 6;99(13):1666-70.

Salminen, E. "Androgen deprivation and cognition in prostate cancer." *Br J Cancer* 2003 Sep 15;89(6):971-6.

Schatzl, G. "High-grade prostate cancer is associated with low serum testosterone levels." *Prostate*. 2001 Apr;47(1):52-8.

Schatzl, G. "Polymorphism in ARE-I region of prostate-specific antigen gene associated with low serum testosterone level and high-grade prostate cancer." *Urology*. 2005 Jun;65(6):1141-5.

Schubert, M. "Late-onset hypogonadism in the aging male: definition, diagnostic and clinical aspects." *J Endocrinol Invest*. 2005;28(3 Suppl):23-7.

Seidman, SN. "Low testosterone levels in elderly men with dysthymic disorder." *Am J Psychiatry* 2002 Mar;159(3):456-9.

Shabsigh, R. "Testosterone therapy in erectile dysfunction." *Aging Male*. 2004 Dec;7(4):312-8.

Shapiro J. "Testosterone and other anabolic steroids as cardiovascular drugs." *Am J Ther*. 1999 May;6(3):167-74.

Shores, MM. "Low serum testosterone and mortality in male veterans: *Arch Intern Med*. 2006 Aug 14-28;166(15):1660-5. (Mortality levels 88 percent higher in men with low testosterone.)

Shores, MM. "Low testosterone is associated with decreased function and increased mortality risk: a preliminary study of men in a geriatric rehabilitation unit." *J Am Geriatr Soc.* 2004 Dec;52(12):2077-81.

Sih, R. "Testosterone replacement in older hypogonadal men: a 12-month randomized controlled trial." *J Clin Endocrinol Metab.* 1997 Jun;82(6):1661-7.

Sigler, LH. "Treatment of angina pectoris by testosterone propionate." *NY State J Med.* 1943:1424-1428.

Slater, S. "Testosterone: its role in development of prostate cancer and potential risk from use as hormone replacement therapy." *Drugs Aging.* 2000 Dec;17(6):431-9.

Smith, JC. "The effects of induced hypogonadism on arterial stiffness, body composition, and metabolic parameters in males with prostate cancer." *J Clin Endocrinol Metab.* 2001 Sep;86(9):4261-7.

Snyder, PJ. "Effect of testosterone treatment on bone mineral density in men over 65 years of age." *J Clin Endocrinol Metab.* 1999 Jun;84(6):1966-72.

Snyder, PJ. "Effect of testosterone treatment in hypogonadal men." *J Clin Endocrinol Metab.* 2000 Aug;85(8):2670-7.

Stattin, P. "High levels of circulating testosterone are not associated with increased prostate cancer risk: a pooled prospective study." *Int J Cancer.* 2004 Jan 20;108(3):418-24.

Swerdloff, RS. "Androgen deficiency and aging in men." *West J Med.* 1993 Nov;159(5):579-85.

Tan, R. S. "Risks of testosterone replacement therapy in aging men." *Expert Opin Drug Saf.* 2004

Tan, RS. "Memory loss as a reported symptom of andropause." *Arch Androl.* 2001Nov-Dec;47(3):185-9.

Tan, RS. "The andropause and memory loss: is there a link between androgen decline and dementia in the aging male?" *Asian J Androl.* 2001Sep;3(3):169-74.

Tang, YJ. "Serum testosterone level and related metabolic factors in men over 70 years old." *J Endocrinol Invest.* 2007 Jun;30(6):451-8.

Teloken, C. "Low serum testosterone levels are associated with positive surgical margins in radical retropubic prostatectomy: hypogonadism represents bad prognosis in prostate cancer." *J Urol.* 2005 Dec;174(6):2178-80.

Tengstrand, B. "Bioavailable testosterone in men with rheumatoid arthritis-high frequency of hypogonadism." *Rheumatology(Oxford)*. 2002 Mar;41(3):285-9.

Tenover, JL. "Male hormone replacement therapy including "andropause." *Endocrinol Metab Clin North Am*. 1998 Dec;27(4):969-87.

Tenover, JL. "Testosterone replacement therapy in older adult men." *Int J Androl*. 1999 Oct;22(5):300-6.

Tenover, JL. "Effects of testosterone supplementation in the aging male." *J Clin Endocrinol Metab*. 1992 Oct;75(4):1092-8.

Tibblin, G. "The pituitary-gonadal axis and health in elderly men: a study of men born in 1913." *Diabetes*. 1996 Nov;45(11):1605-9. (Obesity associated with low testosterone levels.)

Tivesten, A. "Low serum testosterone and high serum estradiol associated with lower extremity peripheral arterial disease in elderly men. The MrOS study in Sweden." *J Am Coll Cardiol*. 2007 Sep 11;50(11):1070-6. (Study of 3,014 men, average age seventy-four years. Low levels of testosterone and high levels of estradiol were independently and positively associated with peripheral artery disease.)

Traish, AM. "Adipocyte accumulation in penile corpus cavernosum of the orchiectomized rabbit: a potential mechanism for veno-occlusive dysfunction in androgen deficiency." *J Androl*. 2005 Mar-Apr;26(2):242-8.

Traish, AM. "The dark side of testosterone deficiency:I.Metabolic syndrome and erectile dysfunction. *J Androl*.2009 Jan-Feb;30(1):10-22.

Traish, AM. "The dark side of testosterone deficiency:II. Type 2 diabetes and insulin resistance." *J Androl*. 2009 Jan-Feb;30(1):23-32.

Traish, AM. "The dark side of testosterone deficiency:III. Cardiovascular disease. *J Androl*.2009 Sep-Oct;30(5):477-94.

Tripathi, Y. "Serum estradiol and testosterone levels following acute myocardial infarction in men." *Indian J Physiol Pharmacol*. 1998 Apr;42(2):291-4.(Men admitted with acute myocardial infarction had elevated estradiol and lower testosterone levels.)

Tsujimura, A. "Bioavailable testosterone with age and erectile dysfunction." *J Urol*. 2003 Dec;170(6 Pt 1):2345-7.

Urban, RJ. "Testosterone administration to elderly men increases skeletal muscle strength and protein synthesis." *Am J Physiol*. 1995 Nov;269(5 Pt 1):E820-6.

van den Beld, AW. "Measures of bioavailable serum testosterone and estradiol and their relationships with muscle strength, bone density, and body composition in elderly men." *J Clin Endocrinol Metab.* 2000 Sep;85(9):3276-82.

van Andel, G. "The impact of androgen deprivation therapy on health related quality of life in asymptomatic men with lymph node positive prostate cancer." *Eur Urol.* 2003 Aug;44(2):209-14.

Vermeulen, A. "Androgen replacement therapy in the aging male—a critical evaluation. *J Clin Endocrinol Metab.* 2001Jun;86(6):2380-90.

Walker, TC. "The use of testosterone propionate and estrogenic substance in the treatment of essential hypertension, angina pectoris and peripheral vascular disease." *J Clin Endocrinol.* 1942;2(9):560-68.

Wang C. "Sublingual testosterone replacement improves muscle mass and strength, decreases bone resorption, and increased bone formation in hypogonadal men: a clinical research center study. *J Clin Endocrinol Metab.* 1996 Oct;81(10):3578-83.

Wang, C. "Transdermal testosterone gel improves sexual function, mood, muscle strength, and body composition parameters in hypogonadal men." *J Endocrinol Metab.* 2000 Aug;85(8):2839-53.

Wang, C. "Long-term testosterone gel treatment maintains beneficial effects on sexual function and mood, lean and fat mass, and bone mineral density in hypogonadal men." *J Clin Endocrinol Metab.* 2004 May;89(5):2085-98.

Wranicz, JK. "The relationship between sex hormones and lipid profile in men with coronary artery disease." *Int J Cardiol.* 2005 May 11;101(1):105-10. (Study used angiograms to measure extent of coronary heart disease.)

Wu, SZ. "Therapeutic effects of an androgenic preparation on myocardial ischemia and cardiac function in 62 elderly male coronary heart disease patients." *Chin Med J (Engl).*1993 Jun;106(6):415-8.

Younes, A. K. "Low plasma testosterone in varicocele patients with impotence and male infertility." *Arch Androl.* 2000

Zmuda, JM. "Longitudinal relation between endogenous testosterone and cardiovascular disease risk factors in middle-aged men. A 13-year follow-up of former Multiple Risk Factor Intervention Trial participants." *Am J Epidemiol.* 1997 Oct 15;146(8):609-17.

Zou, B. "Association between relative hypogonadism and metabolic syndrome in newly diagnosed adult male patients with impaired glucose tolerance or Type 2 diabetes mellitus." *Metab Syndr Relat Disord.* 2004;2(1):39-48.

Zumoff, B. "Abnormal levels of plasma hormones in men with prostate cancer: evidence toward a 'two-disease' theory." *Prostate.* 1982;3(6):579-88. (Low testosterone levels in prostate cancer patients less than sixty-five years.)

Zvara, P. "Nitric oxide mediated erectile activity is a testosterone dependent event: a rat erection model." *Int J Impot Res.* 1995 Dec;7(4):209-19.

Zgliczynski, S. "Effect of testosterone replacement therapy on lipids and lipoproteins in hypogonadal and elderly men." *Atherosclerosis.* 1996 Mar;121(1):35-43.

Estradiol/men

Abbott, RD. "Serum estradiol and risk of stroke in elderly men." *Neurology.* 2007 Feb 20;68(8):563-8.

Abu-Abid, S. "Obesity and cancer." *J Med.* 2002;33(1-4):73-86. (Estradiol levels correlate to body fat mass. Abdominal obesity in men is correlated with heart disease, diabetes, cancer.)

Amin, S. "Estradiol, testosterone, and the risk for hip fractures in elderly men from the Framingham study." *Ann J Med.* 2006 May;119(5):426-33.

Anderson, LA. "The effects of androgens and estrogens on preadipocyte proliferation in human adipose tissue: influence of gender and site." *J Clin Endocrinol Metab.* 2001Oct;86(10):5045-51.

Bosland, MC. "Sex steroids and prostate carcinogenesis: integrated, multifactorial working hypothesis." *Ann NY Acad Sci.* 2006 Nov;1089:168-76.

Carani, C. "Role of estrogen in male sexual behavior: insights from the natural model of aromatase deficiency." *Clin Endocrinol(Oxf).*1999 Oct;51(4):517-24.

Carlsen, CG. "Prevalence of low serum estradiol levels in male osteoporosis." *Osteoporosis Int.* 2000;11(8):697-701.

Ellen, SJ. "Aromatase and prostate cancer." *Minerva Endocrinol.* 2006;31(1):1-12.

Gennari L. "Aromatase activity and bone homeostasis in men." *J Clin Endocrinol Metab.* 2004 Dec;89(12):5898-907.

Giton, F. "Estrone sulfate, a prognosis marker for tumor aggressiveness in prostate cancer." *J Steroid Biochem Mol Biol.* 2008 Mar;109(1-2):158-67.

Ho, CK. "Estrogen and benign prostatic hyperplasia: effects on stromal cell proliferation and local formation from androgen." *J Endocrinol.* 2008 June;197(3):483-91.

Jeong, HJ. "Inhibition of aromatase activity by flavonoids." *Arch Pharm Res.* 1999 Jun;22(3):309-12.

Kampen, DL. "Estradiol is related to visual memory in healthy young men." *Behav Neurosci.* 1996 Jun;110(3):613-7.

Khosla, S. "Estrogens and bone health in men." *Calcif Tissue Int.* 2001 Oct;69(4):189-92.

Kula, K. "Important functions of estrogens in men—breakthrough in contemporary medicine." *Przegl Lek.* 2005;62(9):908-15

Leder, BZ. "Effects of aromatase inhibition in elderly men with low or borderline-low serum testosterone levels." *J Clin Endocrinol Metab.* 2004 Mar;89(3):1174-80.

Matsuda, T. "Relation between benign prostatic hyperplasia and obesity and estrogen." *Rinsho Byori.* 2004 Apr;52(4):291-4.

Mendelsohn, ME. "The protective effects of estrogen on the cardiovascular system." *Am J Cardiol.* 2000 Jun 20;89(12A):12E-17E.

Nuti, R. "Bone metabolism in men: role of aromatase activity." *J Endocrinol Invest.* 2007;30(6 Suppl):18-23.

Sader, MA. "Estradiol improves arterial endothelial function in healthy men receiving testosterone." *Clin Endocrinol (Oxf).* 2001 Feb;54(2):175-81.

Sudhir, K. "Clinical review 110: Cardiovascular actions of estrogens in men." *J Clin Endocrinol Metab.* 1999 Oct;84(10):3411-5.

Singh, PB. "A potential paradox in prostate adenocarcinoma progression: estrogen as the initiating driver." *Eur J Cancer.* 2008 May;44(7):928-36.

Suzuki, K. "Endocrine environment of benign prostatic hyperplasia: prostate size and volume are correlated with serum estrogen concentration." *Scand J Urol Nephrol.*1995 Mar;29(1):65-8.

Tivesten, A. "Circulating estradiol is an independent predictor of progression of carotid artery intima-media thickness in middle-aged men." *J Clin Endocrinol Metab.* 2006 Nov;91(11):4433-7.

Vermeulen, A. "Estradiol in elderly men." *Aging Male.* 2002 Jun;5(2):98-102.

Wynder, EL. "Metabolic epidemiology of prostatic cancer. *Prostate.* 1984;5(1):47-53. (High estrogen and low testosterone found in prostate cancer patients.)

Zumoff, B. "Reversal of the hypogonadotropic hypogonadism of obese men by administration of the aromatase inhibitor testolactone." *Metabolism.* 2003 Sep;52(9):1126-8.

Estrogen and progesterone/women

Adami, HO. "The effect of female sex hormones on cancer survival. A register-based study in patients younger than 20 years at diagnosis." *JAMA.* 1990 Apr 25;263(16):2189-93. (Higher estrogen levels associated with lower mortality.)

Adami, HO. "Female sex hormones and cancer survival" *Lancet* 1994 Sep 10;344(8924):760-1.

Adams, MR. "Inhibition of coronary artery atherosclerosis by 17-beta estradiol in ovariectomized monkeys. Lack of an effect of added progesterone." *Arteriosclerosis.* 1990 Nov-Dec;10(6):1051-7. (Bioidentical progesterone has no detrimental effect on estradiol protection of coronary arteries, unlike Provera.)

Adams, MR. "Medroxyprogesterone acetate antagonizes inhibitory effects of conjugated equine estrogens on coronary artery atherosclerosis." *Arterioscler Thromb Vasc Biol.* 1997 Jan;17(1):217-21. (Provera has negative impact on cardiovascular benefit of estrogens.)

Adamson, DL. "Esterified estrogens combined with methyltestosterone improves emotional well-being in postmenopausal women with chest pain and normal coronary angiograms." *Menopause.* 2001 Jul-Aug;8(4):233-8.

Ahlgrimm, M. "Natural hormone replacement: Individualized treatments vs. 'one-size-fits-all' therapy." *Am J Med.* 1997 Sep;4(7):36-44.

Ahokas A. "Estrogen deficiency in severe postpartum depression: successful treatment with sublingual physiologic 17beta-estradiol: a preliminary study." *J Clin Psychiatry.* 2001 May;62(5):332-6.

Akkad, AA. "Differing responses in blood pressure over 24 hours in normotensive women receiving oral or transdermal estrogen replacement therapy." *Obstet Gynecol.* 1997 Jan;89(1):97-103.

Albertsson, PA. "Beneficial effect of treatment with transdermal estradiol-17-beta on exercise-induced angina and ST segment depression in syndrome X." *Int J Cardiol.* 1996 Apr 19;54(1):13-20.

Alkaersig, N. "Blood coagulation in postmenopausal women given estrogen treatment: comparison of transdermal and oral administration." *J Lab Clin Med.* 1988 Feb;111(2):224-8.

Almeida, OP. "Association between physiological serum concentration of estrogen and the mental health of community-dwelling post menopausal women age 70 years and over." *Am J Geriatr Psychiatry.* 2005 Feb;13(2):142-9.

Almeida,OP. "A 20-week randomized controlled trial of estradiol replacement therapy for women aged 70 years and older: effect on mood, cognition, and quality of life. Neurobiol Aging. 2006 Jan;27(1):141-9.

Aloia, J. "Relationship of menopause to skeletal and muscle mass." *Am J Clin Nutr.* 1991Jan;53(6):1378-83.

Anderson, B. "Estrogen replacement therapy decreases hyperandrogenicity and improves glucose homeostasis: plasma lipids in postmenopausal women with NIDDM." *J Clin Endocrinol Metab.* 1997;82(2):638-43.

Anderson, KE. "The influence of dietary protein and carbohydrate on the principal oxidative biotransformation of estradiol in normal subjects." *J Clin Endocrinol Metab.* 1984 Jul;59(1):103-7.

Andreen, L. "Pharmacokinetics of progesterone and its metabolites allopregnanolone and pregnanolone after oral administration of low-dose progesterone." *Maturitas.* 2006 Jun;54(3):238-44.

Andreen L. "Allopregnanolone concentration and mood-a bimodal association in postmenopausal women treated with oral progesterone." *Psychopharmacology* (Berl). 2006 Aug;187(2):209-21. (Women whose progesterone levels drop develop negative personality changes.)

Angerer, P. "Hormone replacement therapy and distensibility of carotid arteries in postmenopausal women: a randomized, controlled trial." *J Am Coll Cardiol.* 2000 Nov 15;36(6):1789-96.(Vasodilatation effects of estrogens)

Angerer, P. "Influence of 17beta-estradiol on blood pressure of postmenopausal women at high vascular risk." *J Hypertens.* 2001 Dec;19(12):2135-42.

Antonijevic, IA. "Modulation of the sleep electroencephalogram by estrogen replacement in postmenopausal women." *Am J Obstet Gynecol.* 2000 Feb;182(2):277-82.

Archer, DF. "Percutaneous 17beta-estradiol gel for the treatment of vasomotor symptoms in postmenopausal women." *Menopause.* 2003 Nov-Dec;10(6):516-21.

Arenbrecht, S. "Effects of transdermal estradiol delivered by a matrix patch on bone density in hysterectomized, postmenopausal women: a 2-year placebo-controlled trial." *Osteoporosis Int.* 2002;13(2):176-83.

Asthana, S. "High-dose estradiol improves cognition for women with AD: results of a randomized study." *Neurology.* 2001 Aug 28;57(4):605-12.

Badwe, RA. "Serum progesterone at the time of surgery and survival in women with premenopausal operable breast cancer." *Eur J Cancer.* 1994;30A(4):445-8.

Bagur, A. "Hormone replacement therapy increases trabecular and cortical bone density in osteoporotic women." *Medicina* (B Aires). 1996;56(3):247-51.

Bairey Merz, CN. "Hypoestrogenemia of hypothalamic origin and coronary artery disease in premenopausal women: a report from the NHLBI-sponsored WISE study." *J Am Coll Cardiol.* 2003 Feb 5;41(3):413-9. (Low estrogens found in women with heart disease.)

Baker,VL. "Alternatives to oral estrogen replacement. Transdermal patches, percutaneous gels, vaginal creams, rings, implants, and other methods of delivery." *Obstet Gynecol Clin North Am.* 1994 Jun;21(2):271-97.

Baker, ER. "Efficacy of progesterone vaginal suppositories in alleviation of nervous symptoms in patients with premenstrual syndrome." *J Assist Reprod Genet.* 1995 Mar;12(3):205-9.

Balci, H. "Effects of transdermal estrogen replacement therapy on plasma levels of nitric oxide and plasma lipids in postmenopausal women." *Maturitas.* 2005 Apr 11;50(4):289-93.

Barnebei, V. "Plasma homocysteine in women taking hormone replacement therapy: the Postmenopausal Estrogen/Progestin (PEPI) trail." *J. Women's Health Gend Based Med.* 1999 Nov;81(9):1167-72.

Barp, J. "Myocardial antioxidant and oxidative stress changes due to sex hormones." *Braz J Med Biol Res.* 2002 Sep;35(9):1075-81.

Ballard-Barbask, R. "Body weight: estimation of risk of breast and endometrial cancers." *Am J Clin Nutr.* 1996 Mar;63(3 Suppl):437S-41S.

Ballinger, S. "Stress as a factor in lowered estrogen levels in the early menopause." *Ann NY Acad Sci.* 1990;592:95-113.

Barengolts, E. I. "Effects of progesterone on postovariectomy bone loss in aged rats." *J Bone Miner Res.* 1990 Nov;5(11):1143-7.

Barrett-Connor E. "A two-year double-blind comparison of estrogen-androgen and conjugated estrogens in surgically menopausal women. Effects on bone mineral density, symptoms and lipid profiles." *J Reprod Med.* 1999 Dec;44(12):1012-20.

Barlow, D. "Long-term hormone implants therapy-hormonal and clinical effects." *Obstet Gynecol.* 1986 Mar;67(3):321-5.

Battalion, C. "Hormone therapy and ophthalmic artery blood flow changes in women with primary open-angle glaucoma." *Menopause.* 2004 Jan-Feb;11(1):69-77. (Estradiol improves ophthalmic blood flow.)

Baulieu, E. "Progesterone as a neuroactive neurosteroid, with special references to the effect of progesterone on myelination." *Hum Reprod.* 2000 Jun;15(Suppl 1):1-13.

Bech P. "Combined versus sequential hormone replacement therapy: a double-blind, placebo-controlled study on quality of life-related outcome measures." *Psychother Psychosom.* 1998 Jul-Oct;67(4-5):259-65.

Bechilioulis, A. "Endothelial function, but not carotid intima-media thickness, is affected early in menopause and is associated with severity of hot flashes. *J Clin Endocrinol Metab* 2010 Mar;95(3):1199-206.

Bellantoni, M. F. "Effects of oral versus transdermal estrogen on the growth hormone/insulin-like growth factor I axis in younger and older postmenopausal women: a clinical research center study." *J Clin Endocrinol Metab.* 1996 Aug;81(8):2848-53.

Beral, V. "Breast cancer and HRT in the Million Women Study." *Lancet.* 2003 Aug 9;362(9382):419-27. (Synthetic HRT increased breast cancer risk.)

Bergkvist, L. "Prognosis after breast cancer diagnosis in women exposed to estrogen and estrogen-progestogen replacement therapy." *Am J Epidemiol.* 1989 Aug;130(2):221-8. (The relative survival rate was significantly higher in patients who had received estrogen treatment, corresponding to an approximately 40 percent reduction in excess mortality.)

Best, NR. "Effect of estradiol implant on noradrenergic function and mood in menopausal subjects." *Psychoneuroendocrinology.* 1992;17(1):87-93.

Bethea, CL. "Ovarian steroids and serotonin neural function." *Mol Neurobiol.* 1998 Oct;18(2):87-123.

Bhavnani, BR. "Pharmokinetics and pharmadynamics of conjugated equine estrogen: Chemistry and metabolism." *Proc Soc Exp Biol Med.* 1998 Jan;217(1):6-16.

Birge, SJ. "Is there a role for estrogen replacement therapy in the prevention and treatment of dementia?" *J Am Geriatr Soc.* 1996 July;44(7):865-70.

Birge,SJ. "The role of estrogen in the treatment of Alzheimer's disease." *Neurology*. 1997 May;48(5 Suppl 7):S36-41.

Bitran, D. "Anxiolytic effect of progesterone is associated with increases in cortical allopregnanolone and GABBA receptor function." *Pharmacol Biochem Behav*.1993 Jun;45(2):423-8.

Bitran, D. "Anxiolytic effect of progesterone is mediated by the neurosteroid allopregnanolone at brain GABAA receptors."*J Neuroendocrinol*. 1995 May;7(3):171-7.

Blumel, JE. "Effects of transdermal estrogens on endothelial function in postmenopausal women with coronary disease." *Climacteric*. 2003 Mar;6(1):38-44. (Transdermal estrogens cause beneficial vasodilatation.)

Boekhoorn, SS. "Estrogen receptor alpha gene polymorphisms associated with incident aging macula disorder." *Invest Ophthalmol Vis Sci*. 2007 Mar;48(3):1012-7. (Early menopause increases risk of macular degeneration from low estrogens.)

Bolaji, II. "Low-dose progesterone in estrogenised postmenopausal women: effects on plasma lipids, lipoproteins and liver function parameters." *Eur J Obstet Gynecol*. 1993 Jan;48(1):61-8.

Bonduki, CE. "Effect of estrogen-progestin hormone replacement therapy on plasma antithrombin III of postmenopausal women." *Acta Obstet Gynecol Scand*.1998 Jan;48(1):61-8. (Negative impact of synthetic HRT on blood clotting.)

Borgin, N. "Oral treatment of menopausal symptoms with natural estrogens-experience with a new series of estrogens and estrogen-gestagen combinations." *Acta Obstet Gynecol Scand Suppl*.1975;(43):1-11.

Bradlow, HL. "2-hydroxyestrone: the 'good' estrogen." *J Endocrinol*.1996 Sept;150 Suppl:S259-65.

Bradlow, HL. "16 alpha-hydroxylation of estradiol: a possible risk marker for breast cancer." *Ann NY Acad Sci*. 1986;464:138-51.

Brennan, JJ. "Serum concentrations of 17beta-estradiol and estrone after multiple-dose administration of percutaneous estradiol gel in symptomatic women." *Ther Drug Monit*. 2001 Apr;23(2):134-8.

Brenner, DE. "Postmenopausal estrogen replacement therapy on the risk of Alzheimer's disease: a population-based case-control study. *Am J Epidemiol*.1994 Aug1;140(3):262-7.

Brincat,M. "Decline in skin collagen content and metacarpal index after the menopause and its prevention with sex hormone replacement. *Br J Obstet Gynecol*. 1987 Feb;94(2):126-9.

Brincat, M. "Sex hormones and skin collagen content in postmenopausal women." *Br Med J*. 1983 Nov 5;287(6402):1337-8.

Brincat, M. "Subcutaneous hormone implants for the control of climacteric symptoms. A prospective study." *Lancet*. 1984 Jan 7;1(8367):16-8.

Bruning, PF. "Insulin resistance and breast-cancer risk." *Int J Cancer*.1992 Oct 21;52(4):511-6.

Bucolo, C. "Neuroactive steroids protect retinal pigment epithelium against oxidative stress." *Neuroreport*. 2005 Aug 1;16(11):1203-7.

Burger, HG. "The management of persistent menopausal symptoms with estradiol-testosterone implants: clinical, lipid, and hormonal results." *Maturitas*. 1984 Dec;6(4):351-8.

Burger, HG. "Effect of combined implants on estradiol and testosterone on libido in postmenopausal women." *Br Med J*. 1987 Apr 11;294(6577):936-7.

Burry, KA. "Percutaneous absorption of progesterone in postmenopausal women treated with transdermal estrogen." *Am J Obstet Gynecol*. 1999 Jun;180(6 Pt 1):1504-11.

Bush, TL. "Preserving cardiovascular benefits of hormone replacement therapy." *J Reprod Med*. 2000 Mar;45(3 Suppl):259-73.

Bush,TL. "Estrogen use and all-cause mortality. Preliminary results from the Lipid Research Clinics Program Follow-up Study" *JAMA*. 1983 Feb 18;249(7):903-6.

Cacciatore, B. "Randomized comparison of oral and transdermal hormone replacement on carotid and uterine artery resistance to blood flow." *Obstet Gynecol*. 1998 Oct;92(4 Pt 1):563-8.

Cagnacci, A. "Effects of low doses of transdermal 17beta-estradiol on carbohydrate metabolism in postmenopausal women." *J Clin Endocrinol Metab*.1992 Jun;74(6):1396-400.

Campbell, S. "Estrogen therapy and the menopausal syndrome." *Clin Obstet Gynecol*. 1997 Apr;4(1):31-47.

Carey, BJ. "A study to evaluate serum and urinary hormone levels following short and long-term administration of two regimens of progesterone cream in postmenopausal women. *BJOG*. 2000 Jun;107(6):722-6.

Cardoza, L. "The effects of subcutaneous hormone implants during climacteric." *Maturitas*. 1984 Mar;5(3):177-84.

Carette, S. "Fibromyalgia and sex hormones." *J Rheumatol.* 1992 May;19(5):831.

Carlson, CL. "Hormone replacement therapy is associated with higher FEV1 in elderly women." *Am J Respir Crit Care Med.* 2001 Feb;163(2):423-8.

Carr, MC. "The emergence of the metabolic syndrome with menopause." *J Clin Endocrinol Metab.* 2003 Jun;88(8):2404-11. (Obesity associated with low estrogen levels.)

Carranza-Lira, S. "Estrogen therapy for depression in postmenopausal women." *Int J Gynecol Obstet.* 1999 Apr;65(1):35-8.

Castlo-Branco, C. "Circulating hormone levels in menopausal women receiving different hormone replacement therapy regimens. A comparison." *J Reprod Med.* 1995 Aug;40(8):556-60.

Castelo-Branco, C. "Comparative effects of estrogens plus androgens and tibolone on bone, lipid pattern and sexuality in postmenopausal women." *Maturitas.* 2000 Feb 15;34(2):161-8.

Cerquetani, E. "Anti-ischemic effect of chronic estrogen replacement therapy alone or in combination with medroxyprogesterone acetate in different replacement schemes." *Maturitas.* 2001 Sep 28;39(3):245-51. (Adverse cardiovascular impact of Provera)

Chang, KJ. "Influences of percutaneous administration of estradiol and progesterone on human breast epithelial cell cycle in vivo." *Fertil Steril.* 1995 Apr;63(4):785-91.

Chapurlat, RD. "Serum estradiol and sex hormone binding globulin and the risk of hip fracture in elderly women: the EPIDOS study." *J Bone Miner Res.* 2000 Sep;15(9):1835-41.

Chen, FP. "Effects of hormone replacement therapy on cardiovascular risk factors in postmenopausal women." *Fertil Steril.* 1998 Feb;69(2):267-73.

Chen, F. P. "Comparison of transdermal and oral estrogen-progestin replacement therapy: effects on cardiovascular risk factors." *Menopause.* 2001 Sep-Oct;8(5):347-52.

Chen, Y. "The equine estrogen metabolite 4-hydroxyequilenin cause DNA single-strand breaks and oxidation of DNA bases in vitro." *Chem Res Toxicol.* 1998 Sep;11(9):1105-11.

Chetkowski, RJ. "Biologic effects of transdermal estradiol." *N Eng J Med.* 1986 Jun 19;314(25):1615-20.

Chmouliovsky, L. "Beneficial effect of hormone replacement therapy on weight loss in obese menopausal women." *Maturitas.* 1999 Aug 16;32(3):147-53.

Christiansen, C. "Uncoupling of bone formation and resorption by combined estrogen and progesterone therapy in postmenopausal osteoporosis." *Lancet.* 1985 Oct 12;2(8459):800-1.

Christiansen, C. "Bone mass in postmenopausal women after withdrawal of estrogen/progestagen replacement therapy." *Lancet.* 1981 Feb 28;1(8218):459-61.

Christiansen, C. "Prevention of early postmenopausal bone loss: controlled 2-year study in 315 normal females." *Eur J Clin Invest.* 1980 Aug;10(4):273-9.

Cicinelli, E. "Pharmocokinetics and endometrial effects of the vaginal administration of micronized progesterone in an oil-based solution to postmenopausal women." *Fertil Steril.* 1996 Apr;65(4):860-2.

Clemons, M. "Estrogen and the risk of breast cancer." *N Engl J Med.* 2001 Jan 25;344(4):276-85.

Col, NF. "Patient-specific decisions about hormone replacement therapy in postmenopausal women." *JAMA.* 1997 Apr 9;277(14):1140-7.

Colacurci, N. "Effects of hormone replacement therapy on glucose metabolism." *Panminerva Med.* 1998 Mar;40(1):18-21.

Colditz, GA. "The use of estrogens and progestin and the risk of breast cancer in postmenopausal women." *N Engl J Med.* 1995 Jun 15;332(24):1589-93.

Cooper, C. "Matrix delivery transdermal 17beta-estradiol for the prevention of bone loss in postmenopausal women. The International Study Group." *Osteoporosis Int.* 1999;9(4):358-66.

Cowan, LD. "Breast cancer incidence in women with a history of progesterone deficiency." *Am J Epidemiol.* 1981 Aug;114(2):209-17.

Cravioto, M. "Pharmacokinetics and Pharmacodynamics of 25-mg estradiol implants on postmenopausal Mexican women." *Menopause.* 2001 Sep-Oct;8(5):353-60.

Creaseman, WT. "Is there an association between hormone replacement therapy and breast cancer?" *J Womens Health.* 1998 Dec;7(10):1231-46.

Crews, JK. "Antagonistic effects of 17beta-estradiol, progesterone, and testosterone on calcium entry mechanisms of coronary vasoconstriction." *Arterioscler Thrombo Vasc Biol.* 1999 Apr;19(4):1034-40.

Cucinelli, F. "Differential effect of transdermal estrogen plus progestagen replacement on insulin metabolism in postmenopausal women; relation to their insulinemic secretion." *Eur J Endocrinol.* 1999 Mar;140(3):215-23.

Czarnecka, D. "Influence of hormone replacement therapy on quality of life in postmenopausal women with hypertension." *Przegl Lek.* 2000;57(7-8):397-401.

Davis, SR. "Testosterone enhances estradiol's effects on postmenopausal bone density and sexuality." *Maturitas.* 1995 Sep-Oct;61(1-2):17-26.

Davis, SR. "Effects of estradiol with and without testosterone on body composition and relationships with lipids in postmenopausal women." *Menopause.* 2000 Nov-Dec;7(6):395-401.

Decensi A. Effect of transdermal estradiol and oral conjugated estrogen on C-reactive protein in retinoid-placebo trial in healthy women. *Circulation.* 2002 Sep 3;106(10):1224-8. (Transdermal does not raise CRP.)

D'Elia, HF. "Influence of hormone replacement therapy on disease progression and bone mineral density in rheumatoid arthritis." *J Rheumatol.* 2003 Jul;30(7):1456-63.

de Kleijn, MJ. "Hormone replacement therapy in perimenopausal women and 2-year change of carotid intima-media thickness." *Maturitas.* 1999 Aug 16;32(3):195-204.

de Lignieres, B. "Combined hormone replacement therapy and risk of breast cancer in a French cohort study of 3,175 women." *Climacteric.* 2002 Dec;5(4):332-40. (No risk of breast cancer with bioidentical HRT.)

de Lingieres, B. "Biological effects of estradiol-17 beta in postmenopausal women: oral versus percutaneous administration." *J Clin Endocrinol Metab.* 1986 Mar;62(3):536-41.

de Lignieres, B. "Influence of route of administration in progesterone metabolism." *Maturitas.* 1995 Apr;21(3):251-7.

de Lignieres, B. "Differential effects of exogenous estradiol and progesterone on mood in post-menopausal women: individual dose/effect relationship." *Maturitas.* 1982 Apr;4(1):67-72.

Delyani, JA. "Protection from myocardial reperfusion injury by acute administration of 17beta-estradiol." *J Mol Cell Cardiol.* 1996 May;28(5):1001-8.

Deng X. "Correlation between bone mineral density and sexual hormones in healthy Chinese women." *J Environ Pathol Toxicol Oncol.* 2000;19(1-2):167-9.

Dennerstein, L. "Progesterone and the premenstrual syndrome: a double-blind crossover trial." *Br Med J*. 1985 Jun 1;290(6482):1617-21.

Derman, RJ. "Quality of life during sequential HRT—a placebo-controlled study. *Int J Fertil Menopausal Stud*. 1995 May-Apr;40(2): 73-8.

Deutsch, S. "The correlation of serum estrogens and androgens with bone density in the late post menopause." *Int J Gynecol Obstet*. 1987 Jun;25(3):217-22.

Ditkoff, EC. "Estrogen improves psychological function in asymptomatic postmenopausal women." *Obstet Gynecol*. 1991 Dec;78(6):991-5.

Dobs, AS. "Differential effects of oral estrogen vs. oral estrogen-androgen replacement therapy on body composition in postmenopausal women." *J Clin Endocrinol Metab*. 2002 Apr;87(4):1509-16.

Dubrey, RK. "Cardiovascular Pharmacology of Estradiol Metabolites." *J Pharmacol Exp Ther*. 2004 Feb;308(2):403-9.

Dzugan, SA. "Hypercholesterolemis treatment: a new hypothesis or just an accident?" *Med Hypotheses*. 2002 Dec;59(6):751-6.

Erenus, M. "Comparison of effects of continuous combined transdermal with oral estrogen and oragl progestogen replacement therapies on serum lipoproteins and compliance." *Climacteric*. 2001 Sep;4(3):228-34.

Eriksen, B. "Urogenital estrogen deficiency syndrome. Investigation and treatment with special reference to hormone substitution." *Tidsskr Nor Laegeforen*. 1991 Oct;111(24):2949-51.

Eriksen, B. "A randomized, open, parallel-group study on the preventive effect of an estradiol-releasing vaginal ring (Estring) on recurrent urinary tract infections in postmenopausal women." *Am J Obstet Gynecol*. 1999 May;180(5):1072-9.

Eriksen, EF. "Hormone replacement therapy prevents osteoclastic hyperactivity: A histomorphometric study in early postmenopausal women." *J Bone Miner Res*. 1999 Jul;10(7):1217-21.

Ershler, WB. "Age-associated increased interleukin-6 gene expression, late-life diseases, and frailty." *Annu. Rev. Med*. 2000;51:245-70. (Testosterone and estrogen downregulates IL-6 gene expression, a pro-inflammatory cytokine, decreasing inflammation.)

Espeland, M. "Effect of postmenopausal hormone therapy on lipoprotein (a) concentration. PEPI investigators. Postmenopausal Estrogen/Progestin Interventions." *Circulation*. 1998 Mar 17;99(10):979-86.

Ettinger, B. "Low-dose micronized 17beta-estradiol prevents bone loss in postmenopausal women." *Am J Obstet Gynecol.* 1992 Feb;166(2):479-88.

Ettinger, B. "Reduced mortality associated with long-term postmenopausal estrogen therapy." *Obstet Gynecol.* 1996 Jan;87(1):6-12.

Ettinger, B. "Vasomotor symptom relief versus unwanted effects: role of estrogen dosage." *Am J Med.* 2005 Dec 19;118 Suppl 12B:74-8.

Ettinger, B. "Long-term estrogen replacement therapy prevents bone loss and fractures. *Ann Int Med.* 1985 Mar;102(3):319-2. (9,704 patients over sixty-five years old, followed for seven years. Group with estrogen therapy had increased bone density—97 percent had no bone loss at spine; 95 percent had no bone loss at hip.)

Fahraeus, L. "L-norgestrol and progesterone have different influences on plasma lipoproteins." *Eur J Clin Invest.* 1983 Dec;13(6):447-53.

Fahraeus, L. "Estrogens, gonadotrophins and SHBG during oral and cutaneous administration of estradiol-17 beta to menopausal women." *Acta Endocrinol* (Copenh). 1982 Dec;101(4):592-6. (Oral but not topical estrogen increased estrone levels.)

Falconer, C. "Changes in paraurethral connective tissue at menopause are counteracted by estrogen." *Maturitas.* 1996 Jul;24(3):197-204.

Farhat, MY. "The vascular protective effects of estrogen." *FASEB J.* 1996 Apr;10(5):615-24.

Farish, E. "The effects of hormone implants on serum lipoproteins and steroid hormones in bilaterally oophorectomised women." *Acta Endocrinol* (Copenh). 1986 May;106(1):116-20.

Fitzpatrick, LA. "Micronized progesterone: clinical indications and comparison with current treatments." *Fertil Steril.* 1999 Sep;72(3):389-97.

Fitzpatrick, LA. "Comparison of regimens containing oral micronized progesterone or medroxyprogesterone acetate on quality of life in postmenopausal women. A cross-sectional survey." *J Womens Health Gend Based Med.* 2000 May;9(4):381-7.

Fletcher,CD "Long-term hormone implant therapy-effects on lipoproteins and steroid levels in post-menopausal women. *Acta Endocrinol (Copenh).* Mar;111(3):419-23.

Formby, B. "Progesterone inhibits growth and induces apoptosis in breast cancer cells: inverse effects on Bcl-2 and p53." *Ann Clin Lab Sci.*1998 Nov-Dec;28(6):360-9.

Fournier, A. "Breast cancer risk in relation to different types of hormone replacement therapy in the E3N-EPIC cohort." *Int J Cancer.* 2005 Apr 10;114(3):448-54. (The risk was significantly greater with HRT containing synthetic progestins than with HRT containing micronized progesterone, the RR being 1.4 and 0.9, respectively—RR of 1.0 is neutral.)

Fowke, J. "Macronutrient intake and estrogen metabolism in healthy postmenopausal women." *Breast Cancer Res Treat.* 2001 Jan;65(1):1-10.

Freedman, M. A. "Quality of life and menopause: the role of estrogen." *J Womens Health.* 2002 Oct;11(8):703-18.

Frohlich, M. "Effects of hormone replacement therapies on fibrinogen and plasma viscosity in postmenopausal women." *Br. J Haematol.* 1998 Mar;100(3):577-81.

Gambacciani, M. "Hormone replacement therapy: the benefits of tailoring the regimen and dose." *Maturitas.* 2001Dec 14;40(3):195-201.

Gambacciani, M. "Effects of low-dose, continuous combined estradiol and noretisterone acetate on menopausal quality of life in early postmenopausal women." *Maturitas.* 2003 Feb 25;44(2):157-63.

Garnero, P. "Biochemical markers of bone turnover, endogenous hormones and the risk of fractures in postmenopausal women: the OFELY study." *J Bone Miner Res.* 2000 Aug;15(8):1526-36.

Garnett, T. "The effects of plasma estradiol levels on increases in vertebral and femoral bone density following therapy with estradiol and estradiol with testosterone implants." *Obstet Gynecol* 1992 Jun;79(6):968-72.

Garnett, T. "A cross-sectional study of the effects of long-term percutaneous hormone replacement therapy on bone density." *Obstet Gynecol* 1991 Dec;78(6):1002-7.

Gerhard, M. "Estradiol therapy combined with progesterone and endothelium-dependent vasodilation in postmenopausal women." *Circulation.*1998 Sep 22;98(12):1158-63. (Beneficial vascular effect of bioidentical HRT)

Gilligan, DM. "Acute vascular effects of estrogen in postmenopausal women." *Circulation.* 1994 Aug;90(2):786-91.

Gilligan, DM. "Effects of physiological levels of estrogen on coronary vasomotor function in postmenopausal women." *Circulation.* 1994 Jun;89(6):2545-51.

Giuliani, A. "Hormone replacement therapy with a transdermal estradiol gel and oral micronized progesterone. Effect on menopausal symptoms and lipid metabolism. *Wien Klin Wochenschr.* 2000 Jul 28;112(14):629-33.

Godsland, IF. "Effects of postmenopausal HRT on lipid, lipoprotein, and apolipoprotein (a) concentrations: analysis of studies published from 1974–2000. *Fertil Steril.* 2001May;75(5):898-915.

Gorodeski, G. "Impact of the menopause on the epidemiology and risk factors of coronary artery heart disease in women." *Exp Gerontol.*1994 May-Aug;29(3-4):357-75.

Gorsky, RD. "Relative risks and benefits of long-term estrogen replacement therapy: a decision analysis." *Obstet Gynecol.*1994 Feb;83(2):161-6.

Grady E. "Cardiovascular disease outcomes during 6.8 years of hormone therapy: Heart and Estrogen/progestin Replacement Study follow-up." *JAMA.* 2002 Jul 3;288(1):49-57.

Granberg, S. "The effects of oral estriol on the endometrium in postmenopausal women." *Maturitas.* 2002 Jun 25;42(2):149-56.

Greenblatt, R. "Indications for hormone pellets in the therapy of endocrine and gynecological disorders." *Am J Obstet Gynecol.*1988 Feb;57(2):294-301.

Gregoire, AJ. "Transdermal estrogen for treatment of severe postnatal depression." *Lancet.*1996 Apr 6;347(9006):930-3.

Grodstein, F. "Hormone Therapy and Coronary Heart Disease: The role of time since menopause and age at hormone initiation." *J Womens Health.* 2006 Jan-Feb;15(1):35-44.

Grodstein F. "Postmenopausal hormone therapy and mortality." *N Engl J Med.* 1997 Jun 19;336(25):1769-75 (Current hormone users had lower risk of death than never users.)

Grodstein, F. "Postmenopausal estrogen and progestin use and the risk of cardiovascular disease." *N Eng J Med.* 1996 Aug 15;335(7):453-61.

Grodstein, F. "A prospective, observational study of postmenopausal hormone therapy and primary prevention of cardiovascular disease." *Ann Intern Med.* 2000

Grodstein, F. "Postmenopausal hormone use and risk for colorectal cancer and adenoma." *Ann Intern Med.*1998 Dec 19;133(12):933-41.

Guarneri P. "Neurosteroids in the retina: neurodegenerative and neuroprotective agents in retinal degeneration." *Ann NY Acad Sci.* 2003 Dec;1007:117-28. (Importance of hormones to the retina)

Guetta, AA. "The role of nitric oxide in coronary vascular effects of estrogen in postmenopausal women." *Circulation.*1997 Nov 4;96(9):2795-801.

Haines, C. "Effect of oral estradiol on Lp(a) and other lipoproteins in postmenopausal women. A randomized, double-blind, placebo-controlled, crossover study." *Arch Intern Med.* 1996 Apr 22;156(8):866-72.

Haffner, S. "Endogenous sex hormones: impact on lipids, lipoproteins, and insulin." *Am J Med.* 1995 Jan 16;98(1A):40S-47S.

Hall, GM. "A randomized controlled trial of the effect of hormone replacement therapy on disease activity in postmenopausal rheumatoid arthritis." *Ann Rheum Dis.*1994 Feb;53(2):112-6.

Hall, G. "Long-term effects of HRT on symptoms of angina pectoris, quality of life and compliance in women with coronary artery disease." *Maturitas.* 1998 Jan 12;28(3):235-42.

Han, HJ. "Effects of sex hormones on Na+/glucose cotransporter of renal proximal tubular cells following oxidant injury." *Kidney Blood Press Res.* 2001;24(3):159-65.

Hanke, H. "Estradiol concentrations in premenopausal women with coronary heart disease." Coron Artery Dis. 1997 Aug-Sep;8(8-9):511-5. (Low estrogen levels found in women with heart disease.)

Hargrove, JT. "Menopausal hormone replacement therapy with continuous daily oral micronized estradiol and progesterone." *Obstet Gynecol.* 1989 Apr;73(4):606-12.

Hargrove, JT. "An alternative method of hormone replacement therapy using the natural sex steroids." *Infer Repro Med Clin N. Am.* 1995;6:653-74.

Harman, HM. KEEPS: The Kronos Early Estrogen Prevention Study. *Climacteric.* 2005 Mar;8(1):3-12.

Hashimoto, M. "Effects of long-term and reduced-dose HRT on endothelial function and intima-media thickness in postmenopausal women." *Menopause.* 2002 Jan-Feb;5(1):58-64.(Beneficial vascular effects of HRT.)

Haspels, AA. "Endocrinological and clinical investigations in post-menopausal women following administration of vaginal cream containing estriol." *Maturitas.*1981Dec;3(3-4):321-7.

Hayaski, T. "Estriol replacement improves endothelial function and bone mineral density in very elderly women." *J Gerontol A Biol Sci Med Sci.* 2000 Apr;55(4):B183-90.

Head, KA. "Estriol: Safety and efficacy." *Altern Med Rev.* 1998 Apr;3(2):101-13.

Henderson, BE. "Estrogen replacement therapy and protection from acute myocardial infarction." *Am J Obstet Gynecol.* 1988 Aug;159(2):312-7.

Henderson, BE. "Decreased mortality in users of estrogen replacement therapy." *Arch Int Med.* 1991Jan;151(1):75-8.

Henderson,VW. "Estrogen replacement therapy in older women. Comparisons between Alzheimer's disease cases and non-demented control subjects." *Arch Neurol.* 1994 Sep;51(9):896-900.

Henderson, VW. "Cognitive skills associated with estrogen replacement in women with Alzheimer's disease." *Psychoneuroendocrinology.* 1996 May;21(4):421-30.

Henderson, VW. "The epidemiology of estrogen replacement therapy and Alzheimer's disease." *Neurology* 1997 May;48(5 Suppl 7):S27-35.

Herbert-Croteau, N. "A meta-analysis of hormone replacement therapy and colon cancer in women." *Cancer Epidemiol Biomarkers Prev.* 1998 Aug;7(8):653-9.

Hilditch, JR. "A comparison of the effects of oral conjugated equine estrogen and transdermal estradiol-17 beta combined with an oral progestin on quality of life in postmenopausal women." *Maturitas.* 1996 Jul;24(3):177-84.

Hodis, HN. "Estrogen in the prevention of atherosclerosis. A randomized, double-blind, placebo-controlled trial." *Ann Intern Med.* 2001 Dec4;135(11):939-53. (Slower rate of atherosclerosis progression with estradiol therapy.)

Hofseth, LJ. "Hormone replacement therapy with estrogen or estrogen plus medroxyprogesterone acetate is associated with increased epithelial proliferation in the normal postmenopausal breast." *J Clin Endocrinol Metab.*1999 Dec;84(12):4559-65(Synthetic HRT increased breast cancer risk.)

Holland, EF. "Increase in bone mass of older postmenopausal women with low mineral bone density after one year of percutaneous estradiol implants." *Br J Obstet Gynecol.* 1995 Mar;102(3):238-47.

Holland, EF. "The effect of 25-mg percutaneous estradiol implants on the bone mass of postmenopausal women." *Obstet Gynecol.* 1994 Jan;83(1):43-6.

Hollander, LE. "Sleep quality, estradiol levels, and behavioral factors in late reproductive age women." *Obstet Gynecol.* 2001Sep;98(3):391-7.

Iannuzzi-Sucich, M. "Prevalence of sarcopenia and predictors of skeletal muscle mass in healthy, older men and women." *J Gerontol A Biol Sci Med Sci.* 2002 Dec;57(12):M772-7. (Low estradiol and testosterone levels accelerate muscle loss.)

Jacobs, DM. "Cognitive function in non-demented older women who took estrogen after menopause." *Neurology.* 1998 Feb;50(2):368-73.

Janowsky, JS. "Sex steroids modify working memory." *J Cogn Neurosci.* 2000 May;12(3):407-14.

Jarvinen, A. "Steady-state pharmacokinetics of estradiol gel in postmenopausal women: effects of application area and washing." *Br J Obstet Gynecol.* 1997 Nov;104 Suppl 16:14-8.

Jarvinen, A. "Effect of dose on the absorption of estradiol from a transdermal gel. *Maturitas.* 2000 Apr 28;35(1):51-6.

Jassal, SK. "Low bioavailable testosterone levels predict future height loss in postmenopausal women." *J Bone Miner Res.* 1995 Apr;10(4):650-4.

Jochems, C. "Osteoporosis in experimental postmenopausal polyarthritis; the relative contributions of estrogen deficiency and inflammation." *Arthritis Res Ther.* 2005;7(4):R837-43.

Jonas, HA. "Current estrogen-progestin and estrogen replacement therapy in elderly women: association with carotid atherosclerosis." CHS Collaborative Research Group. Cardiovascular Health Study. *Ann Epidemiol.* 1996 Jul;6(4):314-23.

Jung, BH. "Hormone-dependent aging problems in women." *Yonsei Med J.* 2008 Jun 30;49(3):345-51.

Kalantaridou, SN. "Impaired endothelial function in young women with premature ovarian failure: normalization with hormone therapy." *J Clin Endocrinol Metab.* 2004 Aug;89(8):3907-13. (HRT restored endothelial function within six months of treatment.)

Kalkhoff, RK. "Metabolic effects of progesterone." *J Obstet Gynecol.* 1982 Mar 15;142(6 Pt 2):735-8.

Kanaya, A. "Glycemic effects of postmenopausal hormone therapy: the Heart and Estrogen/progestin Replacement Study. A randomized, double-blind, placebo-controlled trial" *Ann Intern Med.* 2003 Jan 7;138(1):1-9. (HRT reduced the incidence of diabetes by 35 percent.)

Karjalainen, A. "Effects of oral and transdermal estrogen replacement therapy on glucose and insulin metabolism." *Clin Endocrinol* (Oxf). 2001Feb;54(2):165-73.

Karlberg, J. "A quality of life perspective on who benefits from estradiol replacement therapy." *Acta Obstet Gynecol Scand.* 1995 May;74(5):367-72.

Kampen, DL. "Estrogen use and verbal memory in healthy post-menopausal women." *Obstet Gynecol.* 1994 Jun;83(6):979-83.

Kawas, C. "A prospective study of estrogen replacement therapy and the risk of developing Alzheimer's disease." The Baltimore Longitudinal Study of Aging. *Neurology.* 1997 Jun;48(6):1517-21.

Keefe, DL. "HRT may alleviate sleep apnea in menopausal women: a pilot study." *Menopause.* 1999 Fall;6(3):196-200.

Khastgir, G. "Hysterectomy, ovarian failure and depression." *Menopause.* 1996 Summer;6(2): 180-1.

Khaw, KT. "Fasting plasma glucose levels and endogenous androgens in non-diabetic postmenopausal women." *Clin Sci.* 1991 Mar;80(3):199-203.

Khosla, S. "Relationship of serum sex steroid levels and bone turnover markers with bone mineral density in men and women: a key role for bioavailable estrogen." *J Clin Endocrinol Metab.* 1998

Khosla, S. "Relationship of volumetric bone density and structural parameters at different skeletal sites to sex steroid levels in women." *J Clin Endocrinol Metab.* 2005 Sep;90(9):5096-103.

Kiel, D. P. "Hip fracture and the use of estrogens in postmenopausal women." The Framingham Study. *N Engl J Med.* 1987 Nov 5;317(15):1169-74.

Kim, S. "Antiproliferative effects of low-dose micronized progesterone." *Fertil Steril.* 1996 Feb;65(2):323-31.

Kimura, D. "Estrogen replacement therapy may protect against intellectual decline in postmenopausal women." *Horm Behav.* 1995 Sep;29(3):312-21.

Kirkengen, AL. "Estriol in the prophylactic treatment of recurrent urinary tract infections in postmenopausal women." *Scand J Prim Health Care.* 1992 Jun;10(2):139-42.

Krasinski, K. "Estradiol accelerates functional endothelial recovery after arterial injury." *Circulation.* 1997 Apr 1;95(7):1768-72.

Klaiber, EL "A critique of the Women's Health Initiative hormone therapy study." *Fertil Steril.* 2005 Dec;84(6):1589-601.

Lafferty, FW. "Postmenopausal estrogen replacement: A long-term cohort study." *Am J Med.* 1994 Jul;97(1):66-77.

Lahdenpera, S. "Effects of postmenopausal estrogen/progestin replacement therapy on LDL particles; comparison of transdermal and oral treatment regimens." *Atherosclerosis.* 1996 May;122(2):153-62.

Lane, G. "Dose dependent effects of oral progesterone on the estrogenised postmenopausal endometrium." *Br Med J.* 1983 Oct 29;(6401):1241-5.

Lauritzen, C. "Results of a 5 year prospective study of estriol succinate treatment in patients with climacteric complaints." *Horm Metab Res.* 1987;19;579-584.

Lemon, H. "Pathophysiologic considerations in the treatment of menopausal symptoms with estrogens: the role of estriol in the prevention of mammary carcinoma." *Acta Endocrinol.* 1980;233:17-27.

Lemon, H. "Reduced estriol excretion in patients with breast cancer prior to endocrine therapy." *JAMA.* 1966 Jun 27;196(13):1128-36.

Leonetti, HB. "Transdermal progesterone cream for vasomotor symptoms and postmenopausal bone loss." *Obstet Gynecol.* 1999 Aug;94(2):225-8.

Leonetti, HB. "Topical progesterone cream has antiproliferative effect on estrogen-stimulated endometrium." *Fertil Steril.* 2003 Jan 79(1):221-2.

Levesque, H. "Estrogen therapy and venous thromboembolic disease." *Rev Med Interne.* 1997;18 Suppl 6:620s-625s (Provera increases risk of blood clots and negates estrogen effects.)

L'hermite, M. "Could transdermal estradiol + progesterone be a safer postmenopausal HRT? A review." *Maturitas* 2008 Jul-Aug;60(3-4):185-201.

Liang, YL. "Effects of estrogen and progesterone on age-related changes in arteries of postmenopausal women." *Clin Exp Pharm Physiol.* 1997 Jun;24(6):457-9. (Improved lipids with HRT. Reduced carotid artery intima-medial thickness in HRT group.)

Liberman, EH. "Estrogen improves endothelium-dependent, flow-mediated vasodilation in postmenopausal women." *Ann Intern Med.* 1994;121:936-941.

Limouzin-Lamothe, M. A. "Quality of life after the menopause: influence of hormone replacement therapy." *Am J Obstet Gynecol.* 1994 Feb;170(2):618-24.

Linzmayer, L. "Double-blind, placebo-controlled psychometric studies on the effects of a combined estrogen-progestin regimen vs. estrogen only on performance, mood and personality of menopausal syndrome patients." *Arzneimittelforschung.* 2001;51(3):238-45.

Lippert, TH. "Estradiol metabolism during oral and transdermal estradiol replacement therapy in postmenopausal women." *Horm Metab Res.* 1998 Sep;70(9):598-600.

Lobo, RA. "Subdermal estradiol pellets following hysterectomy and oophorectomy. Effect upon serum estrone, estradiol, luteinizing hormone, follicle-stimulating hormone, corticosteroid binding globulin-binding capacity, testosterone-estradiol binding globulin-binding capacity, lipids and hot flashes" *Am J Obstet Gynecol.* 1980 Nov 15;138(6):714-9.

Lobo, R.A. "Effects of lower doses of conjugated equine estrogens and medroxyprogesterone acetate on plasma lipids and lipoproteins, coagulation factors, and carbohydrate metabolism." *Fertil Ster.* 2001 Jul;76(1):13-24. (Adverse impact of Premarin and Provera.)

Longcope, C. "Androgen and estrogen metabolism: relationship to obesity." *Metabolism.* 1986 Mar;35(3):235-7.

Luckas, MJ. "The effect of progestagens on the carotid artery pulsatility index in postmenopausal women on estrogen replacement therapy." *Eur J Obstet Gynecol Reprod Biol.* 1998 Feb;76(2):221-4. (Provera negates vascular benefits of estrogen.)

Lufkin, EG. "Treatment of postmenopausal osteoporosis with transdermal estrogen." *Ann Intern Med.* 1992 Jul 1;117(1):1-9.

Lufkin, EG. "Relative value of transdermal and oral estrogen therapy in various clinical situations." *Mayo Clin Proc.* 1994 Feb;69(2):131-5.

Luyer, MD. "Prospective randomized study of effects of unopposed estrogen replacement therapy on markers of coagulation and inflammation in postmenopausal women." *J Clin Endocrinol Metab.* 2001 Aug;86(8):3629-34.

Maki, PM. "Longitudinal effects of estrogen replacement therapy on PET cerebral blood flow and cognition." *Neurobiol Aging.* 2000 Mar-Apr;21(2):373-83.

Manhem, K. "Acute effects of transdermal estrogen in postmenopausal women with coronary artery disease. Using a clinically relevant estrogen dose and concurrent antianginal therapy." *Cardiology.* 2000;94(2):86-90.

Manonal, J. "Effect of oral estriol on urogenital symptoms, vaginal cytology, and plasma hormone level in postmenopausal women." *J Med Assoc Thai.* 2001 Apr;84(4):539-44.

Manson, JE. "Estrogen therapy and coronary-artery calcification." *New Engl J Med.* 2007 Jun 21;356(25):2591-602. (Study with conjugated equine estrogen, lower calcified-plaque burden with estrogen therapy.)

Martorano JY. "Differentiating between natural progesterone and synthetic progestins: clinical implications for premenstrual syndrome and perimenopause management." *Compr Ther.* 1998 Jun-Jul;24(6-7):332-9.

Massafra, C. "Effects of estrogens and androgens on erythrocyte superoxide dismutase, catalase and glutathione peroxidase activities during the menstrual cycle." *J Endocrinol.* 2000 Dec;167(3):447-52.

Mather, KJ. "Preserved forearm endothelial responses with acute exposure to progesterone: A randomized cross-over trial of 17beta-estradiol, progesterone, and 17beta- estradiol with progesterone in healthy menopausal women." *J Clin Endocrinol Metab.* 2000 Dec;85(12):4644-9.

Maxson, WS. "Bioavailability of oral micronized progesterone." *Fertil Steril.* 1985 Nov;44(5):622-6.

Mayeaux, EJ. "Current concepts in postmenopausal hormone replacement therapy." *J Fam Prac.* 1996 Jul;43(1):69-75.

McAuley, J. "Oral administration of micronized progesterone; a review and more experience." *Pharmacotherapy.* 1996 May-Jun;16(3):453-7.

McCrohon, JA. "Hormone replacement therapy is associated with improved arterial physiology in healthy post-menopausal women." *Clin Endocrinol* (England). 1996 Oct;45(4):435-41.

McEwen, BS. "Estrogen actions in the central nervous system." *Endocrinol Review.* 1999 Jun;20(3):279-303.

Meilahn, EN. "Hemostatic Factors and Ischemic Heart Disease Risk among Postmenopausal women." *J Thromb Thrombolysis.* 1995;1(2):125-131.

Mendelsohn, ME. "The protective effects of estrogen on the cardiovascular system." *N Engl J Med.* 1999 Jun 10;340(23):1801-11.

Menon, DV. "Effects of transdermal estrogen replacement therapy on cardiovascular risk factors." *Treat Endocrinol.* 2006;5(1):37-51.

Mercuro, G. "Estradiol-17beta reduces blood pressure and restores the normal amplitude of the circadian blood pressure rhythm in postmenopausal hypertension." *Am J Hypertens.* 1998 Aug;11(8 Pt 1):909-13.

Miller, BE. "Sublingual administration of micronized estradiol and progesterone, with and without micronized testosterone: effect on biochemical markers of bone metabolism and bone mineral density." *Menopause.* 2000 Sep-Oct;7(5):318-26.

Miodrag, A. "Sex hormones and the female urinary tract." *Drugs.* 1988 Oct;36(4):491-504.

Minaguchi, H. "Effect of estriol on bone loss in postmenopausal Japanese women: A multicenter prospective open study." *J Obstet Gynecol Res.* 1996 Jun;22(3):259-65.

Mishell, D. "Clinical study of estrogenic therapy with pellet implantation." *Am J Obstet Gynecol.* 1941

Miyagawa, K. "Medroxyprogesterone interferes with ovarian steroid protection against coronary vasospasm." *Nat Med.* 1997 Mar;3(3):324-7.

Montgomery, JC. "Effect of estrogen and testosterone implants on psychological disorders in the climacteric." *Lancet.* 1987 Feb 7;1(8528):297-9.

Montplaisir, J. "Sleep in menopause: differential effects of two forms of hormone replacement therapy." *Menopause.* 2001 Jan-Feb:8(1):10-6.

Mosca, L. "The role of hormone replacement therapy in the prevention of postmenopausal heart disease." *Arch Intern Med.* 2000 Aug 14-28;160(15):2263-72.

Mureck, AO. "Effect of transdermal vs. oral estradiol administration on the excretion of vasoactive markers in postmenopausal women." *Gynecol Geburtshilfiche Rundsch.* 2000;40:61-7.

Mulnard, RA. "Estrogen replacement therapy for treatment of mild to moderate Alzheimer's disease." *JAMA.* 2000 Feb 23;283(8):1007-15.

Nabulsi, AA. "Association of hormone replacement therapy with various cardiovascular risk factors in post menopausal women. The Atherosclerosis Risk in Communities Study Investigators." *N Engl J Med.* 1993 Apr 15;328(15):1069-75.

Nachtigall, LE. "Estrogen replacement II: A prospective study in the relationship to carcinoma and cardiovascular and metabolic problems." *Obstet Gynecol.* 1979 Jul;54(1):74-9.

Nanda, S. "Effect of estrogen replacement therapy on serum lipid profile." *Aust N Z J Obstet Gynecol.* 2003 Jun;43(3):213-6.

Nasr, A. "Estrogen replacement therapy and cardiovascular protection: lipid mechanisms are the tip of the iceberg." *Gynecol Endocrinol.* 1998 Feb;12(1):43-59.

Nathorst-Boos, J. "Is sexual life influenced by transdermal estrogen therapy? A double blind placebo controlled study in postmenopausal women." *Acta Obstet Gynecol Scand.* 1993 Nov;72(8):655-60.

Nathorst-Boos, J. "Elective ovarian removal and estrogen replacement therapy: effects on sexual life, psychological well-being and androgen status." *J Psychosom Ob Gyn.* 1993

Natrajan, PK. "Estrogen replacement therapy in women with previous breast cancer," *J Obstet Gynecol.* 1999 Aug;181(2):288-95.

Newton, KM. "Estrogen replacement therapy and prognosis after first myocardial infarction." *Am J Epidemiol.* 1997 Feb 1;145(3):269-77.

Nielsen, TF. "Pulsed estrogen therapy in prevention of postmenopausal osteoporosis. A 2-year randomized, double blind, placebo-controlled study." *Osteoporosis Int.* 2004 Feb;15(2):168-74.

Nieto JJ. "Lipid effects of hormone replacement therapy with sequential transdermal 17-beta-estradiol and oral dydrogesterone." *Obstet Gynecol.* 2000 Jan;95(1):111-4.

Nilas, L. "Bone mass and its relationship to age and the menopause. *J Clin Endocrinol Metab.* 1987 Oct;65(4):697-702.

Norman, TR. "Comparative bioavailability of orally and vaginally administered progesterone." *Fertil Steril.* 1991 Dec;56(6):1034-9.

Notelovitz, M. "Suppression of vasomotor symptoms and vulvovaginal symptoms with continuous oral 17beta-estradiol." *Menopause.* 2000 Sep-Oct;7(5):310-7.

Notelovitz, M. "Initial 17beta-estradiol dose for treating vasomotor symptoms." *Obstet Gynecol.* 2000 May;95(5):726-31.

Notelovitz, M. "Effectiveness of Alora estradiol matrix transdermal delivery system in improving lumbar bone mineral density in healthy, postmenopausal women." *Menopause.* 2002 Sep-Oct;9(5):343-53.

Nozaki, M. "Usefulness of estriol for the treatment of bone loss in postmenopausal women." *Obstet Gynecol* (Japan). 1996 Feb;48(2):83-8.

Nozaki, M. "Changes in coagulation factors and fibrinolytic components of postmenopausal women receiving continuous hormone replacement therapy." *Climacteric.* 1999 Jun;2(2):124-30. (Conjugated estrogens disturb blood coagulation.)

Nussmeier, NA. "Hormone replacement therapy is associated with improved survival in women undergoing coronary artery bypass grafting." *J Thor Cardiovasc Surg.* 2002 Dec;124(6):1225-9.

O'Brien, SN. "Differences in the estrogen content of breast adipose tissue in women by menopausal status and hormone use." *Obstet Gynecol.* 1997 Aug;90(2):244-8. (Estrone to estradiol ratio was 2.7-fold higher in postmenopausal women than in premenopausal women.)

O'Connell, MB. "Pharmacokinetic and pharmacologic variation between different estrogen products." *J Clin Pharmacol.* 1995 Sep;35(9 Suppl):18S-24S.

Oger, E. "Assessment of the risk for venous thromboembolism among users of hormone replacement therapy." *Drugs Aging.* 1999 Jan;14(1):55-61. (Negative impact of oral synthetic HRT on clot risk.)

Oger, E. "Hormone replacement therapy in menopause and the risk of cerebrovascular accident." *Ann Endocrinol* (Paris). 1999 Sep;60(3):232-41. (Negative impact of oral synthetic HRT on stroke risk.)

Ohkura, T. "Low-dose estrogen replacement for Alzheimer's disease in women." *J North Am Menop Soc.* 1994

Ohkura, T. "Long-term estrogen replacement therapy in female patients with dementia of the Alzheimer type. 7 case reports." *Dementia.*1995 Mar-Apr;6(2):99-107.

Ohkura, T. "Evaluation of estrogen treatment in female patients with dementia of the Alzheimer's type." *Endocr J.* 1994 Aug;41(4):361-71.

Oldenhave, A. "Hysterectomized women with ovarian conservation report more severe climacteric complaints than do normal climacteric women of similar age." *Am J Obstet Gynecol.* 1993 Mar;168(3 Pt 1):765-71.

O'Meara, ES. "Hormone replacement therapy after a diagnosis of breast cancer in relation to recurrence and mortality." *J Natl Cancer Inst.* 2001 May 16;93(10):754-62. (2,755 women aged thirty-five to seventy-four years who were diagnosed with invasive breast cancer. 174 users of HRT after diagnosis. Study found lower risks of recurrence and mortality in women who used HRT after breast cancer diagnosis than in women who did not.)

O'Sullivan, AJ. "A comparison of the effects of oral and transdermal estrogen replacement on insulin sensitivity in postmenopausal women." *J Clin Endocrinol Metab.* 1995 Jun;80(6):1783-8.

O'Sullivan, AJ. "The route of estrogen replacement therapy confers divergent effects on substrate oxidation and body composition in postmenopausal women." *J Clin Invest.* 1998 Sep 1;102(5):1035-40. (Transdermal estradiol have more beneficial effect on lean body mass and fat mass than oral estrogens.)

Ottosson, U. "Subfractions of HDL cholesterol during estrogen replacement therapy: A comparison between progestogens (Provera) and natural progesterone." *J Obstet Gynecol.* 1985 Mar 15;151(16):746-50.

Pagani-Hill, A. "Estrogen deficiency and risk of Alzheimer's disease in women." *Am J Epidemiol.* 1994 Aug 1;140(3):256-61.

Paganini-Hill, A. "Estrogen replacement therapy and risk of Alzheimer's disease." *Arch Intern Med.* 1996 Oct 28;156(19):2213-7.

Paganini-Hill, A. "The risks and benefits of estrogen replacement therapy: Leisure World." *J Fertil Menopausal Stud*.1995;40Suppl 1:54-62. (7,610 women, mean age seventy-three. Compared estrogen therapy vs. no estrogen therapy. Estrogen group had significantly less cardiac events and lower cardiac fatalities.)

Paganini-Hill, A. "Hormone replacement therapy, hormone levels, and lipoprotein cholesterol concentrations in elderly women." *Am J Obstet Gynecol*.1996 Mar;174(3):897-902.

Pang, SC. "Long-term effects of transdermal estradiol with and without medroxyprogesterone acetate." *Fertil Steril*. 1993 Jan;59(1):76-82.

Pelzer, T. "Estrogen effects in the heart." *Mol Cell Biochem*. 1996 Jul-Aug;160-161:307-13.

Perera, M. "The effects of transdermal estradiol in combination with oral norethisterone on lipoproteins, coagulation, and endothelial markers in postmenopausal women with type 2 diabetes: a randomized, placebo-controlled study." *J Clin Endocrinol Metab*. 2001 Mar;86(3):1140-3.

Petitti, DB. "Noncontraceptive estrogens and mortality: long-term follow-up of women in the Walnut Creek Study. *Obstet Gynecol*. 1987 Sep;70(3 Pt 1):289-93. (Fifty percent reduction in cardiac mortality with estrogen therapy in over six thousand postmenopausal women during ten to thirteen years.)

Polo-Kantola, P. "When does estrogen replacement therapy improve sleep quality?" *Am J Obstet Gynecol*. 1998 May;178(5(:1002-9.

Powers, MS. "Pharmacokinetics and pharmacodynamics of transdermal dosage forms of 17beta-estradiol: comparison with conventional oral estrogens used for hormone replacement." *Am J Obstet Gynecol*. 1985 Aug 15;152(8):1099-106.

Prelevic, GM. "A cross-sectional study of the effects of hormone replacement therapy on the cardiovascular disease risk profile in healthy postmenopausal women." *Fertil Steril*. 2002 May;77(5):945-51. (Transdermal does not raise CRP.)

Psaty, BM. "Hormone replacement therapy, prothrombotic mutations and the risk of incident nonfatal myocardial infarction in postmenopausal women." *JAMA*. 2001 Feb 21;285(7):906-13.

Phillips, S. "Effects of estrogen on memory function in surgically menopausal women." *Psychoneuroendocrinology*. 1992 Oct;17(5):485-95.

Pines, A. "Menopause and ischemic stroke: basic, clinical and epidemiological considerations. The role of hormone replacement." *Hum Reprod Update.* 2002;8(2):161-68

Plu-Bureau, G. "Percutaneous progesterone use and risk of breast cancer: results from a French cohort study of premenopausal women with benign breast disease." *Cancer Detect Prev.* 1999;23(4):290-6.

Prestwood, KM. "The effect of low dose micronized 17beta-estradiol on bone turnover, sex hormone levels, and side effects in older women: a randomized, double-blind, placebo-controlled study." *J Clin Endocrinol Metab.* 2000 Dec;85(12):4462-9.

Prior, JC. "Progesterone as a bone-tropic hormone." *Endocr Rev.* 1990 May;11(2):386-98.

Puder, JJ. "Estrogen modulates the hypothalamic-pituitary-adrenal and inflammatory cytokine responses to endotoxin in women." *Clin Endocrinol Metab.* 2001;86(6):2403-8.

Rasgon, NL. "Estrogen replacement therapy in the treatment of major depressive disorder in perimenopausal women." *J Clin Psychiatry.* 2002;63 Suppl 7:45-8.

Raudaskoski, T. "Insulin sensitivity during postmenopausal hormone replacement with transdermal estradiol and intrauterine levonorgestrel." *Acta Obstet Gynecol Scand.* 1999;78(6):540-5.

Raz, R. "A controlled trial of intravaginal estriol in postmenopausal women with recurrent urinary tract infections." *N Engl J Med.* 1993 Sep 9;329(11):753-6.

Rekers, H. "The menopause, urinary incontinence and other symptoms of the genito-urinary tract." *Maturitas.* 1992 Oct 15(2):101-11.

Ribot, C. "Preventive effects of transdermal administration of 17beta-estradiol on postmenopausal bone loss: a 2-year prospective study." *Gynecol Endocrinol.*1989 Dec;3(4):259-67.

Rice, MM. "Estrogen replacement therapy and cognitive function in postmenopausal women without dementia." *Am J Med.* 1997 Sep 22;103(3A):26S-35S.

Richelson, LS. "Relative contributions of aging and estrogen deficiency to postmenopausal bone loss." *N Engl J Med.* 1984 Nov 15;;311(20):1273-5.

Rigano, A. "Sexuality and well-being in early menopause. Effect of transdermal estradiol therapy." *Panminerva Med.* 2001 Jun;43(2):115-8.

Riis, BJ. "The effect of percutaneous estradiol and natural progesterone on postmenopausal bone loss." *Am J Obstet Gynecol.* 1987 Jan;156(1):61-5.

Rodriguez, C. "Effect of body mass on the association between estrogen replacement therapy and mortality among elderly US women." *Am J Epidemiol.* 2001 Jan 15;153(2):145-52. (300,000 postmenopausal women. All-cause death rates were lower among estrogen users versus never users. Breast cancer mortality did not increase with estrogen use. Cardiovascular mortality decreased by 50 percent with estrogen therapy.)

Roque, M. "Short-term effects of transdermal estrogen replacement therapy on coronary vascular reactivity in postmenopausal women with angina pectoris and normal results on coronary angiograms." *J Am Coll Cardiol.* 1998 Jan;31(1):139-43.

Rosano. GM. "Natural progesterone, but not medroxyprogesterone acetate, enhances the beneficial effect of estrogen on exercise-induced myocardial ischemia in postmenopausal women." *J Am Coll Cardiol.* 2000 Dec;36(7):2154-9.

Rossi, R. "Transdermal 17beta-estradiol and risk of developing type 2 diabetes in a population of healthy, non-obese women." *Diabetes Care.* 2004 Mar27(3):645-9.

Rudolph I. "Influence of a continuous combined hormone replacement therapy (2 mg estradiol valerate and 2 mg dienogest) on postmenopausal depression." *Climacteric.* 2004

Runnebaum, B. "Oral or transdermal estrogen substitution therapy in climacteric?" *Geburtshilfe Frauenheikd.* 1994 Mar;54(3):119-30.

Sacchini, V. "Pathologic and biological prognostic factors of breast cancers in short and long-term hormone replacement users." *Ann Surg Oncol* Apr;9(3):266-71. (1,105 patients. Breast cancers developing during HRT have better prognostic characteristics than seen in HRT nonusers. A trend toward better prognostic characteristics with increasing duration of HRT was seen.)

Sacks, F. "Sex hormones, lipoproteins, and vascular reactivity." *Curr Opin Lipidol.* 1995 Jun;6(3):161-6.

Sauerbronn, AV. "The effects of systemic hormone replacement therapy on the skin of postmenopausal women." *Int J Gynecol Obstet.* 2000 Jan;68(1):35-41.

Savvas, M. "Skeletal effects of oral estrogen compared with subcutaneous estrogen and testosterone in postmenopausal women." *BMJ.* 1988 Jul 30;297(6644):331-3.

Savvas, M. "Increase in bone mass after one year of percutaneous estradiol and testosterone implants in postmenopausal women who have previously received oral estrogens." *Br J Obstet Gynecol.* 1990 Sep;99(9):757-60.

Savvas, M. "Type III collagen content in the skin of postmenopausal women receiving estradiol and testosterone implants." *Br J Obstet Gynecol* 1993 Feb;100 (2):154-6.

Sanada, M. "Substitution of transdermal estradiol during oral estrogen-progestin therapy in postmenopausal women: effects on hypertriglyceridemia." *Menopause.* 2004 May-Jun 11 (3):331-7.

Sandstrom, NJ. "Memory retention is modulated by acute estradiol and progesterone replacement." *Behav Neurosci.* 2001 Apr 115(2):384-93.

Sarrel, PM. "Estrogen actions in arteries, bone and brain." *Sci Am Sci Med.* 1994;1(3):44.

Sarrel, PM. "Vasodilator effects of estrogens are not diminished by androgen in postmenopausal women." *Fertil Steril.* 1997;68(8):1125-27.

Sarti, CD. "Hormone therapy and sleep quality in women around menopause." *Menopause.* 2005 Sep-Oct;12(5):545-51.

Sauerbronn, AV. "The effects of systemic hormone replacement therapy on the skin of postmenopausal women."*Int J Obstet Gynecol* 2000 Jan;68(1):35-41.

Scarabin, PY. "Effects of oral and transdermal estrogen/progesterone regimens on blood coagulation and fibrinolysis in postmenopausal women. A randomized controlled trial." *Arterioscler Thromb Vasc Biol.* 1997 Nov;17(11):3071-8.

Schairer, C. "Menopausal estrogen and estrogen-progestin replacement therapy and breast cancer risk." *JAMA.* 2000 Jan 26;283(4):485-91. (Increased risk with synthetic HRT.)

Schairer, C. "Cause-specific mortality in women receiving hormone replacement therapy." *Epidemiol.* 1997 Jan;8(1):59-65. (Reduction in mortality associated with HRT.)

Schiff, I. "Effects of estrogens on sleep and psychological state of hypogonadal women." *JAMA.* 1979 Nov 30;242(22):2404-5.

Schmidt, J. "Treatment of skin aging with topical estrogens. *Int J Dermatol.* 1996 Sep;35(9):669-74.

Schneider, HP. "Hormone replacement therapy and cancer risks." *Maturitas.* 2002 Aug 30;43 Suppl:S35-42.

Schneider, J. "Effects of obesity on estradiol metabolism; decreased formation of neurotropic metabolites." *Clin Endocrinol Metab.* 1983 May 56(5):973-8.

Schumaker, M. "Local synthesis and dual actions of progesterone in the nervous system: neuroprotection and myelination." *Growth Hormone IGF Res.* 2004;14(Suppl 1):18-33.

Scott, RT. "Pharmacokinetics of percutaneous estradiol: a crossover study using a gel and a transdermal system in comparison with oral micronized estradiol." *Obstet Gynecol.* 1991 May;77(5):758-64.

Seed, M. "The effect of hormone replacement therapy and route of administration on selected cardiovascular risk factors in post-menopausal women." *Fam Pract.* 2000 Dec;17(6):497-507.

Seeger, H. "Effect of medroxyprogesterone acetate and norethisterone on serum-stimulated and estradiol-inhibited proliferation of human coronary artery smooth muscle cells." *Menopause.* 2001 Jan-Feb 8(1):5-9. (Provera has adverse effect on coronary arteries.)

Seeger, H. "Effect of norethisterone acetate on estrogen metabolism in postmenopausal women." *Horm Metab Res.* 2000 Oct;32(10):436-9. (Oral synthetic estrogen increase 16-alpha hydroxyl estrone, associated with increase breast cancer risk.)

Seely, EW. "Estradiol with or without progesterone and ambulatory blood pressure in postmenopausal women." *Hypertension.* 1999 May;33(5):1190-4.

Sendag, F. "Effects of sequential combined transdermal and oral hormone replacement therapy on serum lipids and lipoproteins in postmenopausal women." *Arch Gynecol Obstet.* 2002 Jan 266(1):38-43.

Sesmilo, G. "Inflammatory cardiovascular risk markers in women with hypopituitarism." *J Clin Endocrinol Metab.* 2001 Dec;86(12):5774-81.

Shaywitz, SE. "Effect of estrogen on brain activation patterns in postmenopausal women during working memory tasks." *JAMA.* 1999 Apr 7;28(13):197-202.

Shepherd, JE. "Effects of estrogen on cognition, mood, and degenerative brain diseases." *J Am Pharm Assoc.* 2001 Mar-Apr;4(2):221-8.

Sherwin, BB. "Sex steroids and affect in the surgical menopause: a double-blind crossover study." *Psychoneuroendocrinology.* 1985;10(1):325-35.

Sherwin, BB. "Estrogen and/or androgen replacement therapy and cognitive functioning in surgically menopausal women." *Psychoneuroendocrinology*. 1988;13(4):345-57.

Sherwin, BB. "Estrogenic effects on memory in women." *Am NY Acad Sci*. 1994 Nov 14;(743):213-30.

Sherwin, BB. "Randomized clinical trials of combined estrogen-androgen preparations: effects on sexual functioning." *Fertil Steril*. 2002 Apr;77 Suppl 4:S49-54.

Sherwin, BB. "Sex hormones and psychological functioning in postmenopausal women." *Exp Gerontol*. 1994 May-Aug;29(3-4):423-30.

Sherwin, BB. "Can estrogen keep you smart? Evidence from clinical studies." *J Psychiatry Neurosci*. 1999 Sep;24(4):315-21.

Shilipak, MG. "Estrogen and progestin, lipoprotein (a), and the risk of recurrent coronary heart disease events after menopause." *JAMA*. 2000 Apr 12;283(14):1845-52. (Hormone therapy decreased lipoprotein (a).)

Shulman, LP. "Low-dose transdermal estradiol for symptomatic perimenopause." *Menopause*. 2004 Jan-Feb;11(1):34-9.

Shuster, LT. "Prophylactic oophorectomy in premenopausal women and longterm health." *Menopause Int*. 2008 Sep;14(3):111-6.

Simon, J. "Differential effects of estrogen-androgen and estrogen-only therapy on vasomotor symptoms, gonadotropin secretion, and endogenous androgen bioavailability in postmenopausal women." *Menopause*. 1999 Summer;6(2):138-46.

Simpkins, JW. "Role of estrogen replacement therapy in memory enhancement and the prevention of neuronal loss associated with Alzheimer's disease." *Am J Med*. 1997 Sep 22;103(3A):19S-25S.

Simpkins, JW. "The potential role for estrogen replacement therapy in the treatment of the cognitive decline and neurodegeneration associated with Alzheimer's disease." *Neurobiol*. 1994;15 Suppl 2:S195-7.

Sipila, S. "Effects of hormone replacement therapy and high-impact physical exercise on skeletal muscle in post-menopausal women: a randomized placebo-controlled study." *Clin Sci* (Lond). 2001 Aug;101(2):147-57.

Sitruk-Ware, R. "Oral micronized progesterone. Bioavailability pharmacokinetics, pharmacological and therapeutic implications—a review." *Contraception*. 1987 Oct;36(4):373-402.

Sitruk-Ware, R. "Progestins and cardiovascular risk markers." *Steroids*. 2000 Oct-Nov;65(10-11):651-8. (Provera has adverse cardiovascular effect.)

Slater, CC. "Markedly elevated levels of estrone sulfate after long-term oral, but not transdermal, administration of estradiol in postmenopausal women." *Menopause* 2001 May-Jun;8(3):200-3.

Smith, RN. "Recent advances in hormone replacement therapy." *Br J Hosp Med.* 1993 Jun 2-15;49(11):799-808.

Smith, YR. "Long-term estrogen replacement is associated with improved nonverbal memory and attentional measures in postmenopausal women." *Fertil Steril* 2001 Dec;76(6):1101-7.

Smith W. "Gender, estrogen, hormone replacement, and age-related macular degeneration: results from the Blue Mountains Eye Study." *Aust N Z J Ophthalmol* 1997 May;25 Suppl 1: 513-5.(low estrogen associated with macular degeneration.)

Snabes, MC. "Physiologic estradiol replacement therapy and cardiac structure and function in the normal postmenopausal women: a randomized, double-blind, placebo-controlled, crossover trial." *Obstet Gynecol.* 1997 Mar;16(1):44-6.

Soares, CN. "Efficacy of estradiol for the treatment of depressive disorders in perimenopausal women: a double-blind, randomized, placebo-controlled trial." *Arch Gen Psychiatry.* 2001 Jun;58(6):529-34.

Soares, CN."Efficacy of 17beta-estradiol on depression: is estrogen deficiency really necessary? *J Clin Psychiatry* 2002 May;63(5):451.

Sorensen, MB. "Obesity and sarcopenia after menopause are reversed by sex hormone replacement therapy." *Obes Res.* 2001 Oct;9(10):622-6. (Menopause results in bone loss and increased body fat, both reversed by HRT.)

Sorensen, MB. "Changes in body composition at menopause-age, lifestyle, or hormone deficiency?" *J Br Menopause Soc* 2002 Dec;8(4):137-40.

Spencer, CP. "Effects of oral and transdermal 17beta-estradiol with cyclical oral norethindrone acetate on insulin sensitivity, secretion, and elimination in postmenopausal women." *Metabolism.* 2000 Jun;49(6):742-7.

Stamm W. "A controlled trial of intravaginal estriol in postmenopausal women with urinary tract infections." *N Engl J Med.* 1993 Sep 9;329(11):753-6.

Stampfer, MJ. "Postmenopausal estrogen therapy and cardiovascular disease. Ten-year follow-up from the nurses' health study." *N Eng J Med.* 1991 Sep 12;325(11):56-62. (myocardial infarction mortality 44 percent less with estrogen therapy in 48,470 postmenopausal women followed for ten years.)

Stanczyk, F. "A randomized comparison of non-oral estradiol delivery in postmenopausal women." *Am J Obstet Gynecol.* 1988

Stanczyk, FZ. "Pharmacokinetics of progesterone administered by the oral and parenteral routes." *J Reprod Med.* 1999 Feb;44(2 Suppl):141-7.

Strehlow, K. "Estrogen increases bone marrow–derived endothelial progenitor cell production and diminishes neointima formation. *Circulation.* 2003 Jun 24;107(24):3059-65.

Stefanick, M. "Estrogen, progestogens and cardiovascular risk." *J Reprod Med.* 1999 Feb;44(2 Suppl):221-6.

Stein, DG. "Brain damage, sex hormones and recovery: a new role for progesterone and estrogen?" *Trends Neurosci.* 2001 Jul;24(7):386-91.

Steingold, KA. "A. Comparison of transdermal to oral estradiol administration on hormonal and hepatic parameters in women with premature ovarian failure. *J Clin Endocrinol Metab.*" 1991 Aug;73(2):275-80.

Studd, J. "Ten reasons to be happy about hormone replacement therapy: a guide for patients. *Menopause Int* 2010 Mar;16(1):44-6.

Studd, JW. "Estradiol and testosterone implants." *Baillieres Clin Endocrinol Metab.* 1993 Jan;7(1):203-23.

Studd, J. "Estradiol and testosterone implants in the treatment of psychosexual problems in postmenopausal women." *Br J Obstet Gynecol.* 1977

Studd, J. "The relationship between plasma estradiol and the increase in bone density in postmenopausal women after treatment with subcutaneous hormone implants." *Am J Obstet Gynecol.* 1990 Nov;163(5 Pt 1):1474-9. (8.3 percent increase in bone density per year with pellets)

Stumpf, PG. "Pharmacokinetics of estrogen." *Obstet Gynecol.* 1990 Apr;75(4 Suppl):9S-14S.

Sudhir, K. "Mechanisms of estrogen-induced vasodilation: in vivo studies in canine coronary conductance and resistance arteries." *J Am Coll Cardiol.* 1995 Sep;26(3):807-14.

Sudhir, L. "Estrogen supplementation decreases norepinephrine-induced vasoconstriction and total body norepinephrine spillover in perimenopausal women." *Hypertension* 1997 Dec;30(6):1538-43.

Sugishita, K. "Antioxidant effects of estrogen reduce Ca2+ during metabolic inhibition." *J Mol Cell Cardiol.* 2003 Mar;35(3):331-6.

Sullivan, JM. "Estrogen replacement and coronary artery disease. Effect on survival in postmenopausal women." *Arch Intern Med.* 1990 Dec;150(12):2557-62. (Estrogen use after menopause prolongs survival in patients with coronary heart disease.)

Sullivan, JM. "Practical aspects of preventing and managing atherosclerotic disease in postmenopausal women." *Eur Heart J* (England). 1996;17(Suppl D):32-37.

Sumino, H. "Effect of transdermal hormone replacement therapy on carotid artery wall thickness and levels of vascular inflammatory markers in postmenopausal women." *Hypertens Res.* 2005 Jul;28(7):579-84.

Taaffe, DR. "The effect of hormone replacement therapy and/or exercise on skeletal muscle attenuation in postmenopausal women: a yearlong intervention." *Clin Physiol Funct Imaging* 2005 Sep;25(5):297-304.

Taggart, W. "The effect of site of application on the transcutaneous absorption of 17beta- estradiol from a transdermal delivery system." *Menopause.* 2000 Sep-Oct;7(5):364-9.

Takahashi, K. "Safety and efficacy of estriol for symptoms of natural or surgically induced menopause." *Hum Reprod.* 2000 May;15(5):1028-36.

Takahashi, K. "Long-term hormone replacement therapy delays the age-related progression of carotid intima-media thickness in healthy postmenopausal women." *Menopause.* 2002 Oct 15;49(2):170-7.

Tang, MX. "Effect of estrogen during menopause on risk and age at onset of Alzheimer's disease." *Lancet.* 1996 Aug 17;348(9025):429-32.

Taylor, M. "Unconventional estrogens: estriol, biest, and triest." *Clin Obstet Gynecol.* 2001 Dec;44(4):864-79.

Tchernof, A. "Body fat distribution, the menopause transition, and hormone replacement therapy." *Diabetes Metab.* 2000 Feb;26(1):12-20.

Thom, MH. " Procedures in practice.Hormone implantation." *Br Med J.* 1980 Mar 22;280(6217):848-50.

Thom, MH. "Hormone profiles in postmenopausal women after therapy with subcutaneous implants." *Br J Obstet Gynecol.* 1981 Apr;88(4):426-33.

Tomaszewski, J. "Effect of 17beta-estradiol and phytoestrogen daidzein on the proliferation of pubocervical fascia and skin fibroblasts derived from women suffering from stress urinary incontinence." *Ginekol Pol.* 2003 Oct;74(10):1410-4.

Townsend, PT. "The absorption and metabolism of oral estradiol, estrone and estriol." *Br J Obstet Gynecol.* 1981 Aug 88(8):846-52.

Toy, JL. "The effects of long-term therapy with estriol succinate on the haemostatic mechanism in postmenopausal women." *Br J Obstet Gynecol.* 1978 May;85(5):363-6.

Tremollieres, FA. "Effect of hormone replacement therapy on age-related increase in carotid artery intima-media thickness in postmenopausal women." *Atherosclerosis.* 2000 Nov;153(1):83-8.

Tremollieres, FA. "Withdrawal of hormone replacement therapy is associated with significant vertebral bone loss in postmenopausal women." *Osteoporosis Int.* 2001;12(5):385-90.

Tsuda, K. "Hyperinsulinemia and estrogen-deficiency as risk factors for stroke in women." *Stroke.* 2004 Jun;35(6):e134.

Ulrich, LG. "Quality of life and patient preference for sequential versus continuous combined HRT: the UK Kliofem multicenter study experience. UK continuous combined HRT study investigators." *Int J Gynecol Obstet.* 1997 Oct;59 Suppl 1:S11-7.

van Baal, WM. "Cardiovascular disease risk and hormone replacement therapy. A review based on randomized controlled studies in postmenopausal women." *Curr Med Chem.* 2000 May;7(5):495-517.

Vandenbroucke, JP. "Noncontraceptive hormones and rheumatoid arthritis in perimenopausal and postmenopausal women." *JAMA.* 1986 Mar 14;255(10):1299-303.

van der Linden, MC. "The effect of estriol on the cytology of urethra and vagina post-menopausal women with genitor-urinary symptoms." *Eur J Obstet Gynecol Reprod Biol.* 1993 Sep;51(1):29-33.

Van Erpecum, KJ. "Different hepatobiliary effects of oral and transdermal estradiol in postmenopausal women." *Gastroenterology.* 1991 Feb;100(2):482-8.

Vashisht, A. "A study to look at hormonal absorption of progesterone cream used in conjunction with transdermal estrogen." *Gynecol Endocrinol.* 2005 Aug;21(2):101-5.

Vehkavaara, S. "Effects of oral and transdermal estrogen replacement therapy on markers of coagulation, fibrinolysis, inflammation and serum lipids and lipoproteins in postmenopausal women." *Thromb Heamost.* 2001 Apri;85(4):619-28.

Vermeulen, A. "Sex hormone concentrations in postmenopausal women, relation to obesity, fat mass, age and years postmenopause." *Clin Endocrinol.* 1978 Jul;9(1):59-66.

Vigna, GB. "Simvastatin, transdermal patch, and oral estrogen-progestogen preparation in early-postmenopausal hypercholesterolemic women: a randomized, placebo-controlled clinical trial." *Metabolism.* 2002 Nov;51(11):1463-70.

Vliet, EL. "New insights on hormones and mood." *Menopause Management.* 1993 Jun-Jul;14-16.

Volterrani, M. "Estrogen acutely increases peripheral blood flow in postmenopausal women." *Am J Med.* 1995 Aug;99)2):119-22.

Wagner, JD. "Rationale for hormone replacement therapy in atherosclerosis prevention." *J Reprod Med.* 2000 Mar;45(3 Suppl):245-58.

Wakatsuki, A. "Effect of medroxyprogesterone acetate on endothelium-dependent vasodilation in postmenopausal women receiving estrogen." *Circulation.* 2001 Oct 9;104(15):1773-8. (Negative impact of Provera on blood flow.)

Walsh, BW. "Effects of postmenopausal hormone replacement with oral and transdermal estrogen on high-density lipoprotein metabolism." *J Lipid Res.* 1994 Nov;35(11):2083-93.

Walsh, BA. "17beta-estradiol acts separately on the LDL particle and artery wall to reduce LDL accumulation." *J Lipid Res.* 2000 Jan;41(1):134-41.

Walsh, BA. "17 beta-estradiol reduces tumor necrosis factor-alpha mediated LDL accumulation in the artery wall." *J Lipid Res.* 1999 Mar;40(3):387-96.

Weisberg, E. "Endometrial and vaginal effects of low-dose estradiol delivered by vaginal ring or vaginal tablet." *Climacteric.* 2005 Mar;8(1):83-92.

Weissberger, AJ. "Contrasting effects of oral and transdermal routes of estrogen replacement therapy on 24-hour growth hormone secretion, IGF-I, and GH-binding protein in postmenopausal women." *J Clin Endocrinol Metab.* 1991 Feb;72(2):374-81.

Wieland, S. "Anxiolytic activity of the progesterone metabolite 5 alpha-pregnan-3 alpha-ol-20-one." *Brain Res.* 1991Nov 29 565(2):263-8.

Wiklund, I. "Quality of life of postmenopausal women on a regimen of transdermal estradiol therapy: a double-blind placebo-controlled study." *Am J Obstet Gynecol.* 1993 Mar;168(3 Pt 1):824-30.

Wiklund, I. "Long-term effect of transdermal hormonal therapy on aspects of quality of life in postmenopausal women." *Maturitas.* 1992 Mar;14(3):225-36.

Williams, JK. "Short-term administration of estrogen vascular responses of atherosclerotic coronary arteries." *J Am Coll Cardiol.* 1992 Aug;20(2):452-7.

Williams JK. "Estrogens, progestins, and coronary artery reactivity." *Nat Med.* 1997 Mar;3(3):273-4.

Wolf, PH. "Reduction of cardiovascular disease-related mortality among postmenopausal women who use hormones: evidence from a national cohort. *Am J Obstet Gynecol.* 1991 Feb;164(2):489-94.

Wouters, MG. "Plasma homocysteine and menopausal status." *Eur J Clin Invest.* 1995 Nov;25(11):801-5.

Wren, BG. "Effect of sequential transdermal progesterone cream on endometrium, bleeding pattern, and plasma progesterone and salivary progesterone levels in postmenopausal women." *Climacteric.* 2000 Sep;3(3):155-60.

Wren, BG. "Pharmacokinetics of estradiol, progesterone, testosterone and dehydroepiandosterone after transbuccal administration to postmenopausal women." *Climacteric.* 2003 Jun;6(2):104-11.

Wright, JV. "Comparative measurements of serum estriol, estradiol, and estrone in non-pregnant, premenopausal women; a preliminary investigation." *Altern Med Rev.* 1999 Aug;4(4):266-70.

Xu, H. "Estrogen reduces neuronal generation of Alzheimer's beta-amyloid peptides." *Nat Med.* 1998 Apr;4(4):447-51.

Yaffe, K. "Cognitive decline in women in relation to nonprotein-bound estradiol concentrations." *Lancet.* 2000 Aug 26;356(9231):708-12.

Yates, J. "Rapid loss of hip fracture protection after estrogen cessation: evidence from the National Osteoporosis Risk Assessment." *Obstet Gynecol.* 2004 Mar;103(3):440-6.

Yoneda, T. "Estrogen deficiency accelerates murine autoimmune arthritis associated with receptor activator of nuclear factor-kappa B ligand-mediated osteoclastogenesis." *Endocrinology.* 2004 May;145(5):2384-91.

Zandi, PP. "Hormone replacement therapy and incidence of Alzheimer disease in older women: the Cache County Study" *JAMA.* 2002 Nov 6;288(17):2123-9. (Women on HRT 40 percent less likely to develop

Alzheimer's disease. The longer they were on HRT, the lower their risk.)

Zanger, D. "Divergent effects of hormone therapy on serum markers of inflammation in postmenopausal women with coronary artery disease on appropriate medical management." *J Am Coll Cardiol.* 2000 Nov 15;36(6):1792-802. (Negative impact of oral synthetic HRT on inflammation.)

Zhang, F. "The major metabolites of equilin, 4-hydroxyequilin, autooxidizes to an o-quinone which isomerizes to the potent cytotoxin 4-hydroequilenin-o-quinone." *Chem Res Toxico.* 1999 Feb;12(2):204-13. (Premarin)

Zhu, BT. "Functional role of estrogen metabolism in target cells: review and perspectives." *Carcinogenesis.* 1998 Jan;19(1):1-27.

Zhu, BT. "Is 2-methoxyestradiol an endogenous estrogen metabolite that inhibits mammary carcinogenesis?" *Cancer Res.* 1998 Jun 1;58(11):2269-77.

Testosterone/women

Ahlbom, E. "Testosterone protects cerebellar granule cells from oxidative stress-induced cell death through a receptor mediated mechanism." *Brain Res.* 2001 Feb 23;892(21):255-62.

Barrett-Connor, E. "Interim safety analysis of a two-year study comparing oral estrogen-androgen and conjugated estrogens in surgically menopausal women." *J Reprod Med.* 1999 Dec;44(12):1012-20.

Bernini, GP. "Influence of endogenous androgens on carotid wall in postmenopausal women." *Menopause.* 2001 Jan-Feb;8(1):43-50.(Negative effects on carotid artery associated with low testosterone levels.)

Bernini, GP. "Endogenous androgens and carotid intima-medial thickness in women. *J Clin Endocrinol Metab.* 1999 Jun;84(6):2008-12 (Negative effects associated with low testosterone levels.)

Bird, CE. "Kinetics of testosterone metabolism in normal postmenopausal women and women with breast cancer." *Steroids.* 1978 Oct;32(3):323-35.

Booji, A. "Androgens as adjuvant treatment in postmenopausal female patients with rheumatoid arthritis." *Ann Rheum Dis.* 1996 Nov;55(11):811-5.

Burger, HG. "The management of persistent symptoms with estradiol-testosterone implants: clinical, lipid and hormonal results." *Maturitas.* 1984

Burger, HG. "Effect of combined implants of estradiol and testosterone on libido in postmenopausal women." *Br Med J.* 1987 Apr 11;294(6577):936-7.

Casson. PR. "Testosterone delivery systems for women: Present status and future promise." *Semin Repro Endocrinol.* 1998;16(2):153-9.

Casson, PR. "Effect of postmenopausal estrogen replacement on circulating androgens. *Obstet Gynecol.* 1997 Dec;90(6):995-8.

Davidson, BJ. "Total and free estrogens and androgens in postmenopausal women with hip fractures." *J Clin Endocrinol Metab.* 1982 Jan;54(1):115-20.

Davis, S. "Use of androgens in postmenopausal women." *Curr Opin Obstet Gynecol.* 1997 Jun;9(3):77-80.

Davis, SR. "Effects of estradiol with and without testosterone on body composition and relationships with lipids in postmenopausal women." *Menopause.* 2000 Nov-Dec;7(6):395-401.

Davis, S. "Testosterone deficiency in women." *J Reprod Med.* 2001 Mar;46(3 Suppl 1):291-6.

Davis, SR. "Testosterone enhances estradiol's effects on postmenopausal bone density and sexuality." *Maturitas.* 2008 Sep-Oct;61(1-2):17-26.

Deng, X. "Correlation between bone mineral density and sexual hormones in healthy Chinese women." *J Environ Pathol Toxicol Oncol.* 2000;19(1-2):167-9. (Decrease in bone density associated with low testosterone levels.)

Dimitrakakis, C. "Breast cancer incidence in postmenopausal women using testosterone in addition to usual hormone therapy." *Menopause.* 2004 Sep-Oct;11(5):531-5. (Testosterone use lowers risk of breast cancer.)

Dobs, AS. "Differential effects of oral estrogen vs. oral estrogen-androgen replacement therapy on body composition in postmenopausal women." *J Clin Endocrinol Metab.* 2002 Apr;87(4):1509-16.

Drake, EB. "Associations between circulating sex steroid hormones and cognition in normal elderly women." *Neurology.* 2000 Feb 8;54(3):599-603. (Levels of testosterone correlated positively with verbal fluency.)

Driscoll, I. "Testosterone and cognition in normal aging and Alzheimer's disease: an update." *Curr Alzheimer Res.* 2007 Feb;4(1):33-45. (Testosterone slows progression of Alzheimer's.)

Floter, A. "Effects of combined estrogen/testosterone therapy on bone and body composition in oophorectomized women." *Gynecol Endocrinol.* 2005 Mar;20(3):155-60.

Golden, SH. "Endogenous postmenopausal hormones and carotid atherosclerosis: a case-control study of the atherosclerosis risk in communities cohort." *Am J Epidemiol.* 2002 Mar 1;155(5):437-45.

Goldstat, R. "Transdermal testosterone therapy improves well-being, mood, and sexual function in premenopausal women." *Menopause.* 2003 Sep-Oct;10(5):390-8.

Gower, BA. "Associations among oral estrogen use, free testosterone concentration, and lean body mass among postmenopausal women." *J Clin Endocrinol Metab.* 2000 Dec;85(12):4476-80.

Guay, AT. "Decreased testosterone in regularly menstruating women with decreased libido: a clinical observation." *J Sex Marital Ther.* 2001 Oct-Dec;27(5):513-9.

Jassal, SK. "Low bioavailable testosterone levels predict future height loss in postmenopausal women." *J Bone Miner Res.* 1995 Apr;10(4):650-4.

Kaczmarek, A. "The association of lower testosterone level with coronary artery disease in postmenopausal women." *Int J Cardiol.* 2003 Jan;87(1):53-7.

Mazer, NA. "Transdermal testosterone for women: a new physiological approach for androgen therapy." *Obstet Gynecol Surv.* 2003 Jul;58(7):489-500.

Miller, BE. "Sublingual administration of micronized estradiol and progesterone, with and without micronized testosterone: effect on biochemical markers of bone metabolism and bone mineral density." *Menopause.* 2000 Sep-Oct;7(5):318-26.

Miller, KK. "Androgen deficiency in women." *J Clin Endocrinol Metab.* 2001 Jun;86(6):2395-401.

Montgomery, JC. "Effect of estrogen and testosterone implants on psychological disorders in the climacteric." *Lancet.* 1987 Feb 7;1(8528):297-9.

Penotti, M. "Effects of androgen supplementation of hormone replacement therapy on the vascular reactivity of cerebral arteries." *Fertil Steril.* 2001 Aug;76(2):235-40.

Raisz, EG. "Comparison of the effects of estrogen alone and estrogen plus androgen on biochemical markers of bone formation and resorption in postmenopausal women." *J Clin Endocrinol Metab.* 1995 Jan;81(1):37-43.

Rako, S. "Testosterone deficiency: a key factor in the increased cardiovascular risk to women following hysterectomy or with natural aging?" *J Womens Health.* 1998 Sep;7(7):825-9.

Rohr, UD. "The impact of testosterone imbalance on depression and women's health. *Maturitas*. 2002 Apr 15;41 Suppl 1:S25-46.

Sarrel, PM. "Cardiovascular aspects of androgens in women." *Semin Reprod Endocrinol*. 1998;16(2):121-8.

Sarrel, PM. "Estrogen and estrogen-androgen replacement in postmenopausal women dissatisfied with estrogen-only therapy. Sexual behavior and neuroendocrine responses." *J Reprod Med*. 1998 Oct;43(10):847-56.

Sands, R. "Exogenous androgens in postmenopausal women." *Am J Med*. 1995 Jan 16;98(1A):76S-79S.

Savvas, M. "Skeletal effects of oral estrogen compared with subcutaneous estrogen and testosterone in postmenopausal women." *BMJ*. 1988 Jul 30;297(6644):331-3.

Savvas, M. "Increase in bone mass after one year of percutaneous estradiol and testosterone implants in postmenopausal women who have previously received long-term oral estrogens." *Br J Obstet Gynecol*. 1992 Sep;99(9):757-60.

Sherwin, BB. "Differential symptom response to parenteral estrogen and/ or androgen administration in the surgical menopause." *Am J Obstet Gynecol*. 1985 Jan 15;151(2):153-60.

Sherwin BB. "Androgen enhances sexual motivation in females: a prospective, cross over study of sex steroid administration in the surgical menopause. Psychosom Med. 1985 Jul-Aug;47(4):339-51.

Sherwin, BB. "The role of androgen in the maintenance of sexual functioning in oophorectomized women." *Psychosom Med*. 1987 Jul-Aug;49(4):397-409.

Sherwin, BB. "Affective changes with estrogen and androgen replacement therapy in surgically menopausal women." *J Affect Disord*. 1988 Mar-Apr;14(2):177-87.

Sherwin, BB. "Postmenopausal estrogen and androgen replacement and lipoprotein lipid concentrations." *Am J Obstet Gynecol*. 1987 Feb;156(2):414-9.

Shrifen J. "Transdermal testosterone treatment in women with impaired sexual function and psychological well-being in oophorectomized women." *N Engl J Med*. 2000 Sep 7;343(10):682-8.

Simon, J. "Differential effects of estrogen-androgen and estrogen-only therapy on vasomotor symptoms, gonadotropin secretion, and endogenous androgen bioavailability in postmenopausal women." *Menopause*. 1999 Summer;6(2):138-46.

Simon, JA. "Safety of estrogen/androgen regimens." *J Reprod Med* 2001 Mar;46(3 Suppl):281-90.

Singh, AB. "Pharmacokinetics of testosterone gel in healthy postmenopausal women." *J Clin Endocrinol Metab.* 2006 Jan;91(1):136-44.

Slatar, CC. "Pharmocokinetics of testosterone after percutaneous gel or buccal administration." *Fertil Steril.* 2001 Jul;76(1):32-7.

Sowers, MF. "Testosterone concentrations in women aged 25–50 years: associations with lifestyle, body composition, and ovarian status. *Am J Epidemiol.* 2001 Feb 1;153(3):256-64.

Worboys, S. "Evidence that parenteral testosterone therapy may improve endothelium-dependent and independent vasodilation in postmenopausal women already receiving estrogen." *J Clin Endocrinol Metab.* 2001 Jan;86(1):158-61.

Zumoff, B. "24 hour mean plasma testosterone concentration declines with age in normal premenopausal women." *J Clin Endocrinol Metab.* 1995 Apr;80(4):1429-30.

Breast cancer

Adami, HO. "The effect of female sex hormones on cancer survival. A register-based study in patients younger than 20 years at diagnosis." *JAMA.* 1990 Sep 10;344(8924):760-1.

Adami, HO. "The relation between survival and age at diagnosis in breast cancer." *N Engl J Med.*1986 Aug 28;315(9):559-63.

Badwe, RA. "Serum progesterone at the time of surgery and survival in women with premenopausal operable breast cancer." *Eur J Cancer.* 1994;30A(4):445-8.

Basavilvazo Rodriguez, M. A. "Hormone replacement therapy and breast cancer. A case-control study." *Gynecol Obstet* (Mex). 2004 Jan;72(1):10-5.

Beckmann MW. "Hormone replacement therapy after treatment of breast cancer: effects on postmenopausal symptoms, bone mineral density and recurrence rates." *Oncology.* 2001;60(7):199-206. (HRT reduced recurrence rate.)

Bergkvist, L. "Prognosis after breast cancer diagnosis in women exposed to estrogen and estrogen-progestogen replacement therapy." *Am J Epidemiol.* 1990 Aug;130(2):221-8. (261 women with breast cancer followed for nine years; 40 percent reduction in mortality with estrogen therapy, compared to 6,600 women with breast cancer not on estrogen therapy.)

Birkhauser, M. "Hormone replacement therapy after treatment of breast carcinoma." *Schweiz Med Wochenschr.* 1998 Oct 24;128(43):1675-89.

Chang, KJ. "Influences of percutaneous administration of estradiol and progesterone on human breast epithelial cell cycle in vivo." *Fertil Steril.* 1995 Apr;67(4):785-91.

Cowan, LD. "Breast cancer incidence in women with a history of progesterone deficiency." *Am J Epidemiol.* 1981 Aug;114(2):209-17.

Davelaar, EM. "No increase in the incidence of breast carcinoma with subcutaneous administration of estradiol." *Ned Tijdsch Geneeskd.* 1991

de Lignieres, B. "Combined HRT and risk of breast cancer in a French cohort study of 3175 women." *Climacteric.* 2002 Dec;5(4):332-40. (Showed benefits of transdermal estradiol.)

Dew, JE. A cohort study of hormone replacement therapy given to women previously treated for breast cancer. *Climacteric.* 1998 Jun;1(2):137-42.

Dew, JE. "Tamoxifen, hormone receptors and hormone replacement therapy in women previously treated for breast cancer: a cohort study." *Climacteric.* 2002 Jun;5(2):151-5.

Dimitrakakis, C. "Breast cancer incidence in postmenopausal women using testosterone in addition to usual hormone therapy." *Menopause.* 2004 Sep-Oct;11(5):531-5. (Addition of testosterone to HRT reduced risk breast cancer.)

DiSaia, PJ. "Hormone replacement therapy in breast cancer survivors: a cohort study." *Obstet Gynecol.* 1996 May;174(5):1494-8. (forty-one breast cancer patients on HRT after diagnosis compared to eighty-two breast cancer patients not on HRT after diagnosis. Followed for eleven years; no difference in survival or disease progression in either group.)

DiSaia, PJ. "Breast cancer survival and hormone replacement therapy: a cohort analysis." *Am J Clin Oncol.* 2000 Decp23(6):541-5.

Durna, EM. "Hormone replacement therapy after a diagnosis of breast cancer: cancer recurrence and mortality." *Med J Aust.* 2002 Oct 7;177(7):347-51.

Durna, EM. "Breast cancer in premenopausal women: recurrence and survival rates and relationship to hormone replacement therapy." *Climacteric* 2004 Sep;7 (3):284-91.

Foidart, JM. "Estradiol and progesterone regulate the proliferation of human breast epithelial cells." *Fertil Steril.* 1998 May;69(5):963-9.

Formby, B. "Progesterone inhibits growth and induces apoptosis in breast cancer cells: inverse effects on Bci-2 ad p53." *Ann Clin Lab Sci.* 1996 Nov-Dec;28(6):360-9.

Fournier, A. "Breast cancer risk in relation to different types of hormone replacement therapy in the E3N-EPIC cohort." *Int J Cancer.* 2005 Apr 10;114(3):448-54. (Transdermal estradiol plus bioidentical progesterone produced 10 percent decrease in breast cancer risk.)

Gajdos, C. "Breast cancer diagnosed during hormone replacement therapy." *Obstet Gynecol.* 2000 Apr;95(4):513-8.

Gambrell, RD. "Hormones in the etiology and prevention of breast and endometrial cancer." *South Med J.* 1984 Dec;77(12):1509-15.

Gambrell, RD. "Decreased incidence of breast cancer in postmenopausal estrogen-progestogen users." *Obstet Gynecol.* 1983 Oct;62(4):435-43.

Gambrell, RD "Hormone replacement therapy and breast cancer risk." *Arch Fam Med.* 1996 Jun;5(6):341-8.(256 postmenopausal breast cancer patients, eight- to eighteen-year follow-up, best survival for HRT users. Article quotes fifty studies showing no increased risk of breast cancer with HRT.)

Genazzani, AR. "Controversial issues in climacteric medicine II. Hormone replacement therapy and cancer." International Menopause Society Expert Workshop. *Climacteric* 2001 Sep;4(3):181-93.

Gorins, A. "Hormone replacement therapy in breast cancer patients: a study of 230 patients, with a case-control study." *Gynecol Obstet Fertil.* 2006 Jul-Aug;31(7-8):614-9.

Grodstein, F. "Postmenopausal hormone therapy and mortality." *N Engl J Med.* 1997 Jun 19;336(25):1769-75.

Hammond, CB. "Effects of long term estrogen replacement therapy to neoplasia." *Am J Obstet Gynecol.* 1979 Mar 1;133(5):537-47.

Henderson, BE. "Decreased mortality in users of estrogen replacement therapy." *Arch Intern Med.* 1991 Jan;151(1):75-8.

Holmberg, L. "Preoperative estradiol levels-relation to survival in breast cancer." *Eur J Surg Oncol.* 2001 Mar;27(2): 152-6.

Holli, K. "Low biologic aggressiveness in breast cancer in women using hormone replacement therapy." *J Clin Oncol.* 1998 Sep;16(9):3115-20.

Jernstrom, H. "Hormone replacement therapy before breast cancer diagnosis significantly reduces the overall death rate compared with never-use among 984 breast cancer patients." *Br J Cancer.* 1999 Jul;80(9):1453-8.

Kaufman, DW. Non-contraceptive estrogen use and the risk of breast cancer. *JAMA*. 1984 Jul;80(9):1453-8.

Lando, JW. "Hormone replacement therapy and breast cancer risk in a nationally representative cohort." *Am J Prev Med*. 1999 Oct;17(3)176-80. (5,761 women followed from 1971–1992. No increased risk of breast cancer with HRT.)

Lemon, HM. "Estriol and prevention of breast cancer." *Lancet*. 1973 Mar 10;1(7802):546-7.

Lemon, HM. "Pathophysiologic considerations in the treatment of menopausal patients with estrogens; the role of estriol in the prevention of mammary carcinoma." *Acta Endocrinol Suppl (Copenh)*. 1980;233:17-27.

Lemon, HM. "Antimammary carcinogenic activity of 17-alpha-ethinyl estriol." *Cancer*. 1987 Dec 15;60(12):2873-81.

Marsden, J. "Are randomized trials of hormone replacement therapy in symptomatic women with breast cancer feasible?" *Fertil Steril*. 2000 Feb;73(2):292-9.

Marsden, J. "Randomized HRT trials in breast cancer survivors are justified." *Maturitas* 2003 Oct 20;46(2):107-8.

Magnusson, C. "Prognostic characteristics in breast cancers after hormone replacement therapy." *Breast Cancer Res Treat*. 1996;38(3):325-34. (Better prognostic features with HRT.)

Mason, BH. "Progesterone and estrogen receptors as prognostic variables in breast cancer." *Cancer Res*. 1983 Jun;43(6):2985-90.

Mauvais-Jarvis, P. "Antiestrogen action of progesterone in the breast tissue." *Pathol Biol (Paris)*. 1987 Sep;35(7):1081-6.

Meurer, LN. "Cancer recurrence and mortality in women using hormone replacement therapy: meta-analysis." *J Fam Pract*. 2002 Dec;51(12):1056-62. (Showed reduced recurrence with HRT.)

Mohr, PE. "Serum progesterone and prognosis in operable breast cancer." *Br J Cancer*. 1996 Jun;73(12):1552-5.

Nachtigall, LE. "Estrogen replacement II; A prospective study in the relationship to carcinoma and cardiovascular and metabolic problems." *Obstet Gynecol*. 1979 Jul;54(1):74-9.

Nagai, MA. "Estrogen and progesterone receptor mRNA levels in primary breast cancer: association with patient survival and other clinical and tumor features." *Int J Cancer*. 1994 Nov 1;59(3):351-6.

Nanda, K. "Hormone replacement therapy and the risk of death from breast cancer: a systematic review." *Am J Obstet Gynecol.* 2002 Feb;186(2):325-34. (Reduced mortality with HRT.)

Natrajan, PK. "Estrogen replacement therapy in women with previous breast cancer." *Am J Obstet Gynecol.*1999 Aug;181(2):288-95. (Reduced recurrence rate.)

O'Meara, ES. "Hormone replacement therapy after a diagnosis of breast cancer in relation to recurrence and mortality." *J Natl Cancer Inst.* 2001 May 16;93(10):733-4. (Reduced recurrence and mortality.)

Paganini Hill, A. " Increased longevity in older users of postmenopausal estrogen therapy:the Leisure World Cohort Study."*Menopause.* 2006 Jan-Feb;13(1):12-8.

Peters, GN. "Estrogen replacement therapy after breast cancer: a 12-year follow-up." *Ann Surg Oncol.* 2001 Dec;8(10):826-32. (HRT reduced breast cancer recurrence and increased longevity.)

Plu-Bureau, G. "Progestogen use and decreased risk of breast cancer in a cohort study of premenopausal women with benign breast disease." *Br J Cancer.* 1994 Aug;70(2):270-7.

Plu-Bureau, G. "Percutaneous progesterone use and risk of breast cancer: results from a French cohort study of premenopausal women with benign breast disease." *Cancer Detect Prev.* 1999;23(4):290-6.

Plu-Bureau, G. "Hormone replacement therapy after breast cancer." *J Gynecol Obstet Biol Reprod (Paris).* 2000 May;29(3):292-4.

Rosenberg, L. "Breast cancer and oral contraceptive use." *Am J Epidemiol.* 1984 Feb;119(2):167-76.

Ross, RK. "Effect of hormone replacement therapy on breast and cancer risk: estrogen versus estrogen plus progestin. *J Natl Cancer Inst.* 2000 Feb 16;92(4):328-32.

Sacchini, V. "Pathologic and biological prognostic factors of breast cancers in short- and long-term hormone replacement therapy users." *Ann Surg Oncol.* 2002 Apr;9(3):266-71. (Study included 1,105 postmenopausal patients with breast cancer. Breast cancers developing during HRT had better prognostic characteristics than those seen in HRT nonusers. A trend toward better prognostic characteristics with increasing duration of HRT.)

Salazar-Esquivel, EL. "Infiltrating duct breast carcinoma: the role of estradiol and progesterone receptors." *Gynecol Obstet* (Mex). 1994 Mar;62:85-90.

Schairer, C. "Estrogen replacement therapy and breast cancer survival in a large screening study." *J Natl Cancer Inst.* 1999 Feb 3;91(3):264-70. (Reduced mortality with ERT.)

Schairer, C. "Menopausal estrogen-progestin replacement therapy and breast cancer risks." *JAMA.* 2000 Jan 26;283(4):485-91.

Seifert, M. "Estrogen replacement therapy in women with a history of breast cancer." *Maturitas.* 1999 Jun 21;32(2):63-8.

Sellers, TA. "The role of hormone replacement therapy in the risk for breast cancer and total mortality in women with a family history of breast cancer." *Ann Intern Med.* 1997 Dec 1;127(11):973-80.(HRT not associated with increased risk of breast cancer. HRT reduced overall mortality including overall cancer mortality.)

Stanford, JL. "Combined estrogen and progestin hormone replacement therapy in relation to risks of breast cancer in middle-aged women." *JAMA.* 1995 Jul 12;274(2):137-42. (Reduced breast cancer risk in long-term estrogen therapy >8 years.)

Steinberg, KK. "A meta-analysis of the effect of estrogen replacement therapy on the risk of breast cancer." *JAMA.* 1991 Apr 17;265(15):1985-90.

Ursin, G. "Does menopausal hormone replacement therapy interact with known factors to increase risk of breast cancer?" *J Clin Oncol.* 2002 Feb 1;20(3):699-706. (Better prognosis with estrogen therapy.)

Wile, AG. "Hormone replacement therapy in previously treated breast cancer patients." *Am J Surg.* 1993 Mar;165(3):372-5. (Increased longevity and reduced recurrence.)

Willis, DB. "Estrogen replacement therapy and risk of fatal breast cancer in a prospective cohort of postmenopausal women in the United States." *Cancer Causes Control.* 1996 Jul;7(4):449-57.(Reduced mortality with ERT.)

Wingo, PA. "The risk of breast cancer in postmenopausal women who have used estrogen replacement therapy." *JAMA.* 1987 Jan 9;257(2):209-15. (Estrogen therapy reduced incidence of breast cancer.)

CPSIA information can be obtained at www.ICGtesting.com
Printed in the USA
LVOW110139011011

248693LV00001B/129/P